D0391478

DISCARD

damage noted
moisture, stains
date 9/19 initials P.G.

This Book is Dedicated to

all the patients who have trusted me with their health challenges,
my peers for their wisdom and guidance, and Hugh and Sue Weeks
for their unwavering encouragement.

It wouldn't have been possible without the hard work of my staff:
Juno Thomason, Gina Dickerson, and Michael McCracken.

A special thank-you goes to my persistent and gifted editor,
Betsy Stokes, for your dedication and faith in this project.

And of course, immense gratitude is due my wife and children,
who once again sacrificed time spent with daddy for me to write
an updated edition. Thank you for your love and understanding,
especially when daddy had a "grumpy bad writing day."

This Fourth Edition is Dedicated to

the newest member of our family,
Harris Duboise Murphree.
Welcome to the world, little one.

Many manufacturers and sellers claim trademarks on their unique products. When these trademarks appear in this book and we are aware of them, we have used initial capital letters (e.g., Prozac) for designation.

Patient testimonials are either direct quotes or based on actual experiences as observed by the author. Most patient names have been changed to protect privacy.

ISBN 9780972893831

Fourth Edition

Copyright © 2008 by Rodger H. Murphree II

All rights reserved. No part of this publication may be reproduced, stored in a retrieval system, or transmitted in any form or by any means—electronic, mechanical, photocopying, recording, or otherwise—without the prior written permission of the author.

Printed in the United States of America
by Harrison and Hampton Publishing, Inc.
2700 Rogers Drive, Suite 204, Birmingham, AL 35209

Distributed by Cardinal Publishers Group, Inc.
2402 Shadeland Ave, Suite A, Indianapolis, IN 46219
(317) 352-8200

Editing and book design by Betsy Stokes.

Cover design by Michael McCracken.

Inquiries concerning content of this book may be addressed to the author at 1-888-884-9577 or in Birmingham, (205) 879-2383. Fax: (205) 879-2381.

Visit us at www.TreatingAndBeating.com.

This book and the advice given are intended to help you help yourself. They are not intended to take the place of your physician. Always consult with your prescribing health-care professional before discontinuing any medication.

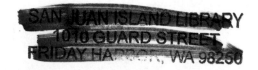
SAN JUAN ISLAND LIBRARY
1010 GUARD STREET
FRIDAY HARBOR, WA 98250

Treating and Beating Fibromyalgia and Chronic Fatigue Syndrome

A STEP-BY-STEP PROGRAM
PROVEN TO HELP YOU GET WELL!

Dr. Rodger H. Murphree

FOREWORD

Wendy Arthur, MD, and Ginger Campbell, MD

Millions of people in the United States suffer from fibromyalgia and chronic fatigue syndrome, yet mainstream medicine offers them little hope beyond marginal control of their symptoms.

Friends, family, and even physicians may think a patient's problems are "all in her head" as she watches her life dissolve into constant pain, overwhelming fatigue, depression, and—maybe the most disabling symptom—mental confusion ("fibro-fog").

In *Treating and Beating Fibromyalgia and Chronic Fatigue Syndrome*, Dr. Murphree provides an extensive investigation into these debilitating conditions. His holistic approach slowly transforms the mind, body, and spirit, restoring normal sleep, decreasing pain, and improving energy. In the past, my (Dr. Arthur's) patients had seen mild to moderate improvement. But with Dr. Murphree's comprehensive approach, I'm seeing energy levels tripled and pain reduced to the point where prescription medicine can be discontinued.

Dr. Murphree's program is grounded in his own clinical experience and passion for nutrition research. Most importantly, it works! Some of the changes he recommends are challenging, but they succeed, because they utilize the body's innate healing abilities.

This is a book about medicine, not miracles, though sometimes Dr. Murphree seems to tap into a little of both. *Treating and Beating* is destined to inspire and educate millions of Americans who just want to feel good again—and their physicians who care for and about them.

CONTENTS

Part Four: Resources

Part Five: Putting it All Together

INTRODUCTION:
MY HEROES

**It was 1971. I can still remember the bright autumn sun
and the glare of the metal bleachers in the stands.**

The air was full of the smell of wet grass. And there I was, holding a brand-new brown-and-white leather football. I was 10 years old and about to meet my hero, Pat Sullivan, star quarterback and Heisman Trophy winner. Like many folks in Alabama, I'd been raised on college football, especially Auburn football.

I loved attending Auburn football games with my dad and watching Pat Sullivan throw 60-yard touchdown passes to his favorite receiver (another hero of mine at the time), Terry Beasley.

I stood in line, holding my new football, clutching it tightly, eagerly waiting to meet my hero. After what seemed like an eternity, dad and I finally made it to the table where Pat was all smiles as he signed my football: "Pat Sullivan #7 War Eagle!"

I slept with that football for several months.

As I grew older, my heroes changed from college-football stars to rock stars: The Police, Sting, Billie Joel, Elton John, Boston, and—as much as I hate to admit it—KISS.

In college, my heroes were the great leaders of our past and present: Washington, Jefferson, Franklin, Lincoln, Kennedy, King Jr., Gandhi, Mother Theresa, and others. I still think highly of these great leaders. But my definition of "hero" has continued to evolve.

My heroes today are the common man and woman, who become extraordinary by doing the day-to-day, mundane, sometimes unpleasant, often unrewarded, and largely unnoticed tasks in life. From taking care of a special-needs child to making time to read to an elderly parent each week—these are acts of heroism.

JAN SANDERSON

One such hero is Jan Sanderson, a single mom with three children, ages 4–8. The youngest, Sam, was born with mild autism. Jan tragically lost her husband, Mike, three years ago in an automobile accident. But despite working full-time, raising three kids alone, and battling periodic fibromyalgia flare-ups, Jan rarely complains.

Jan's budget is tight, so she doesn't have a housekeeper. No maid, no nanny. Just Jan. She wakes up each morning at 5:30, gets the lunches packed and the breakfasts made, and then wakes her children.

It's hard for me to imagine doing all the things Jan must do each day just to get her kids dressed, fed, and off to school. Dressing three children can be a chore, and with Sam, it is often a real challenge. Like in many households, the mornings are usually a whirlwind of activity. I know they are with my three children at my house. But unlike Jan, who does it all by herself, my wife and I share the morning chores.

And anyone with school-aged children knows that the work doesn't end when the children go to school. The kitchen must be cleaned, the house picked up, and then there's the mad dash to get to work on time. Jan teaches third grade, and her students are counting on her. She has the patience of a saint.

After school, she picks up her children, taking John, the oldest, to soccer practice. The other two play nearly while mom grades papers and chats with other parents. Welcome to the single mom's social life! Then it's a quick stop by the grocery store to pick up milk. Then home to fix dinner, help John finish his homework, bathe the kids, clean up the bathroom, lay out the clothes for tomorrow, do a quick load of laundry, and return phone calls.

Time to get the kids to bed! Pajamas on, teeth brushed, read to Sam, then to the middle child, Annette. Lights out. Then clean up the kitchen and answer a few emails from her third-grade parents. Make sure all the doors are locked and the alarm is set. A quick shower and—fingers crossed—a good night's sleep. Because at 5:30 the next morning, it all starts over again.

Jan was in a great deal of pain and on eight different drugs when she first consulted me three years ago. She's worked hard to get healthy and now takes only an occasional sleep aid (Ambien) and Advil. Her fibromyalgia still flares up, especially when she doesn't get enough rest. But being the hero she is, the does whatever it takes to care for her precious children.

Bo Jackson, Kobe Bryant, Peyton Manning, Paris Hilton, and Madonna all pale in comparison to heroes like Jan Sanderson and the thousands of men and women like her who battle fibromyalgia each day and yet find the strength to carry on and even to flourish and thrive. Thank you, Jan, and to all of you who do what it takes to be the best parent, friend, worker, citizen, and fibromyalgia conqueror you can be. You are the reason I do what I do.

PART ONE

YOU'RE
NOT ALONE

Not only do I understand,
but so do many people who feel
just like you do....
and many who only used to!

· 1 ·
I UNDERSTAND

Believe it or not, dear reader, I understand. Even though we most likely have never met, I bet I know something about you. Let's see.

1. **You hurt all over.** Some places more than others, but mostly all over.

2. **You can't sleep at night.** In fact, you've not slept well in years.

3. **Your "get up and go" has long gotten up and went.**

4. **You've been told your illness is all in your head.** You've even started to wonder yourself if you're going crazy. No one seems to have a clue as to why you have so many symptoms that don't seem to have anything to do with each other.

5. **Family and friends have no idea how you really feel.** They all say, "You look fine." You suspect that they secretly convict you of hypochondria or just old-fashioned laziness. You have been urged to just exercise, or lose weight, or take antidepressants. Some people have the laughable idea that you are using an imaginary illness to get attention.

Am I on target? I thought so. You have an illness that's hard to diagnose, harder to "prove," and even harder to endure.

Why can't I handle life anymore?

Maybe physicians have shown ignorance of your condition, or even scorn. If they believe your pain exists at all—and some don't—their first impulse is often to mask your symptoms with prescription drugs. You can end up on a medical merry-go-round, seeing doctor after doctor, ending up more confused and disoriented than ever.

Getting your doctor to listen is hard. Finding one who understands you is even harder. Finding one who knows how to treat you is next to impossible.

I don't even remember what it's like not to hurt!

I understand. No one should suffer alone. But those with fibromyalgia (FMS) or chronic fatigue syndrome (CFS)—or both—often do suffer alone, charting their chaotic and painful courses the best they know how. Perhaps you've visited numerous doctors and taken an assortment of prescription drugs, fad supplements, vitamin regimens, and the latest multilevel herbal remedies promising to cure everything from warts to AIDS. None of them made a difference. No relief. No change. Just more money down the drain. Meanwhile you continue to feel worse each month as your life falls apart.

Listen, I've read those ads in magazines about seemingly magical remedies for fibromyalgia and chronic fatigue. I wish they were true, but your body just doesn't work that way. There's no magic pill. No massage therapy, acupuncture, detox program, colon cleanse, *Candida* treatment, parasite remedy, chiropractic adjustment, or drug will beat fibromyalgia. If there were a magic pill, you'd be well, and I wouldn't be updating this book, yet again.

How do I know which advice to listen to?

I suggest that before you take anyone's advice about treating your fibromyalgia or chronic fatigue syndrome, you see if they pass this three-item test:

1. **Is the advice from someone who actually treats fibromyalgia and CFS patients on a regular basis?** I have held the hand of many a weeping fibro patient as I've assured her that she's not crazy and that she can feel good again. Many so-called fibro "experts" have never treated a fibro patient in their lives. They might have written a book filled with positive thinking, weight-loss plans, and even healthy lifestyle changes. But that just shows how little they really know about fibromyalgia. If a positive outlook, weight loss, and exercise could fix fibro, don't they know that you could have accomplished that long ago? Don't waste your time with their regurgitated, "how-to" advice that you could have come up with on your own.

2. **Is the advice coming from a recognized expert in the field?** I am the author of three critically acclaimed books on the

subject. The one you are holding has been called "the Bible of fibromyalgia." I not only speak to support groups throughout North America but also teach doctors how to more efficiently and effectively treats patients just like you. I have earned the respect of many medical doctors the hard way: results.

3. **After following the advice you're getting, are you healthier?** Are you feeling cured from your pain, fatigue, poor sleep, low moods, and digestive problems?

If you answer "no" to any of these questions, then respectfully offer your "advisor" a copy of this book.

Can you really help me?

You're not sure FMS and CFS can be beat. I understand. But I've successfully treated these illnesses in thousands of patients over the past 14 years. And I can say with confidence, welcome to a new chapter in your life:

• **Your illness is not all in your head.** You're not lazy, crazy, or depressed. (Well, you might be depressed, but if so, it's *because of* your pain, not the cause of it.)

• **My fibromyalgia jump-start program** has helped over 4,000 patients beat fibromyalgia.

• **It's possible for you to start feeling significantly better** within 2–4 week of starting my recommendations.

As the owner and clinical director of an integrative medical practice, I worked with both medical and alternative doctors, using a combination of prescription and nutritional therapies to successfully treat FMS and CFS. I've witnessed firsthand both the positive and negative aspects of drug therapy. I've researched and implemented numerous therapies over the years, keeping what works and discarding what doesn't. Each new patient has brought new challenges and exciting breakthroughs.

These experiences of being "in the trenches" for the past 14 years have uniquely qualified me to write and teach about FMS and CFS. Today I conduct continuing-education seminars for doctors who also want to help people gain freedom from these baffling illnesses. Your illness is my life's calling.

I sold my medical practice and set out to organize and analyze all I'd learned and discovered. I began to aggressively implement specially developed nutritional protocols to yield (often rapid) results without drug therapy. Today, I see irritable bowel syndrome, a common condition associated with FMS, typically corrected within 2–4 weeks of starting my program. Deep restorative sleep, the key to getting well, is often achieved in a matter of a few days. Without drugs.

It sounds too good to be true.

My next step was to write a how-to book on tackling FMS and CFS using my nutritional protocols. I wrote *Treating and Beating* to help people help themselves get well. I didn't want to just program them with another prescription. They needed to understand their own bodies and to hear the stories of other patients who had been where they are. Many needed help explaining their illness to their spouse, parents, kids, friends, or co-workers.

I've often had one patient or another tell me that she feels like I wrote this book specifically about her. So you can stop wondering now if anyone understands. I encourage you to read my book, apply the easy-to-follow recommendations, and see for yourself how good you can feel again.

HOW IT ALL BEGAN

When I first began practicing 19 years ago, I'd never heard of fibromyalgia or chronic fatigue syndrome. They weren't mentioned in any of my medical textbooks.

Then I had a patient referred to me who changed my life forever. Sheila James was suffering from a strange collection of symptoms: diffuse pain throughout her body, headaches, menstrual irregularities, allergies, chronic infections, insomnia, depression, digestive problems, and unrelenting fatigue. After several years of being passed from one doctor to the next, she had recently been diagnosed with fibromyalgia by a local rheumatologist. The doctor couldn't provide her much information on her illness or even much hope of ever being well again. She had read all she could about fibromyalgia (there wasn't much) and knew that traditional medicine had little to offer. Medications recommended to her were mostly for covering up her various symptoms.

A friend had told her about how I had helped her overcome chronic headaches, and Sheila turned to me in desperation. Her symptoms were getting worse, and no one seemed able to help her.

I am embarrassed to admit, I was tempted to dismiss her as a hypochondriac. However, something she said changed my mind: "I've been sick for almost seven years now and I want to feel good again. I used to be so healthy." Hypochondriacs don't want to feel better. Mrs. James honestly wanted to be anywhere but in my office. She was no hypochondriac.

I told her that I didn't know anything about fibromyalgia and didn't know if I could help her. But I promised to do my best to see her get well. Fortunately, I was not aware that there was "no cure" for fibromyalgia. I just did for Mrs. James what I do for all my patients; I treated the whole person from the inside out.

I read everything I could find on FMS and CFS. I reasoned that Mrs. James's body was not properly communicating with itself (known as dysautonomia). Her regulatory system was broken. I began by analyzing her diet and placing her on an allergy-elimination diet. She began to feel better. I then ran some functional medical tests, which revealed insufficient digestion (she had intestinal permeability) and yeast overgrowth. I started her on natural yeast medications and diet restrictions to allow her body to repair her damaged stomach lining. She continued to improve.

I still didn't know a fraction of what I know today about FMS and CFS, but I prescribed vitamins, minerals, and amino acids, and she got better. I developed specific chiropractic adjustments and physical therapies to accommodate her sensitive musculoskeletal pain. The gentler I was, the better she fared.

Three months later, Sheila James was totally well. She no longer had pain, insomnia, fatigue, allergies, or any of her previous symptoms. She was ecstatic, and so was I! I didn't know it at the time, but I was taking the first step of a great adventure.

I continued learning and refining my treatment protocols, as my practice grew almost overnight by dozens of FMS and CFS patients. Some patients got well, but some didn't. Although I was happy with my successes, I was more affected by the failures. I found other chiropractors, nutritionists, massage therapists, and medical doctors who were also searching for answers. It became clear to me that we had to think outside-of-the-box to effectively treat these illnesses. They were not a neatly packaged set of symptoms that fit into an insurance codebook. They demanded a new way of thinking.

Since most of my FMS and CFS patients were on prescription drugs that were making them feel worse, I realized that I needed to have MDs on my team who could help educate patients on which medications were helpful and which ones weren't. By employing and working with medical doctors, I could provide the best of both worlds: prescription drugs along with the natural therapies I'd found to be so helpful.

An integrative approach allowed me to correct nutritional deficiencies alongside judicious use of prescription medication to temporarily relieve some of the worst symptoms. That's when I opened the integrative clinic located on the campus of a major hospital in Birmingham, Alabama. We specialized in combining traditional medical and natural medicine to treat FMS, CFS, and other chronic illnesses.

Four years and thousands of patients later, I realized I needed to pursue a solo practice, one based on my original nutritional foundations. While I valued the relief that prescription drugs can offer, it became clear that the fewer drugs a person was on, the better she fared and the more quickly she improved. Using drugs (or even natural remedies) to cover up FMS and CFS symptoms is clearly a doomed approach. You just can't mask hundreds of symptoms, with new ones cropping up every day! The protocols were becoming too complicated, and the last thing my patients (or their bodies) needed was more stress.

Worse, some of my patients' "symptoms" turned out to be side effects of their drug treatments, and it was getting tough to tell the two apart. For instance, Ambien is a drug commonly used to treat the poor sleep associated with FMS, but its potential side effects include foggy memory and flu-like symptoms. This sounds a lot like fibromyalgia! Today, I try to wean my patients off of the drugs that might be complicating their case, while still accounting for the potential benefits of their prescriptions. Sometimes a safer drug is available. Often a natural remedy works just as well or better.

Since re-entering independent practice, I've successfully treated thousands of patients with high doses of certain vitamins, minerals, amino acids, and other nutrients. This approach is referred to as orthomolecular medicine. It's based solely on biochemistry, manipulating and augmenting chemicals inherent in the body in pursuit of optimal function. By understanding and influencing the natural building blocks of our biochemistry, we can correct or drastically improve the causes of many of our diseases.

I'm firmly convinced that the way to beat your FMS and CFS is to get you healthy. I know this sounds simplistic, yet it's quite intimidating as well. Ultimately, the responsibility is yours. If you've only been taking drugs to manage your symptoms, you've got to make a paradigm shift. You've got to work to uncover and correct any nutritional and/or biochemical deficiencies that may be triggering the causes of your syndrome. If you've just been struggling to do the best with what you know, then you are the perfect potential success story, because you're going to know a whole lot more when we're through!

THE POWER OF NUTRIENTS

No one suffers from a prescription drug deficiency. Nearly all drugs are foreign to the body, and they have potential side effects. Drug therapy can be useful, but covering up symptoms with drugs should only be a short-term, stop-gap solution. It's nutrients that run the body. Every essential chemical in the body—including thyroid hormone, testosterone, estrogen, neurotransmitters (brain chemicals), antibodies, adrenaline, cortisol, and white blood cells—

are built from nutrients: vitamins, minerals, essential fatty acids, and amino acids.

Nutritional deficiencies are common among FMS and CFS patients, and high-dose orthomolecular medicine can consistently correct these deficiencies. Once corrected, a person becomes healthier and healthier until her FMS or CFS is either gone or greatly improved. Unlike drug therapy alone, there is never any danger in getting healthy. Are you safer taking the tranquilizer Klonopin to manage your tight achy muscles or the natural muscle-relaxing mineral, magnesium?

The concept of using nutritional medicine to treat and beat fibromyalgia and chronic fatigue may seem too simplistic, or worse, wishful thinking. But once you give my nutritional protocols a chance, you'll realize that they are safer, often more effective options to drug therapy.

WHAT YOU WILL LEARN FROM THIS BOOK

This book describes fibromyalgia and chronic fatigue syndrome in easy-to-understand language (especially for those with "fibro-fog"). I explain how to diagnose, successfully treat, and overcome these illnesses with my proven step-by-step program. You'll discover....

- who is most likely to develop these illnesses,
- when the illnesses are most likely to occur,
- how the syndromes are diagnosed,
- what underlying conditions are associated with them,
- why traditional medicine alone hasn't been successful in treating FMS and CFS,
- how to feel better in 2–4 weeks than you have felt in years,
- why you can't sleep and how to safely and consistently (99% of the time) solve this problem with natural supplements—within two weeks,
- why certain drugs can actually make you feel worse, causing increased pain, flu-like symptoms, poor memory, anxiety, depression, fatigue, and more[1],

- how my proven program—based on successfully treating thousands of FMS and CFS patients over the past 14 years—corrects causes, not just symptoms,
- why you have "fibro-fog" (a hard time concentrating and remembering things) and how to correct it, usually in 3–4 weeks,
- why you're so tired, even when you're taking stimulants like caffeine and amphetamines (like Ritalin and Adderall), and how to notice a dramatic increase in energy in 2–4 weeks,
- why thyroid tests are usually not accurate, and how to reliably and easily test for low thyroid (hypothyroid) at home and then successfully correct it,
- how to correct general adaptive syndrome so that you don't feel worse before every thunderstorm or after a day of "overdoing it,"
- how prolonged stress eventually overwhelms your adrenal glands and how you can repair them so that you don't "crash" after every stressful event,
- how "leaky gut" can cause food allergies, pain, inflammation, mood disorders, and chronic infections,
- why people with FMS and CFS become depressed and how over-the-counter amino-acid supplements often are more effective, faster working, and safer than prescription medications in treating most cases of anxiety and depression,
- how to beat low moods, anxiety, and depression once and for all,
- why you're in pain and how to reduce or eliminate chronic pain without mind-numbing pain medication—typically within two weeks of supplementing an essential nutrient,
- how your diet affects your health,
- how to finally, successfully treat stubborn allergies and chemical sensitivities,
- how to treat irritable bowel and digestive disturbances, making IBS a distant memory,
- how to lose those unwanted pounds you've gained and increase your metabolism through some clever adjustments to your diet,
- and how to reduce or eliminate your severe reactions to certain chemicals, medications, environments, and even smells.

Thousands of real clinical experiences of trial, error, and consistent success make this book different from others written about FMS and CFS. It's not based only on textbook theories but rather the many patients who have become my living textbook. It's not about coping with illness; it's about overcoming it. I understand what you're going through, and I can't wait to see you on the other side of it!

NOTES

1. Most doctors don't know this information. They've been convinced by drug-company propaganda to push more and more dangerous drugs. You have to learn for yourself which drugs have been proven helpful and which life-threatening drugs should be avoided.

· 2 ·
A GROWING COMMUNITY
OF WELLNESS

These accounts of newfound wellness have come to me from all over: hand-written notes, post-treatment questionnaires, emails, postcards, jotted down phone messages...you name it. And they come from both women and men, business people and stay-at-home parents, those considered to "have it all together" and those on the fringes of society. And isn't that how it should be? Wellness is a gift from God intended for all.

These personal experiences are so inspiring to me. And I want them to inspire you. So I've asked my editor to apply minimal editing to this section, and I've used real names (with permission), except to hide the last name for privacy. I've also listed the geographic location when able.

I know that it's hard to trust someone with your health, especially someone whom you've never met. But consider these many people a part of a new community that welcomes you with open arms. Here are the direct words of just a few of the thousands who have taken that very chance—and thrived to tell about it.

MASSAGE THERAPIST FINDS HOPE
Katie O. in Auburn, Alabama: *I first heard Dr. Murphree speak in 2002. I was officially diagnosed with FMS in 1983 at Mayo Clinic, Jacksonville, Florida. My doctor and physical therapist were multidiscipline-oriented professionals, and they suspected "something systemic" had been going on for several years.*

A year after my diagnosis, I graduated from massage-therapy school and began my career working in a local osteopathic hospital there in Jacksonville. Hands-on treatments for chronic-pain patients were administered daily along with required mild exercises. As I worked with these patients, I learned much about keeping myself in good physical condition with mat exercises and lots of stretching. Keeping a good attitude helped as well, and we encouraged this in the classes. Each patient got 15–20 minutes of massage each afternoon. I noticed such a difference in my pain levels as I kept myself active and really began to think this was a BIG part of the conditioning program for fibros. I also was on a vitamin-mineral supplement and had been for many years.

When Dr. Murphree spoke in Auburn, I decided to give his FMS/CFS supplements a try and have been using them for several years now with very good results. I was also impressed that he included the body/mind connection as well as diet and the Holmes-Rahe Stress Factors scale along with vitamin programs, etc. There is a whole-body connection with FMS/CFS, and the medical profession often misses that.

As a licensed massage therapist of 24 years, I have been privileged to have attended many educational classes that speak to the body-mind connection and try to educate my clients on this so that they can better help themselves with the daily struggle of FMS/CFS. Also, I am delighted that Dr. Murphree speaks about craniosacral therapy and myofascial release! These are two treatments which I have found give me the most relief when my fibro flares. I bless the day the PTs I worked with suggested I take the craniosacral classes. This wonderful modality has helped me help myself and has allowed me to help many patients who were written off by doctors after trying typical therapies with little results. Craniosacral therapy helps balance the stressed nervous system and release long-standing fascial restrictions that may have gotten you into this fibro syndrome in the first place. [Note: see chapter 30, and talk to your massage therapist for more information about these helpful techniques.]

I have been so impressed with the caring attitude of the clinic personnel when I reorder my supplements over the phone, and I'm very thankful for a doctor who has taken a stand on helping people make natural changes in their lifestyle to treat and beat a difficult condition.

I'm going into my 25th year of doing massage therapy, and I am so awed by this fact and privileged for the opportunity to still be doing what I love to do despite my diagnosis of fibromyalgia.

Tammy T., via email: *You have been an absolute godsend to me. I have had fibromyalgia for nearly 14 years (although of course we didn't know what it was back then). Thank you, thank you, thank you!*

SLEEP HELPS HEAL

Emily F. in Australia: *I am 52 years old. The first signs of something wrong started in my mid 30s. I was basically treated as a hypochondriac for the first few years until a new doctor suggested I could have CFS. As it turned out, I was diagnosed with FMS.*

By the time I got my diagnosis, I had already worked out a pretty decent regimen of multivitamins plus extra magnesium and vitamin B. The only meds given by the rheumatologist were antidepressants, but these did very little for the pain and stiffness and added to my woes by slowing down my thinking process, so I took myself off of those.

My regimen grew to include Nurofen and Nurofen Plus at least once per day. In really bad times, I will take Celebrex for a short period of time or paracetamol and ibuprofen on alternate two hours.

I came upon Dr. Murphree's CFS/FibroFormula quite by accident (strangely enough, I was researching angels, and I found Dr. Murphree), and after working out what I was currently paying monthly against the cost of getting his supplements from the United States to Australia, I figured it was worth a go. I am so pleased I did.

The very first thing I noticed was that my sleep patterns improved out of sight! And with this, my body aches lessened. I felt so good, I actually stopped taking anything for a while, but this was a big mistake, as the return of the symptoms has meant a very slow return to feeling good, but I am almost there.

I don't believe I will ever be pain free, but I do believe I will be okay if I keep taking the CFS/FibroFormula on a regular basis—and this is not easy for someone who does not like taking medication of any kind, even vitamins.

I have told my doctor, physical therapist, and chiropractor about the CFS/FibroFormula. It is a shame they are not available over-the-counter here in Australia.

SEROTONIN MAKES ALL THE DIFFERENCE

Veronica V. in Ontario, Canada: *Before I was fortunate enough to come across your web site, I was experiencing mental and anxiety issues that had me thinking I was going crazy. After taking the Brain Dysfunction test, I was so relieved that it was a chemical imbalance. I just lacked some brain chemicals, especially serotonin.*

Although I was suffering FMS pain, the brain dysfunction was much more upsetting to me. I am a health-and-safety trainer, and I would go blank in front of a classroom with no recall of the information I was to teach. I could no longer spell, and the keyboard felt like a stranger under my fingers when trying to write policies and procedures. I was late for sessions, because for the first time in my life, I would get lost regularly.

I have a great life, and yet I was unhappy and depressed most of the time. I started suffering anxiety attacks for no apparent reason. I could not cope with change of any sort. I am a very social person, yet I didn't want to leave the house or have company over. I became a frustrated and angry person.

Two weeks on your FMS protocol, I could think again! Driving was easy again, and I could perform my work. Both the mental and physical symptoms subsided considerably.

Now, 10 months into the program, I am exponentially better than before. The added bonus is that these are one of the few products that I have not developed a tolerance of, and they continue to help me heal. Thank you so much for your dedication and understanding of what we go through.

CONTROL FREAK NEVER GAVE UP

Patricia Z. in Port St. Lucie, Florida: *In retrospect, I believe my body has hosted the unwelcome guest of fibromyalgia for a lot longer than my diagnosis eight years ago. An active person all my life, I suffered more from the restrictions than from the actual pain. In other words, I was depressed. A control freak, I balked at the thought of antidepressants, pain killers, muscle relaxers, and sleeping pills. I like to be in control of my thoughts, pain, and moods. I believe in the in-*

nate intelligence of my body and the chiropractic philosophy. I resented medical doctors telling me if I wanted to get relief I had to take the above. So I researched online and found Dr. Murphree, read his books (still do), and started on the vitamins and minerals he suggested.

Am I fibro free? No. But I am so much better off than I was in the beginning, I am capable of most things in moderation, and I possess all of my wits.

I did find a rheumatologist whom I now see once a year and who will work with me. He admitted recently that he wished more of his patients would quit looking for a miracle drug to take away their pain.

Mental attitude, exercise, chiropractic adjustments, massage, and a good regimen of vitamins are keeping me active. Yes, some days I flare, and when that happens, I allow myself a few minutes for a pity party, drag myself into a hot shower, and get moving, thanking God every day that I do not have a terminal disease as do some.

LIFE IS AN ADVENTURE AGAIN

Jennifer G. in Yakima, Washington: *I battled fibromyalgia for 16 years and tried almost every miracle cure I could find after mainstream medicine failed me. Although nothing helped, I was determined to keep searching, because I knew there would come a day of healing.*

With fibromyalgia, life is not an adventure but a daily survival. My "last ditch" effort led me online to Treating and Beating. I studied the book cover to cover, underlined, highlighted, read and re-read, even though I could barely hold the book open. I got started on the jump-start program on July 1, 2008, and for the first time in years began sleeping through the night and waking up rested!

After four months on the jump start, I am experiencing a great increase in energy and I can actually think clearly. Wow! The pain didn't leave my neck and arms, so I consulted with Dr. Murphree via telephone. After trying a couple more supplements, he suggested a visit to a neurosurgeon. The neurosurgeon discovered herniated discs. I'm not sure what my next step will be, but I know I am getting closer to my day of healing and many new adventures to live.

NOT WANTING TO LIVE ANOTHER DAY

George F. in Baton Rouge, Louisiana: *I am one of the rare males diagnosed with fibromyalgia back in 1991. It started off bearable but got worse over the years. I am 52 years old now and have always been very active outdoors—hunting, fishing, and such.*

Over the past five or six years, I started missing many days at work, sometimes the whole week. I could no longer hunt or fish—just lay in bed taking large doses of pain medications and aspirin by the handful. Without being able to do anything I enjoyed doing, I would start off with tremendous anger which lead to deep depression. I had been through several rheumatologists, both here and in other cities.

I had given up; I could not take it anymore. I went round and round in my head about how much it was going to hurt the ones I love if I took my own life. But I could no longer stand a life like I had.

Then a friend of mine saw Dr. Murphee's book, bought it, and sent it to me. I immediately ordered the starter pack and took it religiously.

Within two weeks, I was feeling better. Now after seven months, I feel 10 years younger. My whole life has changed. I can now do anything and more than most people my age! Thanks to our Lord and Savior for bringing a man like Dr. Rodger Murphree into this world.

FROM DEPRESSION TO FULFILLMENT AGAIN

Mimi M. in Fort Wayne, Indiana: *About two years ago, I had a blood infection. The doctors spent nine weeks figuring out which one it was and treating me. In the meantime, I was in severe pain and could barely walk to the bathroom. I was bedridden for nine weeks! I had just purchased my restaurant and could not work. I had always worked a lot and was always a very active person. Some people called me a workaholic.*

Once they treated me for the infection, I started feeling better, but then I still hurt in my muscles. Sometimes it would be one muscle, then another. It didn't make since to me, and I was very discouraged. So they sent me to a rheumatologist to have him check me and then ran more blood tests, X-rays, an MRI, and a urine test. All the tests came back okay.

I was very upset when he told me I had fibromyalgia. I had never heard of it, and he told me I would never be able to work the hours I had before (usually 60–70 hours a week, plus I did the books for a friend's company, my husband's company, and my own). I was devastated to hear this, and the medication they put me on was worse. I couldn't even think straight, much less do the company books. And when I tried to work in my restaurant, I could only work 3–4 hours at a time. Then I would be in bed the rest of the day and night till the next morning.

After about four times of having a handful of pills ready to swallow and end it all, I decided to get online and do some research. I found this web site [www.TreatingAndBeating.com] and ordered the package of supplements and the book from Dr. Murphree.

My life changed within a month! Now I work seven days a week at my restaurant baking my own pies and cooking my own soups and enjoying my life-long dream of having my own hometown restaurant. I also am still doing the books for three different businesses.

I still have good and bad days, but I can live with that. I also took up canoeing and camping with my husband (a good getaway). I have people tell me all the time I am a miracle. I feel very lucky to have found help, and I have always told people about Dr. Murphree's products, because they work! Thank you very much for being out there for people like me.

LOVED ONES HAPPY FOR HEALING

Pam H. in Bossier City, Louisiana: *This is concerning my sister, Elle Blake. She was diagnosed over a year ago with fibromyalgia. I thank God every day for sending Dr. Murphree to our city. Elle was very doubtful, but she bought the jump-start package.*

Now you have to understand, my sister was in pretty bad shape. She was down for days, no sleep, in so much pain. But after the first day on the jump-start pack, I had my sister back.

She was ready to die she hurt so bad. Now it's been almost two weeks and she is stronger every day. I truly thank God and Dr. Murphree. She is telling everyone she sees about this wonderful miracle.

A BRAND NEW MAN

Eddie C. in Boligee, Alabama: *Today is a great day in my life! I feel like a new man most of the time, and I owe it all to Dr. Murphree and his therapy. I really feel that I am on my way to a full recovery. I now remember more. The pain is much better.*

There were times that I felt completely disconnected from each part of my body. I could not remember anything from one minute to the next. Today my blood pressure is down. My pain is under control. And I thank God for Dr. Murphree. I could write my own book about what Dr. Murphree has done for me. I am very grateful that I found him.

SLEEP RESTORED, PAIN REDUCED

Dale S. in Altoona, Alabama: *I was diagnosed in 1989 with fibromyalgia and have seen four or more doctors in the last five years. I have been on antidepressants, muscle relaxers, and things taken at night and nothing really helped. I have had a lot of pain all over my body especially over the last five years. In 1998, I had lower back surgery and I have had a lot of pain in my right side all the way into my foot.*

I had not been able to sleep well for several years. I was probably waking up every hour or two and not feeling good when I would get up in the morning. I wouldn't take a lot of the medicine that the other doctors prescribed to me, because they made me feel sleepy for about half of the day, so I would just deal with the pain.

About a year ago, I started taking Dr. Murphree's CFS/Fibro vitamins and other supplements and I was feeling better, but I still was not sleeping well. I started seeing Dr. Murphree in December 2003. February 20, 2004, was my fourth visit, and what he has put me on these last two months has helped me a lot. I am sleeping about six hours or so each night, and I am dreaming now and feel much better when I get up. I have more energy and am so thankful for the help that Dr. Murphree has given me.

PAIN FREE IN THREE WEEKS

Ina W. in Birmingham, Alabama: *I have suffered with fibromyalgia for approximately five years and have seen three doctors during* *that time who could never give me a diagnosis. I had taken several drugs and tried different therapies and nothing had helped until I saw Dr. Murphree. Dr. Murphree's book has been most helpful in helping me with my illness and knowing what I should do next, and Dr. Murphree is helpful in suggesting what to read. I would recommend his book and him to anyone. Dr. Murphree gets to the bottom of the problem instead of loading you down with harmful drugs. There is a big lesson to be learned about Dr. Murphree's method in treating fibromyalgia and CFS.*

The day that I entered Dr. Murphree's clinic was a changing day in my life. Not only did he help me tremendously with the pain in my legs and arms but also with my bad menopause symptoms. In three week's time, I was pain free. My menopause symptoms were 90% gone. I feel energetic, vital, and happy and most of all, pain free. Thank you so much Dr. Murphree. I would recommend you and your healing methods to my loved ones and dearest friends.

DID NOT CARE ABOUT LIFE ANYMORE

Lori M. in Florence, Alabama: *When I was first diagnosed with fibromyalgia, I heard many different things about treatment and doctors. The most common was that there really wasn't much that could be done for me except for taking pain medication and/or antidepressants to try to provide some relief from the pain. Everything else pointed to the same conclusion that I would have to accept feeling bad most of the time for the rest of my life. At the age of 40 with a husband, a teenager, and a 7 year old, I could not accept that I would feel like this from now on.*

I began to search for more information and prayed for God to give me wisdom and direction in my search, just as He always does. He led me to Dr. Murphree's book as He answered my prayer. I had no idea when I began reading the book that Dr. Murphree's practice was just 90 minutes away from where I live. I quickly made an appointment and found a practice full of kind, loving, caring people, all eager to see me feel better.

I explained to Dr. Murphree all of my symptoms, the worst being a terrible burning sensation that never went away in my arms and hands. I also described how, because of so much pain and so little energy, I really didn't care about anything. It didn't matter to me if my family was fed, or if my kids had baths, or if their homework was done. I simply felt so bad that nothing mattered to me anymore.

Dr. Murphree got me started on the Fibro/CFS vitamins and 5-HTP, and I began to feel better in just a few days. Within a few weeks, I felt like a new person. From this point on, I have always referred to Dr. Murphree as my "miracle doctor." Finally, I had found someone who was treating the cause of my problem—not just the symptoms. A sweeter, kinder, gentler, more loving doctor could never be found. There are no words or ways to accurately express my or my family's gratitude for giving my life back to me. I am so grateful to God for leading me to such a wonderful person.

There are a number of important men in my life—my husband, my son, and my father—but the next most important man in my life after them is Dr. Murphree, my "miracle doctor."

FINALLY HAS HER LIFE BACK

Sharon G. in Navasota, Texas: *I have fibromyalgia/CFS and was absolutely miserable. I have been to 12 different doctors, tried so many different medications, all to no avail. I saw your book advertised and ordered it. Last July, I started on the CFS/FibroFormula vitamins, digestive enzymes, adrenals, and 5-HTP. I can't take the 5-HTP, but you suggested the melatonin, which helps me sleep through the night.*

I feel so much better since I am off all prescription meds and taking your vitamins and supplements, I actually have a life again. I can work in my yard, go shopping, on long rides, clean my own home, all of which caused me a great deal of pain before taking your products. My husband, Jim, says it is so nice to have his wife back. He is so happy. I am not living in pain 24/7 and can do things with him again. I feel 85%–90% better, and that is such a wonderful gift from you.

If I hadn't found your book, I know I would still be in a great deal of pain and miserable. Thank you so much for taking the time to research these illnesses and help produce these products and for being there any time I need to speak with you, even though I've never been to your office.

SYMPTOMS WERE GETTING WORSE

Becky G. in Andalusia, Alabama: *I have had Fibro for the past 10 years. It has been much worse over the last five years, and I have seen three different doctors.*

I found Dr. Murphree's book and started reading it. It has helped me so much. He explains what to do to get better and not just what it is, as so many other books that I read did.

When I came to see him, I was very sick, having dizzy spells and other issues other than just the pain. I was so tired by 4:00 p.m. that I could hardly go on. Dr. Murphree told me that he could help me, and he has helped me tremendously.

Other doctors told me there was no cure but they could give me something to help with pain. And I had been taking Celebrex and other medications for pain and inflammation. Dr. Murphree has helped me feel so much better by using his supplements and the therapies that he recommends. There are times that I may have pain and soreness, but it doesn't last long, and I can tell that I am better. My family and friends can also tell that I am better. I highly recommend him to others who are suffering.

BACK TO SERVING GOD AND COUNTRY

Father Tim B. in Afghanistan: *I am a chaplain in the United States Air Force. I was diagnosed with fibromyalgia seven years ago. After nearly seven years of problems sleeping, I decided I could no longer handle tossing and turning through the night and the psychological stress of facing bedtime wondering what the night would bring.*

I was surprised by the diagnosis as I thought it was a syndrome that affected only women. I knew something about FMS, because my mother was one of the very early diagnoses after the syndrome was identified. Over the course of the last seven years, my doctors have prescribed many different medications to help me get a good night's sleep. All of them were helpful to a degree or for a period of time. However, none of them allowed me a really deep, good night's sleep, and all of them had unwanted side effects. Last year, I told my doctor I couldn't deal with the "hangovers" anymore in the morning from my medications. He suggested I try Trazodone. While this helped me to get into a fairly deep sleep, there was something better to come along: 5-HTP!

I was at my local natural food store one afternoon when I saw a poster announcing that a doctor from Birmingham was going to be speaking about "treating and beating" fibromyalgia at one of our local universities. My first reaction was skeptical. Would it be possible to "beat FMS?" Yet I figured there may be some new information out there about "treating" it that could be helpful. So, I went.

Dr. Murphree explained how recent research indicated that FMS patients' brains do not create enough serotonin. That intrigued me. I knew serotonin was essential for sleep. Could it be that simple, I wondered? Worth a try, I thought! So, I bought some 5-HTP after the lecture and began taking it according to Dr. Murphree's directions. Within three days, I was sleeping as soundly as when I was in college. No kidding!

That was three months ago. The deep, sound sleep I now experience has contributed significantly to my physical, emotional, and spiritual well-being. As an example: in the military we are required to do physical exercise (running 1.5 miles) three times a week. I could not do this without significant pain that lingered for up to three days, sometimes making it impossible for me to pass my fitness tests. This was stressful emotionally as well as physically. Now, I have no pain from exercising. I'm serious!

As a chaplain, I don't believe in coincidence. I believe God made sure I saw that announcement and attended that lecture. Every night I ask God to bless Dr. Murphree in his important work. Because of him I am better able to do my important work: serving my God and my country!

FROM DISABILITY TO STEADY IMPROVEMENT
Sharon W., via email: *I started seeing doctors in 1995 and finally in 1997 received a diagnosis of fibromyalgia. And then in 2002, I received a diagnosis of CFS. Since 1997, I have been on lots of medication that ran me about $600.00 per month. With my illness I have been in pain all over my body—IBS and severe insomnia due to the pain. In August of 2002, I was placed on disability.*

I had read lots of books on the subject, but it wasn't until I read Dr. Murphree's book that I realized that I could be treated with supplements that were not harmful to my body and weren't as costly. In early 2003, I made an appointment to see Dr. Murphree, and since that time my lifestyle has improved greatly. I have been able to come off all medications, and with taking his FMS/CFS packages and 5-HTP for sleep, I am now back to going to gym and yoga classes. After following his procedures in the book regarding my diet, I no longer have any abdominal pain, and I have lost over 10 pounds and see daily that I continue to improve. His program and book have greatly improved my lifestyle. I tell others to get his book, make an appointment to see him, and he will change their lifestyle like he has done mine.

HAD NOT FELT GOOD FOR YEARS

Lou Ann B. in Elba, Alabama: *I have been suffering with fibromyalgia for about seven years; it actually took two years for me to be diagnosed. I saw several different doctors and they didn't offer much help except pills. If it wasn't a prescription, it was a lot of tests; everything always showed up negative. This was over a course of five years, and I had almost given up. I prayed to God to please give me answers and show me what to do. He did! I saw Dr. Murphree on WSFA [local TV station] and knew that I had to see him. He was speaking in Auburn that night, and I called my husband at work and told him about him, and we went that night.*

His lecture made so much sense. I got a copy of his book and called the next day for an appointment. I had read approximately 10 books, and Dr. Murphree's book was the most helpful—there was no comparison. It was very informative, and I have purchased two to give to friends.

I was on several different medications and wasn't getting any better. I know I would not have gotten better without his help. Within two weeks, I knew I was on the right track. I haven't felt this good in 10 years. Dr. Murphree's guidance with the nutritional aspects was wonderful. His approach is so different from other doctors. He has time for you; he takes your health problems seriously. I have gotten so much helpful advice from him and not a bunch of prescriptions. I know that the Lord sent me to Dr. Murphree, and I thank Him every day for it.

TEARS OF PAIN, DAY AND NIGHT

Debbie H. in Birmingham, Alabama: *I have had fibromyalgia since 1982. I had seen four doctors, and no one had ever heard of it. I was put on lots of medications: Elavil, Celebrex, Tofranil, Vioxx, Xanax, and nothing ever really helped. I had read several book but none were as informative as Dr. Murphree's. I have referred the book to others. There is no comparison with his and others that I have read. His is the BEST!! I had been in pain for so long that I just took pain medications and lived with the tears of hurting all day and night.*

I remember the first day I saw Dr. Murphree. I left with tears in my eyes, not because of pain but because I was not hurting as much. Since I have been going to Dr. Murphree's clinic, it is the first time that I have been pain-free in 20 years. Little did I know that this was only the beginning, I started taking his vitamin supplements, and now I will not go a single day without them. They have reduced my pain by 90%. I would just like to say thanks to Dr. Murphree. My life is a lot better now.

Judy N., via email: *Dr. Murphree was my lifesaver! I am now off all of my medications, and I am pain free with the help of his supplements, vitamins, diet, and myofascial therapy. I plan to stay on his clinical program for the rest of my life. He is a very fine, loving, caring professional who will do his very best to help everyone feel better and enjoy a healthier life.*

Sharon D., via email: *I'd say, along with the adrenal supplements, the CFS/FMS Formula has made the biggest difference in how well I feel. If I miss a few days of either supplement, I start to feel sluggish and run down. I've taken dozens of different supplements over the last few years, but none have seemed to help like the ones Dr. Murphree recommended. I like the convenience of taking a pack in the morning and one in the afternoon. I used to have to carry pills around in my pockets or purse. It was expensive, confusing, and hard to take so many pills each day. Usually I lost interest and simply gave up until another "sure cure" supplement came along.*

Hugh W., via email: *The Inflammation Formulas and CFS/Fibro formula have made a big difference in my pain.*

DOCTOR RECOMMENDED

Dr. Mike Malloy, DC, via email: *This is the best all-around multi-vitamin/mineral formula I've ever used. I'm recommending it to all my Fibro and CFS patients.*

Dr. Steve Willen, DC, in Greensboro, North Carolina (Fibromyalgia Solutions, Center of the Triad): *At Dr. Rodger Murphree's seminar, I was impressed with his knowledge of the fibro patient and nutrition. I have never met a man who knew so much about how nutrition affected the body.*

In the past years of learning from Dr. Murphree, I have been able to build a practice in which I am now confident in the many different scenarios that a Fibro or CFS patient may present. Dr. Murphree has been there for me to answer questions, and he has always answered my emails. These illnesses are very difficult for the patient to have and difficult for the doctors to treat. But it has been the most rewarding experience of treating patients in my 24 years as a doctor. We are changing these people's lives when almost all other methods have failed.

I have literally worn out Dr. Murphree's books, tapes, and CDs by reading or listening to them all the time. His knowledge has given me the confidence to speak to my community about fibromyalgia, and we regularly receive referrals from medical professionals because of our successful care. There are a few times in life that you meet a teacher who can change the course of your life. Dr. Rodger Murphree has been that person. And because of that, I am helping so many others.

Russel L. in Greensboro, North Carolina (a patient of Dr. Willen, above): *Please let me express to Dr. Willen and his staff my thanks for the miracle that has been performed for me. For ten years, I have suffered from pain, fatigue, and hopelessness. Diagnosed with fibromyalgia in 1995, I have seen orthopedic doctors, psychiatrists, therapists, MDs, rheumatologists, and neurologists, only to continue with all the same symptoms. Constantly in a drug stupor from the 12 medications I took daily, I couldn't push forward any longer. I was ready to give up.*

After seeing Dr. Willen and going through the fibromyalgia program, my pain level went from a severe 8–10 down to a 3 or less. A more manageable pain. I have a chance now to actually enjoy life. My sincerest thank you to Dr. Willen and staff for caring about fibromyalgia patients, where other doctors ignore the disease and the symptoms.

Toni K. in Mobile, Alabama: *Having to deal with all the physical and emotional aspects of FMS/CFS can be a frightening and discouraging experience. We must have doctors who stay on the cutting edge of research and who will give this to us in a comfortable way that we can trust. I have always found this in Dr. Rodger Murphree. I thank God for his intelligence and his kindness and willingness to help us.*

Rena B., via email: *Dr. Murphree, I've been on your product for about six months and I just wanted to take a moment and thank you. For the first time in years, I am almost pain free from my fibro symptoms. I am no longer taking Flexeril at night, and I'm off all pain meds during the day. I have my life back, thanks to you.*

No longer do I start my day thinking about how much pain I experience or how little sleep I get. No one else has been able to help me. You are an answer to my prayers. I tell everyone I meet with fibro symptoms to check out your website and try the products. Again, thank you.

POWER WALKER GAINING GROUND
(No name provided), via email: *Since I've been taking these vitamins for CFS, I'm doing so much better (80%–85%). I am able to function a lot better during the day and able to think clearly. I still have fatigue when doing yard work; I'm not able to do it like I did about three years ago. But I'm back to power walking (about two miles a day). I hope to increase this in the next couple of months.*

Thank you for all your help and the excellent vitamin formulas. I stopped taking my other ones! Yours are so much better and act fast.

LEARNING THE ART OF RELAXING
Linda M., via email: *I cannot thank you enough for all your help. In the past four weeks, I have gone from being nearly incapacitated to functioning like a human once again. There are a lot of struggles that I know I will continue to endure, but the hope I have been given will get me through it all. Thank you also for being a great listener and a compassionate person. It shows that you do truly care about your patients.*

My family is very thankful as well. My husband has his wife back, and our kids have their mother back. I know where I have been—I was sick. It was such a scary time. I lost myself during that time. I never want to experience that low again. I'm truly thankful for each and every day even more so now than before. Our trials should make us stronger, and this one definitely did. My family is much closer now. We've really had to rethink a lot of things and make changes—taking a long, hard look at ourselves and reprioritizing. It is so easy to let the not-so-important things take over your life—until it is too late.

I'm thankful now that I know what is wrong with me. I've struggled for years with this—this time being the worst episode ever. My biggest fear became going to a doctor and being told everything was normal. It happened so often, being so sick I could hardly function, feeling as if I had the flu over and over.

It was so hard to hear that all my lab work was normal. That hurt me more than it helped. Pretending it didn't exist certainly didn't make it go away. I just think of all the doctors out there who failed me. I'm not a complainer. When I am sick, I am really sick. And I don't like to be sick. I'd much rather be healthy and feel well and enjoy life. Life's too short to waste. I pushed myself so hard when I felt so tired and exhausted, because I thought I had to. I thought I had to pretend like the sickness didn't exist because no one else could "see" it. I know that all that pushing did nothing but make things worse.

Sometimes, I find myself feeling mournful for the person I used to be who was full of energy—always busy with something, accomplishing so much. Learning to slow down and pace myself has been a definite battle. I am a perfectionist at heart, and that isn't something I can easily change. I don't do well just "relaxing." I will have to learn that art.

Standing up for myself will be very hard. I know I'll face many obstacles at work. I've always been so dependable and efficient at my job and therefore have been asked to do numerous extra duties. Saying no will be the hardest. However, If I don't, it will have a great impact not only on me, but my whole family. I will be back to work in a few weeks, and I am trying to get ready for that. I've already given up one big extra duty, which will be a big load off of my shoulders.

At the front of your book, you mentioned that this is your life's purpose. Thank you so much for devoting so much of your time to help people like me. I thank God that I was able to find you. I had basically lost hope. I am grateful that I was led to the right answers and eventually to your website. And I want you to know that my husband went to work the next day after my first visit to your office and had to draw the diagram of the serotonin bank for several people. He is obviously happy to have a diagnosis for his wife's illness! Thanks again for all that you and your staff do to help people.

SO HARD TO EXPLAIN THE PAIN

Belinda S. in Anniston, Alabama: *On April 12, 2006, I walked into the office of Dr. Rodger Murphree. I felt as if I had hit rock bottom with all the pain in my body. I had been to every type of doctor that you could think of: general doctors, endocrinologists, rheumatologists, ENTs.*

And I never got any better. All I was told was that I had fibromyalgia. In January 2006, I started gaining weight rapidly, and that alone made my symptoms even worse. There would be times when I would tell my husband or family, "I HURT!" It was so hard to explain the pain that was all over my body.

The day I started seeing Dr. Murphree, I felt hope again. He started me out on the jump-start program along with adrenal cortex, digestive enzyme, Liver Detox, and 5-HTP to help me with the sleep I was not getting. Juno, his nurse, was excellent also and has been there for me every step I've made.

Dr. Murphree found that I was also having thyroid problems, and he is still working on this with me. But in three months, I have lost 42 pounds! Now I feel 100% better and am feeling like I am getting my life back.

I am still seeing Dr. Murphree and can not imagine not having him to turn to when I have questions or concerns. So many times, he has called just to check on me.

Now, looking back over those horrible months, I thank God every day for bringing Dr. Murphree into my life! It is amazing the progress he has brought me through. I would like to say thank you from the bottom of my heart to Dr. Murphree and Juno! I can't imagine what condition I would be in right now without having them to guide me through and take such good care of me.

OVERMEDICATED AFTER HEART ATTACK

Mike M. in Tuscaloosa, Alabama (my graphic designer and webmaster): *I had a heart attack almost two years ago, and I'll never forget the reaction of the cardiologist on my first visit to him after getting out of the hospital. I had just given him a list of the vitamins and minerals that I was going to be taking, and he jumped up off of his chair in shock and said, "Don't take ANY of that!" He did say that I'd have to take all this other medicine the rest of my life to control my cholesterol and blood pressure, etc.*

But I talked to an old friend of mine who had been a vascular surgeon for over 20 years and also to Dr. Murphree. They both agreed that I was being overmedicated. I could tell that the drugs were affecting my memory and mood. Needless to say, I never went back to that cardiologist again. I will NOT have a doctor who doesn't understand basic nutrition and uses the "cookbook" method of healing. I weaned myself off of the drugs with the side effects and have been following Dr. Murphree's protocols for heart health. I have spent hours and hours researching this myself as I now feel that you can't just let the medical doctors put you on the "drug track."

You really have to take control of your own health, and I can't think of a better partner to have in that endeavor than Dr. Murphree. I work on his website and newsletters and always learn so much during the process. I am also privy to emails that are sent in by his patients, and I see a constant flow of thanks from those he has helped. It's very, very rare to see any negative responses, and he is very good about being available (unlike most doctors) through email and working with the individual to find solutions that work.

FROM DESPAIR TO THRIVING LIFE

Betsy S. in Austin, Texas (my editor and book designer): *I was one of Rodger's original guinea pigs. Lucky enough to be living in his* *hometown when I contracted fibromyalgia, I turned to him as my last hope. He turned out to be my best hope.*

My editing career was just taking off at that time when my body went through a physical crash from which I may never fully recover. I had to quit my job as a full-time editor because I got so sick, and my husband and I postponed starting a family. I tried working part-time, but even that was too much for me. I would come home from a day of editing (not exactly heavy lifting) and fall asleep on the bed fully dressed, including my shoes.

Most of my coworkers were genuinely concerned, but more than a few accused me of "trying to get attention." Ha! Oh yeah, I looooved losing my job, frustrating my husband to no end, and being terrified that I would be too sick to ever have children.

My family did everything they could to help me get better, including getting me in to see the best-of-the-best MDs in my area, many of whom were family friends. An antidepressant from my rheumatologist worked wonders for me, and I thought that I had been cured.

But I soon grew weary of the horrible side effects of debilitating heartburn, crazy sleep patterns, and lack of any "real" emotions. I wasn't hurting as badly, but I couldn't feel true joy or even true sorrow anymore. I began to lose touch with myself, to put it naturopathically. When I heard about Dr. Murphree, I made an appointment, and suddenly I went from seeing many doctors who had little idea what was wrong with me to just one who knew what was wrong before I told him!

And today, his protocols are more effective than ever. When I started under his care in 1999, it wasn't uncommon to hear, "Let's see if this will work for you." Now he's able to say, "This has worked for many, many people just like you." He's constantly refining, keeping records, pursuing true causes, tossing what doesn't work, and continuing to test what does. I swear he's going to go to his grave quoting some double-blind, placebo-controlled breakthrough study. And then calling me to tell me how he's going to work it into his next chapter!

Now I have a thriving editing business, two beautiful children, and a husband who lights up as I tell him how great I feel again each day. No longer Dr. Murphree's patient, I am honored to be his editor. His treatments—along with lots of prayer and support—turned my life around. I am also a type-1 diabetic and have a lot of health challenges. But I can honestly say that my FMS is in remission. I am no longer on an antidepressant, and I don't even need 5-HTP any more. I only continue the high-potency multivitamins and minerals and an occasional sleep aid.

I thank the Lord God, Who has transformed me through His love. And Rodger has plainly been an instrument of healing in my life. He helped teach me to wait on my body to heal itself and to trust that it wants to be well. Heck, I would edit his books for free. (That's a joke, Doc!)

WITNESSES MIRACLES EVERY DAY
Juno T. in Homewood, Alabama (my nurse and office manager):
I have two children, four grandchildren, a husband, and a full-time job. I am 53 years old and take no prescription medication, thanks to Dr. Murphree. I have worked for him over six years now. For three years, I was the IV nurse in the medical practice that Dr. Murphree owned. Although we do not do IVs in this clinic, patients enjoy the same benefits by taking their supplements on a daily basis.

One of his patients, Mr. Harris, was unable to walk and was mobile only by wheelchair. He had considered closing his business due to his poor health. Mr. Harris began a regimen of chelation IVs and supplements. Within just a few weeks, he was walking with no assistance. Now he has added to his business, and he functions normally.

Another patient, Mrs. Mann, came to us using a walking cane. Her medical doctors had no idea what was wrong with her. Dr. Murphree put her on an elimination diet and a regimen of supplements. She found that she was allergic to dairy, wheat, and several other foods. She no longer needs her cane, and in a year she lost 71 pounds. She now lives a normal, healthy lifestyle. She is once again able to enjoy her grandchildren and her life. I still keep in contact with her each month when she orders her supplements.

I could tell you many more stories about the endless list of patients who *find their miracles, working with Dr. Murphree to get their lives back. Many of his patients have recovered from debilitating illnesses that seemed to be hopeless. Working with Dr. Murphree is the most rewarding experience I have ever had.*

PART TWO

FIXING WHAT WENT WRONG

We can't change the past,
but at least we can
make sense of it together.

· 3 ·
THE PAIN-FATIGUE SPECTRUM

If you have presented your symptoms yet to any doctor who has been paying attention, you've likely received a diagnosis (or at least a suggestion) of either fibromyalgia (FMS) or chronic fatigue syndrome (CFS). In fact, one doctor might have suspected one of these, and another doctor might have suspected the other. How do you determine which illness you actually have? Or do you perhaps have symptoms of both? Or maybe you don't fully qualify for either diagnosis but you are certainly on your way there.

PLOT YOUR SPOT ON THE SPECTRUM

In order to place yourself on the pain-fatigue spectrum, you'll need to think hard about your actual symptoms. Are you truly fatigued (have to literally drag yourself out of bed in the morning) or are you just overtired? If you were able to get a good night's sleep, would it help at all? Or would you wake up just as tired as when you lay down? If you have true CFS, then you are more tired than you could have *ever* imagined you could be and still function.

Think about your pain. Are you just achy because you've been pushing yourself too hard? Would a good massage and a weekend away solve your problem? Or does your body hurt *all* the time, standing or lying down, waking or sleeping, enjoying yourself or in stress? Those with true FMS don't even remember what it's like not to hurt.

Then, consider your other symptoms. Do you seem to be constantly fighting off colds, as if your immune system isn't working right? Then you're leaning more toward CFS. Do you not remember the last time you slept all night? You're leaning toward FMS. See the graphic on the next page for a simple way to visualize where you fit on the pain-fatigue spectrum.

Place a dot on the horizontal line below to indicate where you think you fall on the pain-fatigue spectrum. Most patients lean more one way than the other.

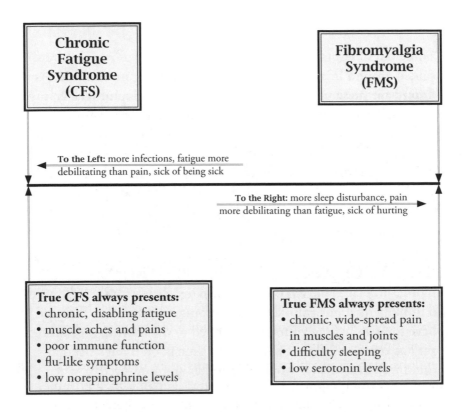

· 4 ·
FIBROMYALGIA SYNDROME

"Some days I couldn't even remember the names of my children. I walked around in a fog, and the pain was getting unbearable. As I drifted further and further away from my friends and family, my doctors insisted that there was nothing wrong with me."

The illness known as fibromyalgia syndrome (FMS) is characterized by diffuse muscle pain, poor sleep, and often, unrelenting fatigue. Individuals with fibromyalgia may also experience headaches, anxiety, depression, poor memory, numbness and tingling in the extremities, cold hands and feet, irritable bowel syndrome, lowered immune function, and chemical sensitivities. Over 10 million Americans suffer with fibromyalgia; ninety percent of them are women between 25 and 45 years old.

It's pronounced FIY-bro-my-AL-jia. The word is derived from the Greek "algia," meaning pain; "myo," indicating muscle; and the Latin "fibro," referring to the connective tissues of ligaments and tendons. So basically, fibromyalgia means "pain in the muscles, ligaments, and tendons." It's a syndrome by definition: a group of signs and symptoms that occur together and that characterize a particular illness.

HISTORY OF FIBROMYALGIA

Symptoms similar to those associated with FMS were reported as early as 1736 by Guillaume de Baillou, who coined the term "rheumatism" to describe muscle aches and pains as well as rheumatic fever. "Fibrositis" was coined by Gowers in 1904 and was not changed to "fibromyalgia" until 1976. Smythe laid the foundation of modern FMS in 1972 by describing widespread pain and tender points. The first sleep electroencephalogram study was performed in 1975, and the first controlled clinical study with validation of known symptoms and tender points was published in 1981. This same study also proposed the first data-based criteria. The important concept that FMS and similar conditions are interconnected was proposed in 1984. The first American College of Rheumatology (ACR) criteria were published in 1990.

FIBROMYALGIA AND CFS

Fibromyalgia shares several symptoms with chronic fatigue syndrome (CFS). One study comparing 50 CFS patients with 50 FMS patients found the symptoms of low grade fever (28%), swollen lymph nodes (33%), rash (47%), cough (40%), and recurrent sore throat (54%) to be the same for both syndromes. Another study comparing CFS patients with FMS patients showed that the brain-wave patterns, tender points, pain, and fatigue were virtually identical in both groups. Still, I've found some distinct differences between the two syndromes. Those with true fibromyalgia suffer from fatigue but always list poor sleep and diffuse muscle pain as their primary complaints. They consistently demonstrate symptoms associated with low serotonin levels: poor sleep, increased pain, irritable bowel, brain fog, anxiety, and depression.

Although both of these illnesses have their own unique symptoms and separate criteria for diagnostic purposes, they're really different sides of the same coin. Patients can be anywhere on the scale between FMS and CFS. Most patients share some of the symptoms associated with both syndromes and fall somewhere in the middle.

DIAGNOSIS OF FIBROMYALGIA

There is currently no diagnostic test to confirm the presence of fibromyalgia. The diagnosis is usually reached after ruling out other neurological, autoimmune, endocrine, musculoskeletal, immunological, and mental disorders. Patients have typically had the illness at least seven years and been seen by a dozen different doctors before they're diagnosed with FMS.

The ACR's current criteria for defining fibromyalgia syndrome includes a history of widespread pain lasting more than three months and the presence of at least 11 (out of a possible 18) tender points. Pain is considered to be "widespread" when it affects all four quadrants of the body; that is, you must have pain in both your right and left sides as well as above and below the waist to be diagnosed with fibromyalgia.

The ACR reports that 2–4% of the population suffers from fibromyalgia, but this estimate is much too low. The main problem with the ACR criteria is that many individuals with FMS meet some but not all of them. Most of these individuals have other symptoms associated with FMS not explicitly outlined in the ACR criteria. They may have insomnia, irritable bowel, fatigue, mental confusion, and only four of the 18 trigger points. Or they may have insomnia, fatigue, and five reproducible tender points.

I like to say "anything that can go wrong in a FMS patient, will." FMS patients have a wide variety of complaints, and some of them can be quite bizarre: *Dr. Murphree, have you ever heard of getting dizzy when eating peanut butter on your bagels?* or *I tingle all over, including my tongue. Is this normal?* It's easy to see how doctors could be skeptical of FMS. Some rationalize that only a mental illness could produce so many different and seemingly unrelated symptoms. And some choose to ignore FMS and CFS, despite the guidelines of the ACR and of other notable studies published in various distinguished medical journals. Other physicians accept FMS as an entity, but they don't know much about diagnosing it and even less about treating it.

SYMPTOMS OF FIBROMYALGIA

A more complete list of FMS symptoms would include much more than trigger points:

• **Sleep disturbances:** Sufferers may not feel refreshed, despite getting adequate amounts of sleep. They may also have difficulty falling asleep or staying asleep.

• **Stiffness:** Body stiffness is present in most patients. Weather changes and remaining in one position for a long period of time contribute to the problem. Stiffness may also be present upon awakening.

• **Headaches and facial pain:** Headaches may be caused by

associated tenderness in the neck and shoulder area or soft tissue around the temporomandibular joint (TMJ).

- **Abdominal discomfort:** Patients may suffer from irritable bowel syndrome (IBS), which involves digestive disturbances, abdominal pain and bloating, constipation, and diarrhea.

- **Poor digestion:** Individuals with FMS may suffer from poor digestion and assimilation of their foods, as evidenced by the fact that the majority of them have a deficiency in certain amino acids, which are usually obtained from protein-rich foods. Low levels of five amino acids—histidine, methionine, tryptophan, isoleucine, and leucine—and low urinary levels of norepinephrine and dopamine have been identified in FMS patients with an accuracy of 81%.

- **Irritable bladder:** An increase in urinary frequency and a greater urgency to urinate may be present.

- **Numbness or tingling:** Known as parethesia, symptoms include a prickling or burning sensation in the extremities.

- **Chest pain:** Muscular pain at the point where the ribs meet the chest bone may occur.

- **Cognitive disorders:** The symptoms of cognitive disorders may vary from day to day. They can include "spaciness," memory lapses, difficulty concentrating, word mix-ups when speaking or writing, and clumsiness.

- **Environmental sensitivity:** Sensitivities to light noise, odors, and weather are often present, as are allergic reactions to a variety of substances. Substantial overlap exists among chemical sensitivity, fibromyalgia, and chronic fatigue syndrome, as they are all really based on the same disorder. Certain chemicals are more likely to cause the onset of chemical sensitivity and chronic illness: gasoline, kerosene, natural gas, pesticides (especially chlordane and chlorpyrifos), certain solvents, new carpet, paints, glues, fiberglass, carbonless copy paper, fabric softener, formaldehyde, carpet shampoos and other cleaning agents, combustion products (from poorly vented gas heaters, overheated batteries, etc.), perfumes, deodorants, and various medications. A sluggish detoxification system, allergic reactions, neurological mediated sensitivities, and opportunistic pathogens may also contribute to chemical sensitivity.

- **Disequilibrium:** Difficulties in orientation may occur when standing, driving, or reading. Dizziness and balance problems may also be present.

- **Allodynia:** Fibromyalgia suffers have a lower than average pain threshold (allodynia). They perceive pain that would normally not be felt by healthy individuals. This can be caused by low levels of certain neurotransmitters (brain chemicals) including serotonin, norepinephrine, and dopamine.

- **Central sensitization/hyperalgesia:** This occurs when the nerve cells that supply the brain become more excitable, overamplifying sensations of pain. When you have FMS, a bumped knee, a stubbed toe, or even a playful poke from a friend can take your breath away or still be felt hours later.

OTHER SYMPTOMS

Carol Jessop, MD, reports that a sample of close to 1,000 of her FMS patients showed the following:

- 100% had muscular pain.
- Nearly all suffered from poor sleep and fatigue.
- Most were battling depression.
- 40% had cold hands and feet with poor circulation, known as Raynaud's syndrome.
- 24% had anxiety.
- 10% had an elevated temperature.
- 65% had a low temperature, suggesting low thyroid and metabolism.
- 86% had low blood pressure, suggesting dysautonomia and poor adrenal function.
- 85% had white spots on their nails, suggesting low zinc and poor digestion or malabsorption.

- 40% had a tender thyroid.
- 18% had swollen lymph nodes (I see a larger percentage of patients with this), suggesting immune dysfunction.
- 73% had irritable bowel syndrome.
- Half suffered from severe headaches, usually associated with low magnesium and thyroid/adrenal hormones.
- 18% had dry eyes, suggestive of allergies.
- 12% suffered from osteoarthritis.
- 7% had rheumatoid arthritis.
- 82% tested positive for yeast in their stool cultures.
- 30% had parasites in their stool sample.
- 60% had irregular periods, suggestive of poor nutrition.
- 25% had temporomandibular joint (TMJ) syndrome.
- 15% had endometriosis, suggestive of estrogen dominance and/or liver dysfunction.
- 30% had restless leg syndrome, suggestive of low magnesium.
- 40% had multiple chemical sensitivity, suggestive of liver dysfunction.
- 25% had interstitial cystitis.
- 15% had an irritable bladder.
- 75% had mitral valve prolapse.

Just as interesting are the symptoms that her patients had before developing FMS. These symptoms, listed below, suggest a chronic malabsorption (digestion) problem. This, as we'll discuss in chapter 12, can lead to all sorts of deficiencies in essential nutrients and finally to FMS:

- 58% had constipation.
- 80% had bloating, gas, and/or indigestion.
- 40% had heartburn.
- 89% had irritable bowel syndrome.

FIBROMYALGIA IS NOT ARTHRITIS
The pain of fibromyalgia may be erroneously presumed to be joint arthritis or an autoimmune connective disorder. However, unlike

arthritis, there is usually no joint pain or inflammation. Instead, FMS sufferers have generalized muscle and soft-tissue pain that appears gradually and becomes worse with additional physical, emotional, or mental fatigue. The soft tissue and muscles of the neck, shoulders, rib cage and chest, lower back, and thighs are especially vulnerable.

Because rheumatologists were the first to officially acknowledge and classify FMS, they became the medical "experts" on the syndrome. They specialize in diseases of the joints, muscles, and connective tissue, such as rheumatoid arthritis, osteoarthritis, Sjögren's syndrome, and lupus. The rheumatologist's treatment of choice for theses illnesses involves an ever-increasing amount of potentially dangerous drugs as the disease progresses. Fibromyalgia sufferers rarely benefit from long-term drug therapy, so they are often worse off for following a rheumatologist's instructions. And their illness doesn't really "progress" like arthritis can. It often comes and goes, and FMS can, in fact, be reversed!

This misunderstanding presents an unfortunate predicament for those with FMS. Most family doctors don't know what to do with them and simply refer them to a rheumatologist. Of course it usually takes months to be seen by such a specialist, who orders a battery of blood

> The ACR has previously admitted on their web site that the drugs they commonly recommend have little benefit on average.
>
> Four controlled trials have evaluated the efficacy of amitriptyline (Elavil) in the treatment of fibromyalgia, and the longest trial showed no benefit when compared to placebo. Furthermore, the overall degree of benefit was found to be relatively small in relevant outcomes such as improvement in pain, fatigue, and sleep. In addition, 95% of Elavil-treated patients experience side effects. Long-term, follow-up observations of FMS patients treated with drug therapy indicated that their clinical findings did not change appreciably after 15 years.
>
> The ACR reports that, furthermore, use of anti-anxiety benzodiazepines (such as Klonopin and Xanax), corticosteroids (such as Medrol and prednisone), and nonsteroidal anti-inflammatory agents (such as Mobic, Celebrex, and Bextra) have been shown to be ineffective and should be generally avoided. For more details on how traditional drug therapy alone offers little long-term relief for fibromyalgia and may actually make your condition worse, see chapter 6.

tests, the results of which "look fine." The patient next hears, "I think you have fibromyalgia. Here are some sleeping pills, muscle relaxants, antidepressants, and nerve pills. Good luck. I'll see you in four months." You guessed it; I'm not a fan of the typical rheumatological approach to treating fibromyalgia.

CLINICAL SIGNS

Whatever the initial cause, fibromyalgia symptoms are thought to arise from a miscommunication among nerve impulses of the central nervous system. FMS patients typically display certain clinical signs:

• **Low levels of the neurotransmitter serotonin.** Neurotransmitters are chemicals that relay, amplify, and coordinate electrical signals between a nerve cell and another cell.

• **A four-fold increase in nerve growth factor (NGF),** a specific type of peptide. Peptides are short molecules formed from the ordered combination of various amino acids.

• **Elevated levels of substance P.** The exposure of pain receptors to NGF leads to elevated levels of this neurotransmitter, which is found in spinal fluid. Increased substance P lowers a person's pain threshold. The longer a person has fibromyalgia, the worse this condition can become. Where before the illness, she could stand for long periods without pain, perhaps now she can barely tolerate the pressure of her feet on the floor.

• **Dysfunction of the hypothalamus-pituitary-adrenal (HPA) axis.** This condition is not fully understood, but we know that this imbalance creates inconsistencies in communication among certain cells, disrupting the body's ability to maintain homeostasis. Many of the most common fibromyalgia symptoms (including widespread muscle pain, fatigue, poor sleep, gastrointestinal problems, and depression) regularly occur in people with various hormonal disorders, including those manifested by HPA-axis dysfunction. I believe that suppression of the HPA axis begins with *chronic stress,* and several studies have demonstrated this. And a survey by The Fibromyalgia Network reports that 62% of their respondents list physical or emotional stress as the initiating factor in their fibromyalgia.

> *Q: So, what caused my fibromyalgia?*
>
> A: I wish I had an easy answer for you. But FMS can be caused by any combination of several factors:
>
> • hypothalamus-pituitary-adrenal axis (HPA) dysfunction
> • trauma, especially whiplash
> • emotional, physical, or mental stress (see ch. 9)
> • low thyroid function
> • low serotonin states
> • adrenal dysfunction
> • chronic viral, mycoplasma, or bacterial infections
> • endocrine disorders
> • sleep disorders

THE HPA AXIS

As described above, the HPA axis is comprised of the hypothalamus, the pituitary gland, and the adrenal glands. The pituitary gland is responsible for releasing many important hormones, and you'll see more about it throughout this book. You'll learn a lot about the **adrenals** in chapter 11.

As for the **hypothalamus,** its main function is homeostasis, or maintaining the body's status quo. Because of its broad sphere of influence, the hypothalamus could be considered the body's master computer. It receives and transmits messages with the nervous and circulatory systems, keeping continuous tabs on the state of the body. It must be able to initiate compensatory changes if anything drifts out of line. The hypothalamus regulates many bodily functions:

• **Blood pressure:** this is often low in those with fibromyalgia.
• **Digestion:** bloating, gas, indigestion, and reflux are common in FMS patients.
• **Circadian rhythms (the sleep/wake cycle):** this is consistently disrupted in FMS cases.
• **Sex drive:** loss of libido is a common complaint for FMS patients.

- **Body temperature:** this is often low in FMS patients.
- **Balance and coordination:** FMS patients typically have balance and coordination problems.
- **Heart rate:** mitral valve prolapse (MVP) and heart arrhythmias are a common finding in FMS patients.
- **Sweating:** it's not unusual for FMS patients to experience excessive sweating.
- **Adrenal hormones:** these are consistently low in FMS patients.
- **Thyroid hormones and metabolism:** Recent studies show that over 43% of FMS patients have low thyroid function. It's also estimated that those with FMS are 10 to 250,000 times more likely to suffer from thyroid dysfunction.

A VICIOUS CYCLE

Once the nightmare of fibromyalgia is jump-started, whatever the underlying cause, it begins to spin out of control, and a vicious cycle takes over.

1. Chronic stress disrupts the HPA axis, leading to allodynia (lowered pain threshold) and chronic pain.
2. Chronic pain disrupts the circadian rhythm (normal sleep/wake cycle).
3. Dysfunction in the circadian rhythm results in poor sleep.
4. Poor sleep reduces growth hormone production, leading to poor repair of damaged muscle fibers, poor memory, fatigue, suppressed immune function, and more pain.
5. Increased pain further disrupts sleep and leads to depletion of stress-coping chemicals, including serotonin.
6. A reduction in serotonin causes an increase in substance P, which enhances pain receptors, creating even more pain.
7. Poor sleep and ongoing stress lead to fatigue, mood disorders, irritable bowel syndrome (IBS), adrenal fatigue, decreased DHEA, possibly thyroid dysfunction, and lowered resistance to stress.
8. Decreased stress-coping abilities leads to lowered immune function, and lowered blood volume from adrenal dysfunction leads to further fatigue.

In chapters 8 and 9, we'll explore more thoroughly how stress can lead to HPA-axis dysfunction, fibromyalgia, and CFS.

FOR FURTHER READING AND RESEARCH

- G.K. Adler, "Neuroendocrine Abnormalities in Fibromyalgia," *Current Pain and Headache Reports* 6 (2002): 289–298.
- M. Altamus et al., "Abnormalities in Response to Vasopressin Infusion in Chronic Fatigue Syndrome," *Psychoneuroendocrinology* 26(2) (2001): 175–88.
- M. Biondi and A. Picardi, "Psychological Stress and Neuroendocrine Function in Humans: the Last Two Decades of Research," *Psychotherapy and Psychosomatics* 68 (1999): 114–150.
- D. Buskila D et al., "Increased Rates of Fibromyalgia Following Cervical Spine Injury," *Arthritis and Rheumatism* 40(3) (1997): 446–52.
- M. Calis M et al., "Investigation of the Hypothalamo–pituitary–adrenal Axis (HPA) by 1 Microg ACTH Test and Metyrapone Test in Patients with Primary Fibromyalgia Syndrome," *Journal of Endocrinological Investigation* 27(1) (2004): 42–6.
- D.T. Chalmers et al., "Molecular Aspects of the Stress Axis and Serotonergic Function in Depression," *Clinical Neuroscience* 1 (1993): 122–8.
- G.K. Endresen, "Mycoplasma Blood Infection in Chronic Fatigue and Fibromyalgia Syndromes," *Rheumatology International* 23(5) (2003): 211–15.
- *Fibromyalgia Network Newsletter* October 1999: 1–3.
- D. Goldenberg, "Fibromyalgia and its Relationship to CFS, Viral Illness and Immune Abnormalities," *Journal of Rheumatology* 16(S19) (1989): 92.
- S. Harding, "Sleep in Fibromyalgia Patients: Subjective and Objective Findings," *American Journal of the Medical Sciences: Fibromyalgia* 315(6) (1998): 367–76.
- W. Jeffries, "The Present Status of ACTH, Cortisone, and Related Steroids in Clinical Medicine," New England Journal of Medicine 253 (1995): 441–6.
- J.F. Lopez et al., "Serotonin 1a Receptor mRNA Regulation in the Hippocampus After Acute Stress," *Biological Psychiatry* 45: 943–7.
- J.C. Lowe et al., "Effectiveness and Safety of T3 (Triiothyroxine) Therapy for Euthyroid Fibromyalgia: a Double–blind Placebo–controlled Response–driven Crossover Study," *Clinical Bulletin of Myofascial Therapy* 2(2/3) (1997a): 31–58.
- H. Moldofsky H, "Fibromyalgia, Sleep Disorder and Chronic Fatigue Syndrome, " CIBA Symposium, 173 (1993): 262–79.
- *Nutrition Reviews* 52(7) (1994): 249.
- A. Okifuji and D.C. Turk, "Stress and Psychophysiological Dysregulation in Patients with Fibromyalgia Syndrome," *Applied Psychophysiology and Biofeedback* 27(2) (2002): 129–41.
- D. Rudman, "Growth Hormone, Body Composition, and Aging," *Journal of the American Geriatrics Society* 33 (1985): 800–7.
- I. Russell et al., "Serum Serotonin in FMS and Rheumatoid Arthritis and

Healthy Normal Controls," *Arthritis and Rheumatism* 36(9) (1993): S-2231.

- I.J. Russell, "Elevated Cerebrospinal Fluid Levels of Substance P in Patients with the Fibromyalgia Syndrome," *Arthritis and Rheumatism* 37(11) (1994): 1593–601.

- I.J. Russell, "Neurohormonal Aspects of Fibromyalgia Syndrome," *Rheumatic Diseases Clinics of North America* 15 (1989): 149–168.

- H. Selye, "The General Adaptation Syndrome and Diseases of Adaptation," *Journal of Clinical Endocrinology and Metabolism* 6 (1946): 117–230.

- S.R. Smitherman, "Peripheral and Central Sensitization in Fibromyalgia: Pathogenetic Role," *Currant Pain and Headache Report* (4) (2002): 259–66.

- T.L. Wisniewski et al., "The Relationship of Serum DHEA–S and Cortisol Levels to Measures of Immune Function in Human Immunodeficiency Virus–related Illness," *American Journal of the Medical Sciences* 305(2) (1993): 79–83.

- C.J. Woolf, "Nerve Growth Factor Contributes to the Generation of Inflammatory Sensory Hypersensitivity," *Neuroscience* 62 (1994): 327–31.

- F. Wolfe et al., "The American College of Rheumatology 1990 Criteria for the Classification of Fibromyalgia," *Arthritis and Rheumatism* 33 (1990): 160–72.

- M. Yunus et al., "Interrelations of Biochemical Parameters and Classification of FMS," *Journal of Musculoskeletal Pain* 3(4) (1995): 15–24.

· 5 ·
CHRONIC FATIGUE SYNDROME

Chronic fatigue syndrome (CFS), also known as chronic fatigue immune dysfunction syndrome (CFIDS), is a disabling condition affecting approximately 500,000 Americans. And research conducted by the Centers for Disease Control and Prevention (CDC) indicates that fewer than 20% of CFS patients in this country have even been diagnosed. Needless to say, it's not rare. Patients are usually women in their 40s and 50s, but anyone can develop CFS. Though much less common in children, the syndrome can manifest in childhood, particularly during the teen years.

Unlike someone with fibromyalgia, CFS patients may have normal serotonin levels and little trouble sleeping. But if you have true chronic fatigue syndrome, you're often still fatigued, no matter how well you sleep.

SIGNS OF CFS
Patients with CFS typically have a compromised immune system, elevated blood antibodies, intermittent sore throats, and tender lymph nodes. CFS can affect any part of the body, including the central nervous system, the brain, the blood, muscles, joints, the GI tract, and the immune, digestive, and lymph systems.

DIAGNOSIS OF CFS
No one knows exactly what causes CFS; there's just no specific diagnostic test for it. And since many illnesses can cause incapacitating fatigue, doctors must rule out other conditions before finally diagnosing CFS in a patient. Some studies following CFS sufferers over time reveal that though some cases improve with time, most patients remain functionally impaired for at least several years.

SYMPTOMS OF CFS

CFS is marked by extreme fatigue—lasting at least six months—that isn't just due to exertion and isn't substantially relieved by rest. Naturally, this fatigue causes a significant reduction in daily activities. In addition to fatigue, CFS includes eight characteristic symptoms:

• postexertional malaise (relapse of symptoms after physical or mental exertion)
• unrefreshing sleep
• substantial impairment in memory and/or concentration
• muscle pain
• pain in multiple joints
• headaches of a new type, pattern, or severity
• sore throat
• tender neck or armpit lymph nodes

Patients also report various nonspecific symptoms, including weakness, irritable bowel syndrome (IBS), dizziness, bloating, gas, indigestion, irregular heartbeat, nausea, night sweats, mood disorders (depression, irritability, anxiety, or panic attacks), shortness of breathe, tingling sensations, flu-like symptoms, chemical sensitivities, allergies, poor immune function, and insomnia. Neurally mediated hypotension (low blood pressure upon rising) is common in CFS patients, as is dysautonomia (dysfunction of the autonomic nervous system), which occurs in about 96% of cases. Those with CFS also tend toward sinus, upper respiratory, or other infections, which linger and return.

The symptoms can be quite severe. CFS can be as disabling as multiple sclerosis, lupus, rheumatoid arthritis, or congestive heart failure! The severity of symptoms varies from person to person and can also change over time.

MEDICAL CONDITIONS SIMILAR TO CFS

The main difference between CFS and the conditions below is that CFS has unrelenting fatigue as its main and most pronounced symptom. Other illnesses can cause chronic fatigue as a symptom, but they usually begin with at least one other primary complaint.

These illnesses can each be clinically defined by either a set of symptoms or a diagnostic test, and they should be ruled out or successfully treated before a diagnosis of CFS is seriously considered.

Illnesses to Rule Out Before Treating CFS

Autoimmune Disorders
- Behçet's syndrome
- dermatomyositis
- lupus
- polyarteritis
- polymyositis
- Reiter's syndrome
- rheumatoid arthritis
- Sjögren's syndrome
- vasculitis

GI Disorders
- celiac disease
- Crohn's disease
- irritable bowel syndrome
- sarcoidosis
- ulcerative colitis

Blood Disorders
- anemia
- hemochromatosis

Endocrine/Hormonal Disorders
- Addison's disease
- Cushing's syndrome
- diabetes mellitus
- hyperthyroidism
- hypothyroidism
- ovarian failure
- panhypopituitarism

Malignancies/Cancer
- Hodgkin's disease
- lymphoma

Sleep Disorders
- sleep apnea
- narcolepsy

Neuromuscular Disorders
- fibromyalgia
- muscular dystrophies
- multiple sclerosis
- myasthenia gravis

Infections
- subacute infections
- bacterial endocarditis
- chronic brucellosis
- mononucleosis
- hepatitis
- HIV infection
- Lyme disease
- occult abscess
- poliomyelitis/post-polio syndrome
- tuberculosis
- parasitic infection
- fungal infection

Other Conditions
- major depressive disorders
- bipolar affective disorders
- schizophrenia
- obesity
- alcohol or substance abuse
- reactions to prescribed medications

SIMILAR BUT NOT THE SAME

Since CFS shares many similarities with FMS, some researchers have suggested that they are the same illness. One early study comparing 50 CFS patients with 50 FMS patients showed the following symptoms to be the same for both groups: low-grade fever

(28%), swollen lymph nodes (33%), rash (47%), cough (40%), and recurrent sore throat (54%). Another study comparing CFS patients with FMS patients showed that the brain-wave patterns, tender points, pain, and fatigue were virtually identical in both groups.

But chronic fatigue syndrome is not really the same as fibromyalgia; remember from chapter 3 that they are two ends of one spectrum, two sides of one coin. But they are still distinct. To quickly distinguish a CFS patient from one with FMS only, your doctor can run an EBV panel (see more about this blood test on p. 457).

But you don't need a lab test to diagnose CFS. Its symptoms are generally consistent. The CFS patient usually has chronic infections (sinusitis, upper respiratory, urinary tract infections, colds, flu, etc.) and gets at least two bad infections a year. She will usually have chronic or intermittent sore throats, swollen lymph nodes, and periodic fevers. These states aren't as typical of FMS patients. And while a CFS patient may ache all over, FMS patients can usually point to specific areas that are the most troublesome.

Simply put, if it's tough for you to get out of bed each day, you suffer from diffuse body aches, and you have frequent infections, then you either have CFS or you're at high risk for developing it.

CFS AND SLUGGISH LIVER
Many CFS patients will also have a sluggish liver (more likely than in those with FMS). Evidence of a sluggish liver includes strange or opposite reactions to medications (you take something to put you to sleep and it wakes you up instead, or a little goes a loooong way). Other signs include intolerance to caffeine, alcohol, and odors such as perfumes, gasoline, smoke, and cleaners. This intolerance tends to worsen over time.

A history of elevated liver enzymes on past blood tests also indicates a sluggish liver. Of course, anyone with hepatitis or fatty liver also has a sluggish liver, and long-term prescription-medication therapies can also create this condition, independent of CFS.

A sluggish liver can cause severe chemical sensitivities that complicate the use of even the purist nutritional supplements. So nutritional therapy must be started slowly. Be patient with yourself. Slow and steady wins the race!

POSSIBLE CAUSES OF CFS

No one knows for certain what causes CFS, but it appears to be triggered by a number of factors. These causes include infectious agents (viruses, bacteria, mycoplasma, fungi, etc.), mental or physical stress, oxidative stress, autonomic nervous system dysfunction, hormonal abnormalities, nutrient deficiencies, autoimmune abnormalities, and allergies.

Unfortunately and in spite of evidence, some physicians believe that CFS is principally a component of a psychological disorder (basically, that you're crazy). Others view it only as a symptom of other problems (viewed similarly to anemia and high blood pressure) and not a syndrome in itself.

Indeed, no primary cause has been found that explains all cases of CFS. But a number of experts believe that CFS is caused by a combination of initiating factors that overwhelm a person's stress-coping abilities. These factors may include:

• genetic factors
• brain abnormalities
• inability of the self-regulating mechanisms, especially the autonomic nervous system and the hypothalamus-pituitary-adrenal (HPA) axis
• a hyper-reactive immune system
• viral, bacterial, fungal, mycoplasma, or other infectious agents, including the Epstein-Barr virus (EBV)

EPSTEIN-BARR VIRUS

Several studies have focused on identifying an infectious agent as the cause of CFS, and the EBV has received a lot of attention over the past two decades.

In 1985, reports in the *Annals of Internal Medicine* described a mysterious severe viral epidemic that gripped the Lake Tahoe region of California. This epidemic of what we now know as CFS was presumed to be caused by the Epstein-Barr virus, since the National Institutes of Health (NIH) confirmed elevated levels of EBV antibodies in those afflicted. (Now we know that EBV is only one of many viruses associated with CFS.)

EBV, a member of the herpes group of viruses, has the ability to establish a lifelong latent presence in the body after an initial infection. Fortunately, a healthy immune system can keep this latent virus in check. For instance, the EBV causes the debilitating disease of the teen years, infectious mononucleosis or "mono." Mono is marked by debilitating fatigue, fever, sore throat, and swollen lymph glands. Caused by the Epstein-Barr virus, it usually lasts from three to six weeks.

But not everyone who carries the virus develops mono. In fact, over 90% of Americans have been exposed to EBV by age 20. Some of these individuals develop mono; others simply experience flu-like symptoms for a few days. But most show no symptoms at all as their immune system fends off the attacking virus.

It was once thought that mono patients produced sufficient antibodies to keep them immune from future EBV infection, but recent research has helped change this line of thinking. Interestingly, it's now believed that individuals who developed mono are slightly more susceptible to recurrent EBV than the general population.

Physicians and researchers began to recognize the incidence of recurrent EBV as early as 1948. Reports continued to appear throughout the '50s and '60s, but it wasn't until the late 1970s that studies were published describing persistent EBV infection characterized by intermittent fever, muscle and joint aches, sore throats, and debilitating fatigue.

By the mid 1980s, numerous studies had seemed to correlate these symptoms directly with reactivation of latent EBV. The disorder was dubbed chronic Epstein-Barr virus (CEBV) syndrome. Unlike mono, the condition did not seem to be self-limiting. It would come and go, or never fully go away. Describing it as "the flu from hell," patients experienced physical and mental exhaustion. Other symptoms varied, usually including extreme fatigue, weakness, depression, muscle and joint aches, sore throat, swollen lymph glands, headache, and low-grade afternoon fever. In addition, many patients reported impaired memory, difficulty concentrating, disturbed balance, anxiety, irritability, and insomnia. These symptoms usually fluctuated in severity from month to month, and even day to day. Periods of wellness were often followed by relapse, as patients attempted to resume normal activities or exercise.

This chronic EBV syndrome is known today as CFS. Sadly, a compromised immune system allows the virus to reemerge in a frustratingly persistent manner. A variety of immune system abnormalities have been observed in CFS cases, and there is little argument that a disturbed immune system plays a central role in the syndrome.

CYTOMEGALOVIRUS

Although not as common as EBV, cytomegalovirus (CMV) is estimated to infect close to 75% of adults in Western nations, with the incidence in Asia and Africa approaching 100%. In the majority of cases, primary exposure produces no clinical illness, but like all herpes viruses, CMV remains latent in the body for life. During times of immune suppression, CMV can become reactivated and produce symptoms very similar to EBV. In fact, 10–15% of all mononucleosis cases appear to be caused by CMV, not EBV. For the most part, however, CMV produces observable illness in two groups: infants and immune-suppressed adults.

Both CMV and EBV can infect the central nervous system, causing a wide range of neurological symptoms ranging from confusion and memory loss to inflammation of the brain (encephalitis) and a common nervous system disorder known as Guillain-Barré syndrome.

CMV is also known to infect the gastrointestinal tract. A common occurrence, it might go unnoticed. But for the unlucky few, intestinal permeability (leaky gut syndrome) and malabsorption can result. Current research even suggests that the virus may contribute to ulcers, colitis, and cancer of the colon.

The majority of physicians who actively treat CFS agree that correcting immune dysfunction is perhaps the most important priority in any CFS treatment plan.

POOR IMMUNITY

I, like many other specialists, do believe there is an infectious agent or agents involved in CFS. Plainly, something foreign is interacting with a compromised immune system. And that something is possibly causing the weakening of immunity itself. The question is: Is that agent (be it virus, bacteria, fungus, mycoplasma, or a combination of these) latent or acute? Some researchers suggest that CFS is caused not by a reactivated virus but rather an infection that attacks the body, causes immune abnormalities, and is then eliminated.

The theory, though not based on hard evidence, does have some supporting observations. For instance, in up to 80% of cases, CFS starts suddenly with a flu-like condition. And outbreaks of CFS occurring within the same household, workplace, and community have been reported, though most have not been confirmed by the CDC. Perhaps the most important evidence for previous acute infection is that CFS patients typically have elevated levels of antibodies to many fatigue-causing substances, including Lyme disease, Candida (yeast infection), herpes virus type 6 (HHV-6), human T-cell lymphotropic virus (HTLV), EBV, measles, Coxsackie B viruses, cytomegalovirus, and parvovirus B19 (fifth disease).

In one study, some patients, particularly those with severe CFS symptoms, had higher-than-normal numbers of infection-fighting white blood cells known as CD8 killer T cells, which launch attacks on invading viruses and other disease-causing microorganisms. These same people had lower-than-normal levels of another white blood cell known as the suppressor T cell, which helps to shut down the immune response once the invading organisms have been killed. As a consequence of these imbalances, their immune system could have become persistently overactive and produced fatigue, muscle aches, and other symptoms of CFS.

The most consistently observed abnormality is a decreased number or activity of natural killer (NK) cells, which are used by the body to destroy cells infected with cancerous or viral toxins. Read more about immune-system cells in chapter 17.

CHRONIC CYTOKINE SECRETION

One intriguing theory is that various triggering events, such as stress or a viral infection, may lead to the chronic expression of cytokines and then to CFS. Cytokines are small, secreted proteins that regulate immunity, inflammation, and the development of blood cells. The body releases them when they are needed, in response to stress, and they usually act just for a short time.

Administration of some cytokines in therapeutic doses is known to cause fatigue, but no characteristic pattern of chronic cytokine secretion has ever been identified in CFS patients. In addition, some investigators have noted clinical improvement in patients with continued high levels of circulating cytokines; if a causal relationship exists between cytokines and CFS, it is likely to be complex.

ALLERGIES

Several studies have shown that CFS patients are more likely to have a history of allergies than are healthy controls. A history of allergies, then, could be one predisposing factor for CFS. But it cannot be the only one, since not all CFS patients have them.

OVERWHELMING STRESS

The majority of patients report some preceding moderate to serious physical stress (such as a chronic viral infection) or emotional event (often an episode of depression or chronic mental stress). Some experts theorize that such events, especially in people with certain neurological and genetic abnormalities, may overwhelm a person's ability to regulate her own homeostatic self-regulating systems.

I believe there is a great deal of truth to this idea (though admitting so may not endear me to those who believe that CFS is the result entirely of an infectious agent). I do believe that infectious agents can and do trigger CFS, but stress and infection go hand in hand. Stress weakens the body's immune system, and an overtaxed immune system is quite stressful.

HPA-AXIS DYSFUNCTION

Some researchers are investigating abnormalities in CFS patients of the brain system known as the hypothalamus-pituitary-adrenal axis. This system produces or regulates hormones and brain chemicals that control important functions, including sleep, response to stress, and depression. It's our self-regulating, homeostatic system.

The HPA axis is a major part of the neuroendocrine system, which controls reactions to stress. It regulates various body processes such as digestion, the immune system, and metabolism, and it's generally suppressed in CFS patients.

CORTISOL DEFICIENCY

A number of studies on CFS patients have observed deficiencies in cortisol levels, a stress hormone produced in the hypothalamus. Cortisol suppresses inflammation, increases stamina, boosts mental and physical energy, and coordinates cellular immune activation.

Cortisol deficiency may be why CFS patients consistently demonstrate a severely compromised resiliency to stress. (Although stress is commonly thought of as resulting from emotional or psychological causes, certain infections may cause severe unrelenting internal biochemical stress.)

As a diagnostic marker for CFS, however, individual cortisol levels aren't useful. Typically, the altered cortisol levels noted in CFS cases fall within the accepted range of normal, and only the average between cases and controls reveals a distinction.

> Q: So what's the real cause of CFS? I must know what's making me feel this way!
>
> A: As with so many complex chronic illnesses, CFS may be caused and aggravated by a wide variety of environmental and physiological challenges. Whether the cause is one described here or something else entirely is not definitively known. But, I bet that you care even more about getting well than you do about how you got sick. Read on in this book to uncover some key health strategies that have consistently yielded clinical improvement in the majority of my patients suffering with CFS.

BRAIN ABNORMALITIES AND OXIDATIVE STRESS

Some of the symptoms of CFS, such as impaired cognition, may result from brain abnormalities. Several studies have reported significantly more abnormalities on MRI among CFS subjects relative to controls.

Other studies have revealed lesions within the brains of CFS patients, and Single Photon Emission Computed Tomography (SPECT) scanning has repeatedly demonstrated a decrease of blood flow in the brain. In one study, decreased regional cerebral blood flow throughout the brain was observed in 80% of CFS patients!

These observations may explain the "brain fog," poor mental clarity, and fatigue associated with CFS. They might also demonstrate CFS's association with oxidative (free radical) stress. Oxidative stress is a general term used to describe the level of damage to a cell, tissue, or organ caused by the reactive oxygen species (ROS) These very small, highly reactive molecules can affect any cell or system, including the brain. Most ROS come from normal internal bodily reactions, but external sources include first- and secondhand cigarette smoke, environmental pollutants, excess alcohol, asbestos, ionizing radiation, and bacterial, fungal, or viral infections.

Supporting this oxidative-stress theory is the fact that antioxidant therapy has been proven helpful in the treatment of CFS. In one study involving CFS patients who required bed rest following mild exercise, 80% were deficient in Coenzyme Q10 (CoQ10), a potent antioxidant.

After three months of supplementing with 100 mg. of CoQ10, 90% of the patients had a reduction or disappearance of clinically measured symptoms, and 85% had decreased post-exercise fatigue.

ABNORMALITIES IN NEUROTRANSMITTERS

Other research has reported that some patients with CFS have abnormally high levels of serotonin, a neurotransmitter (chemical messenger in the brain). Such elevated levels in the brain are associated with fatigue. Yet other studies report that deficiencies in dopamine and norepinephrine, other important neurotransmitters, may play a role in CFS. You'll read more about neurotransmitters in later chapters.

ALL IN YOUR HEAD?

Still, some physicians contend that CFS is nothing more than a psychological, or worse, psychosomatic, disorder. To support their views, they might reference this statement from the CDC:

Due in part to its similarity to chronic mononucleosis, CFS was initially thought to be caused by a virus infection, most probably Epstein-Barr virus (EBV). It now seems clear that CFS cannot be caused exclusively by EBV or by any single recognized infectious disease agent. No firm association between infection with any known human pathogen and CFS has been established. CDC's four-city surveillance study found no association between CFS and infection by a wide variety of human pathogens, including EBV, human retroviruses, human herpesvirus 6, enteroviruses, rubella, Candida albicans, and more recently the Borna disease virus and Mycoplasma. Taken together, these studies suggest that among identified human pathogens, there appears to be no causal relationship for CFS. However, the possibility remains that CFS may have multiple causes leading to a common endpoint, in which case some viruses or other infectious agents might have a contributory role for a subset of CFS cases.

True, not any one virus has been significantly linked with CFS, but much more research is warranted, especially investigating the combined effects of herpes viruses and other infections. When researchers include CMV, EBV, and herpes simplex viruses in their evaluations, CFS patients are found to have significantly higher viral antibody levels than do healthy controls.

When researchers find no consistent elevations of EBV antibody levels and then conclude that viruses do not play a role in CFS, they are like firefighters who ignore the billowing smoke on the horizon, insisting that there must be no fire, since they can't see it yet. And no matter how many times the smoke invariable leads to fire, they refuse to make the connection.

FOR FURTHER READING AND RESEARCH

- I. Bou-Holaigah et al., "The Relationship Between Neurally Mediated Hypotension and the Chronic Fatigue Syndrome," *JAMA* 274 (1995): 961–7.
- D. Buchwald et al., "A Chronic Illness Characterized by Fatigue, Neurologic and Immunologic Disorders, and Active Human Herpes Virus Type 6 Infection," *Annals of Internal Medicine* 116(2) (1992): 103–13.
- M.S. Demitrack et al., "Evidence for Impaired Activation of Hypothalamic-pituitary-adrenal Axis in Patients with Chronic Fatigue Syndrome," *Journal of Clinical Endocrinology and Metabolism* 73 (1991): 1224–34.
- J.D. Hamilton, "Cytomegalovirus and Immunity," *Monographs in Virology* 12 (1982).
- G.P. Holmes et al., "A Cluster of Patients with a Chronic Mononucleosis-like Syndrome. Is EBV the Cause?" *JAMA* 257 (17) (1987): 2297.
- M. Ichise et al., *Nuclear Medicine Communications* 13 (1992): 767–72.
- W. Judy, Presentation to the 37th Annual Meeting of the American College of Nutrition, Southeastern Institute of Biomedical Research, 1996.
- G. Kennedy et al., "Increased Plasma Isoprostanes and Other Markers of Oxidative Stress in Chronic Fatigue Syndrome," *Journal of Thrombosis and Haemostasis* 1(Suppl 1) (2003): 0182.
- A.L. Komaroff, "The Physical Basis of CFS," *The CFIDS Research Review* 1(2) (2000b): 1–3:11.
- P.K. Peterson et al., "Chronic Fatigue Syndrome in Minnesota," *Minnesota Medicine* 74 (1991): 21–6.
- H. Selye, "The General Adaptation Syndrome and the Diseases of Adaptation," *Journal of Clinical Endocrinology* 6 (1946): 117.
- R. B. Schwartz et al., "Detection of Intracranial Abnormalities in Patients with Chronic Fatigue Syndrome: Comparison of MR Imaging and SPECT," *American Journal of Roentgenology* 162 (1994): 935–41.
- A. Wilson et al., "Longitudinal Study of Outcome of Chronic Fatigue Syndrome," *British Medical Journal* 308 (1994): 756–9.

PART THREE

YOUR PATH
TO HEALING

It's not a simple road,
but with each new insight,
it's becoming easier to tread.

· 6 ·
WHY CONVENTIONAL MEDICINE ALONE
CAN'T BEAT YOUR ILLNESS

"Today's standard, AMA-approved medicine is rooted
in treating symptoms, rather than causes. Its dependence
on drugs and surgery is ruinously expensive to patients,
insurance companies, and society as a whole."
—Derrick Lonsdale, MD, *Why I Left Orthodox Medicine*

Conventional medical treatments of FMS and CFS focus on
controlling various symptoms. Physicians generally rely on pain
medications of various sorts, muscle relaxants and tranquilizers,
antidepressants, and nonsteroidal anti-inflammatory medicines.
Unfortunately, as you already know, these drugs rarely yield lasting
results.

Traditional Western medicine has evolved from the early days of
blood draining and magic potions, to become the most sophisticated, powerful, prosperous, and revered health care industry in the
world. The judicious use of antibiotics has saved millions of lives.
Laparoscopic surgery, MRIs, CAT scans, heart-lung machines, synthetic insulin, and other cutting-edge developments have helped
improve the lives of millions of people around the world. Doctors
are able to use an ever-growing arsenal of tools to diagnose and
then effectively treat whatever ails you.

As a result, we expect nothing short of miracles from our doctors.
When we are sick, we want to feel better. Not tomorrow or next
week, but right now (myself included)! This instant gratification
begins as a child when we are told: "Take your medicine. It will
make you feel better." And most of the time, it does. Strep throat
is usually no match for good old antibiotics. And don't even think

about treating type-1 diabetes without insulin therapy. And if your appendix is about to rupture, a chiropractor isn't going to be a lot of help, unless he knows a good surgeon.

But conventional medicine has its limits, and our quick-fix society has gotten out of hand. So much of modern medicine is about covering up our symptoms with drugs, rather than treating the causes that are to blame for the symptoms. This is like trying to mop the wet kitchen floor while ignoring the leaky roof!

Many drugs are associated with side effects, and the majority don't actually cure anything. Treating symptoms doesn't translate to better health. We've got to stop thinking, "just stop the pain," and start thinking, "let's fix the problem." Or else we just won't make any progress at all toward true wellness. Consider this quote from John R. Lee, MD:

> "Most over-the-counter, and almost all prescribed, drug treatments merely mask symptoms....Drugs almost never deal with the reasons why these problems exist, while they frequently create new health problems as side effects of their activities."

That said, there's no need to suffer if you can safely avoid it! Short-term use of drugs to mask unwanted symptoms is certainly appreciated by both patient and doctor. But FMS and CFS are not short-term illnesses. And drugs used to treat these syndromes can lead to dependence and further complications. One drug's side effects can initiate new symptoms, which must then be treated by more drugs!

A BIG-MONEY BUSINESS

Americans now spend over $200 billion a year on prescription drugs, and this spending continues to increase by an average of 12 percent each year. And drugs are now the fastest growing part of the staggeringly high American health-care bill.

Profits are soaring for drug companies, as the top 10 companies reported combined profits of $35.9 billion dollars in 2002. This is more than all the rest of the 490 Fortune-500 companies put together! These same 10 companies spent $36 billion on advertising and marketing in 2002. It seems the more they advertise, the more they rake in.

They aren't bashful about saturating the TV, radio, newspapers, and magazines with reasons why you need to be taking their pills. "Having trouble sleeping?" the TV commercial asks at 3 a.m. "Ask your doctor if _____ is right for you. This drug isn't for everyone." The truth is, some of these drugs aren't for anyone! Each year, Americans consume five billion sleeping pills, and 15,000 Americans die from them.

Many individuals, affected by drug advertising, dutifully request the drug from their doctor, whether or not the doctor would have normally thought of it herself. For instance: "I want the latest, greatest, blood-pressure pill"—even when the new drug costs three times more than older hypertensive drugs, performs only a fraction better (and then only in certain cases), and is associated with a five-fold increased risk of heart attack. Sometimes the "best" medicine isn't the best medicine. Whatever happened to lifestyle changes? Well, in today's managed-care setting where an office visit lasts an average of seven minutes, a prescription is quicker than lifestyle coaching.

But drugs have to be expensive, right? All that money for research and development has to come from somewhere. *Don't believe it.* In reality, in 2002 (the date of an extensive nonprofit investigation), only about 14% of Fortune 500 drug-company revenues were applied toward research and development. Over 30% were devoted toward marketing and administration. Around 17% was received as profit.[1] The Families USA, a nonprofit organization, reports that the former CEO of Bristol-Meyers Squibb made $74,890,918 in 2001. This doesn't include his $76,095,611 of unexercised stock options. The chairman of Wyeth pharmaceuticals made over $40 million dollars, exclusive of an additional $40 million in stock options![2] Remember this when you wonder why your health-insurance premiums continue to rise.

Pharmaceutical companies know that in order to make a profit, they must do one of three things: create new illnesses (such as heartburn, erectile dysfunction, social anxiety disorder, or shyness) for their new drugs to treat; get patients to ask for newer, more expensive drugs; or have doctors write more prescriptions, preferably for more expensive "me-too" drugs.

What are "me-too" drugs? They are newer, more expensive versions of older drugs. Between 1998 and 2002, the FDA approved 415 new drugs. Only 14% of these newly approved drugs were actually uniquely different or innovative in their design. The other 86% were old drug formulas masquerading as new innovative therapies. You see, drug companies hoping for FDA approval are only required to prove that new drugs are safe, not that they are more effective than older drugs.[3]

"In this profit-driven world of medicine, I did not often hear the executives talk of cures. Instead, they focused like honeybees circling a picnic cake on products for what they called chronic disorders. These were drugs that did not cure but 'managed' disease as patients took them once a day for the rest of their lives."

—Melody Peterson, former medical reporter for the *New York Times*, author of *Our Daily Meds*[12]

Dr. Marcia Angell, former editor of The *New England Journal of Medicine,* discusses these "me-too" drugs in her book, *The Truth About the Drug Companies.* Take, for instance, the drug Nexium (perhaps you already do). Its creator, AstraZeneca, had been relying on the drug Prilosec for a significant portion of its yearly profits—$6 billion—in 2000.

However, Prilosec was going to lose its patent in 2001, and the folks at AstraZeneca were probably experiencing some heartburn at the thought. Faced with the potential for significant revenue loss, the company simply took one of the two patentable metabolites (chemicals) out of Prilosec and remarketed it as the new and improved Nexium. This "purple pill" then became the original TV drug, as we can all recall. And even though a one-month supply of Nexium costs almost nine times that of the over-the-counter version of Prilosec ($180 compared to $23), the public and their doctors have happily gone along for the ride. The truth? Studies show that both drugs work equally well at reducing stomach acid.[4]

Also consider clot-dissolving medications, which can be lifesaving if given at the onset of a heart attack. There are three different ones on the market. The most prescribed one (tissue plasminogen activator) costs $3,500 for a single dose; the least prescribed one costs $250. Studies show no difference in their effectiveness. It's not quality that's driving these increased prescriptions; it's marketing.

TECHNIQUES OF GREED

So how do drug companies get doctors to prescribe similarly made yet more costly new drugs? Partly through the assault of marketing giveaways by more than 80,000 drug reps who gave away $11 billion worth of free samples.[5] (This amounts to one drug rep for every doctor in the United States.) Bottom-line results clearly show that free samples, vacation "workshop" retreats to posh resorts, and free "educational" gourmet dinners do in fact sway the opinions of doctors. Even more effective, of course, is cash. It's not unusual for drug companies to pay doctors hundred of thousands of dollars a year in "consulting fees." In 2005, drug companies paid for hundreds of millions of dollars and up to 80% of the costs of all doctors' continuing-education classes.[6] Many doctors are paid handsomely to speak on behalf of the drug companies at conferences held at vacation destinations. Through the promise of increased wealth, the drug companies continue to persuade and even brainwash many conventional medical doctors. And as we've already seen, it works.

> "The result of all those attractive women in short skirts armed with pseudoscience invading the practices of doctors is that Americans are over-medicated, taking far too many drugs, most of which they don't even need, and they are paying too much for them."
>
> —Jerome Kassirer, MD,
> distinguished professor,
> Tufts University School of Medicine[7]

Of course, drug companies must aggressively court both doctors and patients alike because their drugs don't even work for most people. Dr. Allen Rose, a top executive at GlaxoSmithKline, reports that drugs work for as few as 25% of those who take them.[8,9]

In fact, drug companies spend more money on lobbying than does any other industry. There are now two drug lobbyists for every member of Congress.[10]

Not only are drug companies seeking out chronic diseases to "manage," they're creating new diseases to market, too. In 2003, the magazine Medical Marketing and Media ran an article by Vince Parry who was happy to report that pharma-

"I'm not that hopeful for any real change....They have bought politicians and doctors. They've looked at everyone and anyone who could stand in their way and they've thrown money at them. The only hope we have is a grassroots revolution that will make the politicians decide they love votes more than drug company money."

—Dr. Marcia Angell, MD, former editor, New England Journal of Medicine.[11]

ceutical companies were taking the "art of branding a condition" to ever higher levels of expertise. The focus on developing new disorders (diseases) was apparently all the buzz in the industry.[13]

MEDICAL MYTHS ARE KEEPING US SICK

The American Medical Association, American Heart Association, American Diabetes Association, and other conventional medical organizations continue to promote the medical myth that prescription drugs are safer and more effective than more natural alternatives. Unfortunately, while conventional medical doctors are writing record numbers of prescriptions each year, the health of our nation continues to decline. The Centers for Medicare and Medicaid reports that the nation spent $140.6 billion in the year 2000 on prescription drugs.[14] And of course this number escalates each year. It is estimated that over 3 billion prescriptions were written last year.[15]

But even though the United States spends more money on health care per capita than does any other country in the world, The World Health Organization in 2000 ranked the U.S. health-care system first in both responsiveness and cost, but 37th in overall performance and 72nd in overall health (among 191 member nations included in the study).[16]

DANGEROUS DRUGS

In January 1999, Business Week reported on the fourth leading cause of hospitalizations: damage from FDA-approved drugs. This affects 2.2 million people a year at a cost of $5 billion. Americans are dying—one every three to five minutes—from the effects of FDA-approved pharmaceutical drugs...used as directed![17] In fact, iatrogenic (accidentally doctor-induced) illnesses take the lives of over 780,000 Americans each year.[18] This makes conventional medicine the number one cause of death in the United States, beating out heart disease and cancer! (And this number is conservative, since only 5–20% of all iatrogenic events are ever reported.)[19]

It's estimated by some experts that adverse drug reactions affect as many as 5 million Americans each year.[20] This is assuredly a conservative estimate. The average U.S. citizen filled 12 prescriptions in 2006,[21] and over a lifetime of drug taking, he or she has a 26% chance of being hospitalized from a drug injury. Yet these same drugs—taken as directed—kill over 270 Americans each day. This is comparable to a commercial jet going down on a daily basis! **The very drugs that are being used to treat various illnesses are causing more American deaths in one year than occurred in the entire Vietnam War.**[22]

Still, medical drug use continues to increase in the United States. Americans now spend over $250 billion a year on prescription drugs, more than the gross domestic product of most countries in the world. Drugs are now the fastest growing part of the staggeringly high American health-care bill. In fact, Americans spend more on drugs than do all the people in Australia, Canada, France, Germany, Italy, Japan, Spain, Brazil, Argentina, Mexico, New Zealand, and the United Kingdom combined![23]

And many of these prescriptions aren't safe at all. For instance, calcium channel blockers—used to treat high blood pressure and heart disease—actually increase the risk of stroke and heart attack five times, according to Dr. Curt Furberg, Wake Forest School of Medicine.[24] And Propulsid—a drug used to treat GERD (gastroesophageal reflux disease) and gastroparesis (delayed emptying of the stomach, usually found in type-2 diabetics)—has caused severe heart-rhythm abnormalities. In June 1998, the FDA issued a statement reporting 38 deaths in the United States from people taking Propulsid: "Due to reports of serious heart arrhythmias and deaths in people taking Propulsid (Cisapride), the label had been changed to reflect these dangers."[25]

Perhaps more subtle, but certainly serious, are drug-induced nutritional deficiencies.[26] Although these can be corrected early, they often aren't, because conventional medicine tends to gloss over such "minor" concerns.

CONVENTIONAL MEDICINE AND FMS OR CFS

With so many different symptoms, it's no surprise that fibromyalgia and CFS patients are typically taking 6–12 different prescription drugs. Lyrica, Elavil, Klonopin, Paxil, Effexor, Xanax, Trazadone, Neurontin, Zanaflex, Ambien, Lunesta, Cymbalta, and Provigil have all been heralded as "the drug" for fibromyalgia. Some of these are helpful, some worthless, and some really dangerous.

Drug management alone typically fails to yield lasting relief from the most common fibromyalgia and CFS symptoms, and patients' and doctors' optimism over a new drug treatment eventually gives way to this sad reality. Oh well, a new drug with an even larger marketing budget is on the horizon. (Forgive my cynicism. I've just seen this situation so many times!)

Many of the most commonly prescribed drugs for fibromyalgia have side effects that are similar or identical to the symptoms of FMS and CFS. These similarities can cause a lot of confusion when doctors are trying to determine the effectiveness of treatment. Ambien, for instance, can cause flu-like symptoms, achy muscle pain, sore throat, and fatigue. Sounds like CFS, doesn't it?

Tranquilizers are often prescribed for restless leg syndrome; achy, tight muscles; and sleep problems. But these drugs deplete the sleep hormone melatonin, which then leads to a disruption of a person's circadian rhythm (sleep-wake cycle). Instead of promoting deep restorative sleep, these drugs prevent it!

It's important to realize that your drug or drugs may be causing or contributing to some or all of your symptoms. I spend a great deal of time with my new patients reviewing and discussing their current drugs—how they interact with each other, and the potential side effects. I often find that by asking the right question, I can help the patient realize that her symptoms began or worsened soon after the drug treatment began.

Sometimes, though, I do find drug-induced symptoms that began months after the start of the drug treatment. Drugs deplete essential nutrients that the body needs to properly function, but it can take weeks, months, or even years for the drug to fully deplete the nutrient and for you to see the side effects surface.

Still, not everyone can be drug free, and most of my patients are on at least one prescription medication. But the least offensive drug

---

The Perfect Storm

Drugs that deplete CoQ10, magnesium, and B vitamins create the perfect storm for those with FMS and CFS. Here's why:

CoQ10 provides the spark for cellular energy. Without adequate CoQ10, the body's energy is drastically reduced, and this can trigger a whole host of unwanted health problems. Many drugs deplete CoQ10, and individuals with FMS or CFS are often low in CoQ10 already.

Magnesium is perhaps that most important mineral in the body. It helps regulate the neurotransmitters. It naturally relaxes tight, achy muscles and corrects constipation (which is a common sign of magnesium depletion). Seventy percent of the population is deficient in this mineral, including around 90% of FMS patients. Low magnesium can cause high blood pressure, mitral valve prolapse, tight and achy muscles, muscle spasms, constipation, chronic headaches, migraines, anxiety, depression, fatigue, irregular heartbeats, insomnia, hair loss, confusion, and more.

Folic Acid is one of the most potent antidepressants known. Lowered levels of this important B vitamin can cause depression, insomnia, heart problems, high blood pressure, and GI disorders.

Vitamin B6 is involved in more bodily functions than any other vitamin. It regulates the production of neurotransmitters, serotonin, dopamine, and norepinephrine. Low levels of B6 can cause anxiety, depression, insomnia, tingling in the hands and feet, lowered immune function, fluid retention, and chronic headaches.

should be used—sparingly—and only to manage symptoms unresponsive to more natural therapies.

A study conducted by the Mayo Foundation for Medical Education and Research demonstrates the need for FMS and CFS treatment beyond drug therapy. Thirty-nine patients with FMS were interviewed about their symptoms. Twenty-nine were interviewed again 10 years later. Of these 29 (mean age 55 at second interview), all had persistence of the same FMS symptoms. Moderate to severe pain or stiffness was reported in 55% of patients, moderate to a great deal of sleep difficulty was noted in 48%, and moderate to extreme fatigue was noted in 59%. These symptoms showed little change from earlier surveys. The surprising finding was that 79% of the patients were still taking medications to control symptoms. We can conclude that the medications weren't making a significant impact.

Conventional medical treatments for FMS and CFS is a controversial topic, and I certainly have no desire to offend the many brilliant medical doctors out there. Still, in my experience, most traditional doctors continue to rely on prescription medications to treat fibromyalgia, even though their own studies show them to be ineffective and potentially dangerous. They still just don't get it. Those with fibromyalgia and CFS are sick and they want to feel well, not drugged.

Just *try* to find a doctor who really knows anything about these illnesses. Most

"Four controlled trials have evaluated the efficacy of Amitriptyline [Elavil] in fibromyalgia.…the longest trial showed no benefit when compared to placebo. Furthermore, the overall degree of benefit was found to be relatively small in relevant outcomes such as improvement in pain, fatigue, and sleep.

"Use of anti-anxiety medications Benzodiazepines, corticosteroids, and nonsteroidal anti-inflammatory agents, and pain medications have been shown to be ineffective and should be generally avoided.

"Our best therapies Amitriptyline and Cyclobenzaprine could not be distinguished from placebo after three months of therapy. Long-term, follow-up observations indicated that clinical findings for patients with FMS did not change appreciably after 15 years."

—American College of Rheumatology web site

don't. It's even harder to find one who is having any lasting success treating these illnesses. How many folks with fibromyalgia get well under the care of a traditional rheumatologist? I speak to fibromyalgia support groups across North America, and I can tell you what the answer is: very few. The three-month wait for a new patient appointment typically ends in a two-hour interview and exam followed by a 10 minute visit to discuss test results, and then several prescription drugs and a follow-up appointment every 3–6 months.

And let's face it, those with fibromyalgia are medical misfits, they don't usually respond to medications like other folks. The ACR has, like many physicians, thrown up their hands and admitted they have little if anything to offer for those suffering from fibromyalgia. They focus more on helping their patients "cope." At least they're honest about their limitations.

ARGUMENTS AGAINST NATURAL APPROACHES

Many conventional doctors are quick to ridicule nutritional therapies, even though these therapies have consistently shown themselves effective in treating fibromyalgia. This prejudice just doesn't make sense.

The usual accusation is that "there are no controlled studies...." But actually, there are numerous studies that validate the use of nutritional supplements to manage and often correct the symptoms of poor health. There are over 1,000 studies demonstrating the positive effects of various supplements and foods in the treatment of hypertension alone. And hundreds of studies demonstrate magnesium's benefits in treating high blood pressure, angina, heart arrhythmias, chronic pain, muscle spasms, anxiety, mitral valve prolapse, and fatigue.

Dr. Janet Travell, White House physician for Presidents John F. Kennedy and Lyndon B. Johnson, and Professor Emeritus of Internal Medicine at George Washington University, co-wrote *Myofascial Pain and Dysfunction: The Trigger Point Manual,* which is acknowledged as the authoritative work on muscle pain. In one chapter alone, Dr. Travell references 317 studies showing that problems such as hormonal, vitamin, and mineral deficiencies can contribute to muscle pain and soreness.

And modern medicine itself, despite the millions of dollars spent to promote it's superiority over other forms of health care, is largely an art—with a lot of unproven science. The Office of Technology Assessment, under the authority of the Library of Congress, published a year-long study entitled "Assessing the Efficacy and Safety of Medical Technology." The study showed that only 10–20 percent of all present-day medical practice have been shown to be beneficial by scientific controlled clinical trials. The study concluded that the vast majority of medical procedures now being utilized routinely by physicians are "unproven."

Or how about, "Nutritional supplements aren't regulated and therefore are dangerous." Too much might make you queasy, but no one dies from taking vitamins, minerals, and other essential nutrients! The same can't be said about drug therapy.

The great physician Oliver Wendell Holmes once said, "A medicine…is always directly hurtful; it may sometimes be indirectly beneficial. I firmly believe that if most of the pharmacopoeia [prescription drugs] were sunk to the bottom of the sea, it would be all the better for Mankind and all the worse for the fishes."

For instance, calcium-channel blockers, used to treat high blood pressure and heart disease, actually increase the risk of stroke and heart attack. Propulsid, a drug used for reflux and gastroparesis, has caused severe heart-rhythm abnormalities. The original warning read, "Due to reports of serious heart arrhythmias and deaths in people taking Propulsid (Cisapride), the label had been changed to reflect these dangers. In June of 1998, the FDA issued a statement reporting 38 deaths in the United States from people taking Propulsid." I'll stick with my over-the-counter digestive enzymes, thanks.

Let's examine some drugs commonly used to treat fibromyalgia. Along with information on the drugs, I list some possible side effects. Your experiences may differ from what's described, but be sure to read about the drugs you're taking. See if they might be causing some of your symptoms. If you suspect they are, work with your doctor to slowly wean off of them. If they were helping, you can always start them again.

NSAIDs

Nonsteroidal anti-inflammatory drugs (NSAIDs) can be helpful, especially when used for inflammation that comes from traumatic injuries (sprains, strains, accidents, etc.). They can also be effective in relieving pain and inflammation associated with chronic pain syndromes including all forms of arthritis and some cases of FMS. However, long-term use of these medications can cause a host of unwanted side effects, and NSAIDs do not actually correct the cause of pain. In fact, they can accelerate joint destruction and cause intestinal permeability, which leads to more inflammation.

You might have heard of how drug company Merck pulled its NSAID **Vioxx** off the market. They were responding to the results of a long-term (18-month) clinical trial that revealed that some patients developed serious heart problems while taking the drug. The data that ultimately persuaded the company to withdraw the drug indicated 15 cases of heart attack, stroke, or blood clots per thousand people each year over three years, compared with 7.5 such events per thousand patients taking a placebo.

One of the FDA's own scientists, Dr. David Graham, estimated that Vioxx has been associated with more than 27,000 heart attacks or deaths linked to cardiac problems. There is disagreement within the FDA over these findings, but they are still staggering to consider.

Potential side effects of drugs like Vioxx: Vioxx is what doctors call a "COX-2 inhibitor." These drugs were developed to reduce pain and inflammation without the risk of ulcers and other—potentially deadly—gastrointestinal side effects posed by aspirin and similar medications. But in solving one serious problem, COX-2 inhibitors might be causing another. By blocking COX-2 enzymes, Vioxx reduced the risk of internal bleeding but also kept COX-2 enzymes from doing the important work of counteracting COX-1 enzymes, which narrow the blood vessels. The blood vessels were then remaining too narrow, increasing the chances of a dangerous blood clot forming.

Other COX-2 inhibitors, including **Celebrex** and **Bextra,** are being linked to an increased risk of heart attack and stroke. It may be a matter of time before all COX-2 inhibitor drugs are pulled from the market.

And the really sad news is that although Vioxx did apparently protect the stomach as intended, other COX-2 inhibitors do not. Celebrex and Bextra have turned out to be no safer to the stomach than older NSAIDs. And studies show that neither drug alleviates pain any better than the older medicines.

Plus, the COX-2 inhibitors cost close to $3.00 per pill. Over-the-counter pain relievers, in contrast, cost pennies a dose. Other NSAIDs are safer than COX-2 inhibitors. These include **Mobic** (meloxicam), **Motrin** (ibuprofen), **Daypro** (oxaprozin), and **Naprosyn** (naproxen). But still, unless nothing else works to control your pain, NSAIDs shouldn't be used for any extended period of time.

Potential side effects of other NSAIDS: A person taking NSAIDs is seven times more likely to be hospitalized for gastrointestinal adverse effects. The FDA estimates that 200,000 cases of gastric bleeding occur annually and that this leads to 10,000 to 20,000 deaths each year. **NSAIDs more than double a person's risk of developing high blood pressure, possibly leading to more medication.** In one study, 41% of those who had recently started on medication to lower their blood pressure were also taking an NSAID.

NARCOTIC ANALGESICS

These pain-relieving medications, which act on the central nervous system, are extremely effective in relieving acute and chronic pain. Unfortunately, they eventually lose their effectiveness as your body becomes "tolerant" of them. If these analgesics worked long-term, I'd be recommending them. However, the person taking these medications finds that she has to take an ever-increasing dose to get any relief. Before she knows it, her body is addicted to a potentially life-threatening drug. Typically, another drug or additional drugs are then tried, and the process continues until the person becomes zapped of her vitality, living hour to hour in accordance with her medication schedule.

Narcotic analgesics include **Ultram** (tramadol), **Lortab** (hydrocodone), **Darvocet** (propoxyphene and acetaminophen), the **Duragesic patch** (fentanyl), **Percocet** (oxycodone and acetaminophen), **Vicodin** (hydrocodone and acetaminophen), **Zerlor** (dihydrocodeine, acetaminophen, and caffeine), and others. Ultram, which is less addictive, has been considered the best choice for those with FMS if a narcotic pain medication is truly necessary. **However, many are not recommending Ultram due to its risk for causing seizures.** Taking Ultram along with SSRI antidepressants increases the risk.[27]

Other side effects include cold, clammy skin; severe confusion; convulsions; diarrhea; severe dizziness; severe drowsiness; increased sweating; low blood pressure; nausea or vomiting; severe nervousness or restlessness; pinpoint pupils in the eyes; difficulty breathing; slow heartbeat; stomach cramps or pain; and severe weakness. These can happen to either you or any baby you are breastfeeding. More rare side effects include hallucinations, severe swelling in the face, and unusual bruising and/or bleeding.

Withdrawing from these medications can be a traumatic experience in itself, especially after your body has begun to build up a tolerance and expects to keep getting the drug. When the drug treatment stops, you could experience body aches; diarrhea; a fast heartbeat; a fever, runny nose, or sneezing; nausea or vomiting, nervousness or irritability; shivering or trembling; stomach cramps; trouble sleeping; or weakness, among other symptoms.

SLEEP AIDS

Ambien (zolpidem) has been a very popular prescription medications in the United States. **Lunesta** (eszopiclone) is a similar sleep aid. Both are short-acting, designed to last four–six hours. If a patient takes a half-dose before bed, then he can take an additional half-dose if needed in the middle of the night. The newer Ambien CR tries to avoid this midnight redosing, however, by including a slower-release layer designed to last all night. Even though the literature on Ambien suggests that most patients don't build up a tolerance, many do. But other patients do well on Ambien, and it does promote deep restorative sleep.

An Actual Case Study

Nicole had been suffering with fibromyalgia for almost 11 years. When she first consulted me, she was taking Klonopin (for anxiety), Lyrica (nerve pain), Celebrex (body pain), Norvasc (high blood pressure), Paxil (depression), Ambien (sleeplessness), and others—nine different medications in all!

We discovered together that her **Klonopin** was depleting her body's natural sleep hormone, melatonin, and contributing to her depression, fatigue, and short-term memory loss.

The **Lyrica** wasn't helping, and many of its side effects seemed to be making her worse. She weaned off this medication over a two-month period. A lot of her side effects, which she had thought were new symptoms, disappeared once she was completely off the Lyrica—including the chronic achy low-back pain, the poor memory, her low moods, and her low energy.

The **Celebrex** were most likely causing her high blood pressure. (Did you know that's a potential side effect? In fact, regular use of NSAIDs more than doubles a person's risk of high blood pressure.) When she quit the Celebrex, she didn't notice that her pain was any worse for it.

Within a few weeks, she was able to discontinue the potentially deadly calcium-channel-blocking drug **Norvasc.** (These types of drugs increase the risk of heart attack and stroke five fold.) She immediately noticed more energy.

The **Paxil** was no longer helping her depression, and it had likely caused her 30-pound weight gain. She stayed it, however, for six months while we built up her stress-coping savings account (she had been under a great deal of stress for a long time, and a recent hysterectomy had been her body's last straw). She then weaned off the Paxil over a two-month period. She lost 20 pounds in the following months! She lost nearly 10 in the first month on my elimination diet (see ch. 12).

The **Ambien** might have been contributing to her short-term memory loss; it is a common side effect. It might also have been contributing to her depression, fatigue, and even diffuse muscle pain. Within a few weeks of starting my fibromyalgia jump-start protocol, Nicole began consistently sleeping through the night without it.

Over the next two months, she saw continual improvement in her pain, fatigue, depression, anxiety, and poor memory. Her IBS disappeared within two weeks.

Nicole still has some "fibro flare" days with pain and fatigue, but she is 80% better and still on the mend!

Sonata (zaleplon) is designed to last for only four hours; this helps prevent morning hangover. I've not found it to be very effective, though, since most of my patients have trouble sleeping through the night, not just with getting to sleep.

Medications other than sleep aids (such as antidepressants and tranquilizers) can also be used to encourage sleep. Each one works differently.

Potential side effects of sleep aids: short-term memory loss, fuzzy thinking, sedation, next-day hangover, mood disorders (anxiety and depression), flu-like symptoms, muscle aches, incoordination, dizziness, diarrhea, and others. Long-term use can lead to other symptoms, including upset stomach, joint pain, upper respiratory-tract infection, sore throat, urinary infection, and heart palpitations. Don't these symptoms sound a lot like those of FMS/CFS? If you do choose a sleep aid, familiarize yourself with its side effects, as they might show up later and appear at first to be unrelated.

These drugs, like most, are processed by the liver, so those with sluggish liver function should use them with caution.

ANTIDEPRESSANTS

Selective serotonin re-uptake inhibitors (SSRIs), such as **Zoloft** (sertraline), **Paxil** (paroxetine HCl), **Celexa** (citalopram), **Prozac** (fluoxetine), and **Luvox** (fluvoxamine), work by increasing the brain's use of the neurotransmitter serotonin. (Serotonin deficiency is linked to anxiety, depression, lowered pain tolerance, poor sleep, and mental fatigue.)

Trazadone (desyrel) blocks the re-uptake of the neurotransmitters serotonin and norepinephrine. It reduces anxiety and promotes deep sleep. I've found this drug helpful when the preferred natural therapies (outlined in chapter 16) don't work, though it can cause early-morning hangover.

Tricyclic antidepressants, such as **Elavil** (amitriptyline), **Pamelor** (nortriptyline), and **Sinequan** or **Adapin** (doxepin), block the hormones serotonin and norepinephrine, producing a sedative effect. Elavil was one of the first drugs to be studied in the treatment of

FMS. It can be very helpful in reducing the pain associated with FMS, but it has several potential side effects. It is also prone to lose its effectiveness over time. It does promote deep restorative sleep.

The latest overly hyped fibromyalgia drug, **Cymbalta** is designed to re-uptake norepinephrine. All of us in the fibromyalgia community welcome any and all drugs that provide long-term symptom relief with minimal side effects. And Cymbalta might work for you. Unfortunately, the majority of my FMS patients report very little benefit on it, even after months.

Lastly, the future of fibromyalgia treatment might lie in **Milnacipran**. Similar to **Effexor** and Cymbalta—all three block the re-uptake of norepinephrine—it might offer relief for some, and I hope so. But I've learned not to listen to the hype and to wait and see what science says instead.

> **Cymbalta** might become the next FDA-approved drug for treating fibromyalgia specifically. Other drugs have been used to treat the illness, obviously, but none could legally be marketed specifically for that purpose until **Lyrica** gained approval—see more about Lyrica at the bottom of page 105.

Potential side effects of antidepressants: Upset stomach, constipation, headache, heartburn, diarrhea, rash, muscle pain, mental confusion, hostility, swelling in the arms or legs, dizziness, nightmares, drowsiness, fatigue, chest pain, anxiety, nervousness, sleeplessness, weakness, changes in sex drive, impotence, tremors, difficulty in urinating, sensitivity to light, dry mouth, loss of appetite, nausea, itching, weight gain, hair loss, dry skin, bronchitis, abnormal heart rate, twitching, anemia, low blood sugar, low thyroid function, blurry vision, and early-morning hangover. Don't these sound a whole lot like the symptoms of FMS/CFS?

All antidepressants are partially or wholly broken down in the liver, and this can create liver dysfunction in patients with a sluggish liver. Elavil commonly causes weight gain. Some of my patients have gained 50 or more pounds in 3–6 months on the drug.

Harvard Medical School's Dr. Joseph Glenmullen recently reported on the many dreadful side effects associated with conventional anti-depressant medications. His report included neurological disorders, sexual dysfunction (in up to 60% of users), debilitating withdrawal symptoms (including hallucinations, electric shock–like sensations, dizziness, nausea, and anxiety), and decreased effectiveness in about 35% of long-term users.

Another frightening "side effect" is a suspected link between SSRI use and suicide in teenagers and children. Drug regulators have recommended that Paxil not be newly prescribed to anyone under age 18. Some regulators believe the risk extends to adult patients, as well.

TRANQUILIZERS

Soma (carisprodol) is a muscle relaxant that acts on the central nervous system. The most common complaint is its sedating nature. It can be helpful, especially if there is a great deal of muscle guarding or chronic unrelenting tightness, but it does not promote deep, restorative sleep. **Flexeril** (cyclobenzaprine) is a muscle relaxant chemically similar to the antidepressant **Elavil**. It is quite sedating and does promote deep, restorative sleep. **Baclofen** (lioresal) is a muscle relaxant similar to the natural neurotransmitter GABA. It does not promote deep, restorative sleep. **Zanaflex** (tizanidine) is a muscle relaxant that has gained some popularity among physicians treating FMS. It is sedating but does not promote deep, restorative sleep.

Potential side effects of tranquilizers: Fatigue, rapid heartbeat, slow heart action, vomiting, dizziness, depression, breathing difficulties, chest tightness, trembling, low blood pressure, weakness, nausea, headache, weight gain, and insomnia. Zanaflex has been associated with liver failure and liver injury; at least three individuals have died from taking it.

BENZODIAZEPINES

These medications are usually used as anti-anxiety medication, and they include **Xanax** (alprazolam), **Klonopin** (clonazepam), **Ativan** (lorazepam), **Restoril** (temazepam), **BuSpar** (buspirone hydrochloride), **Tranxene** (clorazepate dipotassium), **Serax** (oxazepam), **Librium** (chlordiazepoxide), **Tegretol** (carbamazepine), **Valium** (diazepam), **Trileptal** (oxcarbazepine), **Seroquel** (quetiapine), **Risperdal** (risperidone), and **Symbyax** (olanzapine and fluoxetine HCl).

Benzodiazepines are addictive, and patients build up a tolerance so that the drugs eventually lose effectiveness as a sleep aid. Addiction may occur in as little as two weeks.

The big problem with these medications, though, are the side effects, many of which mirror the symptoms of fibromyalgia and CFS. And they don't promote deep, restorative sleep, so they are definitely not worth the risk.

Benzodiazepines depress the central nervous system and act on the neurotransmitter GABA (gamma-amino butyric acid). GABA acts as a calming chemical as it transmits messages from one cell to another. So directly or indirectly, these drugs influence almost every brain function and most other bodily systems, including those of the nervous, neuromuscular, endocrine, and gastrointestinal systems. It's no wonder their side effects are so severe.

Benzodiazepines should be weaned off, starting as soon as possible. Be sure to work with a medical doctor as you wean off, and take it slow to avoid terrible withdrawal symptoms.

Potential side effects of benzodiazepines: Poor sleep; seizures; mania; depression and suicidal thoughts; tinnitus (ringing in the ears); transient amnesia; dizziness; agitation; disorientation; low blood pressure; nausea or vomiting; fluid retention; muscular incoordination and tremors; sexual dysfunction; prolonged drowsiness or a trance-like state; fatigue; headaches; body aches and pains; chills; runny nose; cough; congestion; difficulty breathing; feelings of discouragement, sadness, or emptiness; diarrhea; difficulty swallowing; vision and voice changes; and a host of others.

The crippling side effects and addictive nature of these drugs have been known for at least 40 years, yet doctors continue to prescribe them at an ever-increasing rate, especially for seniors. Surveys show that over 5.6 million adults over the age of 65 are now taking benzodiazepines. A mouth-dropping 50% of all women 60 and older will be prescribed a benzodiazepine drug.

And since addiction often occurs within four weeks of starting these drugs, the majority of these folks are now dependent on them.

Tolerance to the hypnotic (sleep) effects of these drugs may occur within one week. Symptoms of tolerance are identical to drug-withdrawal symptoms and may include anxiety, panic, severe insomnia, muscle pain and stiffness, depression, suicidal thoughts, rage, heart and lung problems, and agoraphobia (extreme fear of public or crowded spaces).

> How tragic to live a productive, active life, only to become addicted to a life-draining, mind-numbing drug. If you are a senior on a benzodiazepine for your fibromyalgia, I encourage you to seek out other options with your doctor's help.

Tragically, only 10%–30% of people are able to successfully stop taking these drugs. The rest are addicted for life.

ANTICONVULSANT DRUGS

GABA inhibitors such as **Gabitril** (tiagabine HCl) and **Neurontin** (gabapentin) are anticonvulsant medications originally used to control seizures. They are now being used to block nerve-related pain (neuralgia), including pain caused by herpes zoster. These medications are also prescribed with some success for chronic headaches. I've not found them to be helpful, though, for the diffuse extremity pains associated with FMS. They do not promote deep, restorative sleep and can cause many of the same symptoms associated with CFS and FMS. Most patients can wean off these medications with no problems.

Turn the page to learn some frightful truths about the marketing of Neurontin.

Neurontin for Everything!

When clinical studies revealed that Warner-Lambert's new epilepsy drug, Neurontin, was generally ineffective and potentially dangerous (it worsened the symptoms of 5%–10% of those who tried it), their shareholders weren't happy.

Executives at Warner-Lambert decided to expand sales beyond the limited epilepsy patients to those suffering such chronic conditions as attention deficit disorder (ADD), mood disorders, migraines, and other illnesses. In order to save time and money, they decided not to actually test Neurontin's effectiveness on any of these illnesses. Instead of clinical trials, they spent their time hatching a promotion strategy.

To convince doctors (some unsuspecting, some willing to be deceived) of their patients' need for the drug, the company sent doctors to a Chateau Elan (a luxury resort outside of Atlanta, Georgia) while treating them to an all-expense-paid extended weekend with tickets to the 1996 Olympics. They dined in four-star restaurants, lounged by the pool, played golf, and got their daily spa treatments. For the makers of Neurontin, it was a small price for the intended payoff.

During this time, the doctors were exposed to constant Neurontin-to-treat-everything brainwashing "information."

In her book, *Our Daily Meds,*[28] Melody Peterson quotes one of the sales executives pushing Neurontin, who left a voice message to the medical liaisons: "When we get out there, we want to kick some ass. We want to sell Neurontin on pain. All right? And monotherapy and everything we can talk about. That's what we want to do." John Ford, a senior marketing executive for Parke-Davis, had this to say at a sales meeting: "Neurontin for pain, Neurontin for monotherapy, Neurontin for bipolar, Neurontin for everything." Ford went on to rally his sales troops to encourage doctors to prescribe the drug in higher and higher doses (which of course, would yield higher and higher profits).

Again from *Our Daily Meds,* Mr. Ford is quoted: "I don't want to see a single patient coming off Neurontin before they've been up to at least 4,800 milligrams per day. I don't want to hear that safety crap either."

To further promote Neurontin to unsuspecting doctors, the company paid Medical Education Systems, Inc. over $160,000 to create dozens of "scientific" articles endorsing Neurontin. After the professional writers were finished, doctors received $1,000 each to sign off on them. Then they were circulated to others in the field.

Doctors were also hired to give "dinner talks" where other doctors received continuing education credit for attending a Neurontin propaganda pitch over a free gourmet meal at the best restaurants in town. These meet-and-greet events were lucrative for the doctor spokesperson who presented there; some earned as much as $100,000 a year, just for wining and dining—and of course, pushing Neurontin for everything.

Not taking any chances, Parke-Davis applied another scheme, paying doctors to actually prescribe Neurontin. The company sets up an "experimental trial" and pays doctors $350 for each patient place on the drug. More money is added if the doctor keeps the patient on the drug when the trial ends. One thousand doctors signed up.

Meanwhile, legitimate research and unbiased trials continued to report that Neurontin had little if any benefit for the conditions it was being promoted for.[29]

In 2004, pharmaceutical giant Pfizer (which owns Warner-Lambert and Parke-Davis) pleaded guilty to marketing Neurontin for uses unapproved by the federal government. They were fined $430 million, including a $240 million criminal fine, the second largest in a health-care fraud prosecution. (Of course, Pfizer's 2003 revenue was $45.1 billion, so this was merely a drop in the bucket.)

Not convinced that at least some folks at Pfizer aren't out for your best interests? Consider this: a study done in the late 1900s showed Neurontin ineffective for diabetic nerve pain. Then Michael Rowbotham, marking team leader, wrote this in a 2000 email: "I think we can limit the potential downsides of the…study by delaying the publication for as long as possible.…It will be more important to how WE write up the study."[30] The study's scientific manager, Beate Rodes, wrote in an email that she had been told, "we should take care not to publish anything that damages Neurontin's marketing success." And a Scandinavian study clearly demonstrated that Neurontin was no better than a sugar pill in treating diabetic nerve pain.

Given the facts surrounding the faulty data and outright lies in marketing Neurontin, should we be leery of Pfizer's new drug Lyrica, which is being hyped as the next wonder treatment for fibromyalgia?

Pfizer's anticonvulsant **Lyrica,** the first FDA-approved drug for the treatment of fibromyalgia, is very similar to Neurontin. The two compounds share similar mechanisms of action, but Lyrica is supposed to be as effective as Neurontin but at lower doses, which hopefully means lower side effects. Still, Lyrica is associated with all the same side effects as Neurontin.

Some say the Lyrica doesn't work well enough to have warranted

FDA approval. In 2004, reviewers recommended against approving the drug, citing its side effects. But the FDA approved it anyway. Pfizer then asked the FDA to expand the approved uses of Lyrica to include the treatment of fibromyalgia, and the agency did so in June 2007.

Is Lyrica effective? According to clinical trials, patients taking Lyrica reported that their pain fell, on average, about two points on a 10-point scale, compared with one point for patients taking a placebo. Not a big effect, to say the least.

Roughly 30% of patients reported that their pain fell by at least half, compared with 15% of those taking a placebo. While a 50% reduction in pain is impressive, remember that it occurred in only three out of ten patients who took Lyrica. And half of those could have been under the placebo effect. Still, for those who can't get their pain under control any other way, Lyrica is certainly an option. But you must go into treatment aware of the potential risks. Here are excerpts from just a couple of emails I have received from people who tried Lyrica and reported to me about it. The first is from Lydia T., a registered respiratory therapist.

When Lyrica was approved, I was the first in my doctor's practice, at the door, ready to try it. Unfortunately, the drug tried me. One 25-mg. dose, and...I couldn't think, my vision was severely blurred, my speech slurred to the point my husband determined I'd had a stroke. I couldn't walk...After notifying the doctor, he assured my husband....

I have absolutely NO memory of anything 30 minutes after taking that pill....I looked my daughter directly in the fact from about 12 inches away and had no idea who she was. According to [my husband and daughter], I had absolutely no affect [emotions] and didn't say a word....

They took me home, put me to bed, and I stayed there for two days, barely eating and sleeping between waking in horrible pain....So it only made me worse, but I'm grateful it does help a few of us, and I'm grateful most of all for the commercials that validate that we're out here, we're normal people, and we are in pain."

Another email is from Mary R. in Tampa, Florida, who wrote to tell me about her experience with Lyrica:

The drug helped me sleep deeply, although I was never really refreshed by my sleep. Slowly but inexorably, even on this low dose, my pain did not improve but worsened over the year.

I developed incredible muscle stiffness; the muscles in my back often felt like they were set in concrete. I could not bend forward an inch upon getting up in the morning. Eventually, I felt that perhaps what I thought were worsening fibromyalgia symptoms were actually Lyrica side effects. I decided to give myself a birthday present and stop taking Lyrica.

This was a terrible mistake. In my enthusiasm, I neglected to ask my physician how to discontinue Lyrica. I just stopped. Not good.

First 24 hours, nothing. Just a normal day except that I got out of bed and could instantly touch my toes again. I was delighted! During the second 24 hours, I began to feel uneasy and "flu-ish." On the third night after discontinuing the drug, I felt like I had walked off a cliff.

I experienced high agitation and anxiety—was totally unable to rest or sleep. My heart pounded as if it would leap from my body. My chest was tight, and I felt unable to breathe. I hurt from head to toe, experienced awful tingling in my legs, arms, and hands. The itching was terrible, especially around my neck and shoulders. I was nauseated and completely unable to eat.

These symptoms continued for two weeks, in greater and lesser intensity. I made one trip to the ER, sure that I must be having a heart attack. I was terrified. The ER doctor was confident that it was Lyrica, saying that it was a really hard drug to withdraw from. I'll vouch for that!...

I would never encourage anyone to take this medication. I am almost two months past this awful episode in my life, but I am still struggling with the aftermath.

Pfizer wasted no time in promoting Lyrica for the treatment of fibromyalgia. They spent $46 million in the first nine months of 2007 alone. But their commercials are certainly not public-service announcements just for the common good. No way. Pfizer fully intends to gain back every penny they've spent—and more. Following the FDA approval, online investment research forecaster Datamonitor had this to say about the potential for drug-company profits due to fibromyalgia: "foresees a dramatic rise in market value resulting from an upsurge in diagnosis and treatment rates. Estimated at $367m in 2006 in the US….the market is forecast to grow to $1.7 billion in 2016. Polypharmacotherapy [the use of multiple drugs] will become common place in fibromyalgia management."

On the bright side, Pfizer's multimillion-dollar public-relations campaign should also help the general public become more knowledgeable about fibromyalgia. Plenty of my patients are thankful for the validation that the commercials seem to provide. Lydia T., quoted above, wrote, "on the other hand, just the advertisements have been such a boon to the education of those who simply don't believe, as if fibromyalgia is a disease made up by Disney cartooners. I've actually heard and seen people watch the commercial, look at me and say: 'ooooohhh!' "

Topamax (topiramate) is used primarily for adjunctive therapy for tonic-clonic seizures. It is also used to treat anxiety disorders.

Potential side effects of anticonvulsant drugs: prolonged drowsiness or a trance-like state; dizziness; weakness; blurry or double vision; fluid retention; muscular incoordination, balance changes, clumsiness, and accidental injury; long-term ophthalmic problems (abnormal eyeball movements and disorders); tremors; rapid weight gain or severe weight loss; severe back pain; constipation and painful, uncontrollable, or difficult urination; muscle aches; memory loss; weakness; depression, confusion, dementia, and delusions; difficulty breathing or speaking; itching; involuntary muscle twitching; serious rash; runny nose; swelling; stabbing or tingling pain; seizures; and even rarely, coma.

> Don't some of these side effects sound like some of the symptoms of FMS/CFS, too? That's one reason that drug therapy can be so frustrating for my patients. It's nearly impossible to figure out what the drug is helping and what it's causing.

Topamax can also cause "serious eye damage and/or blindness." This is a quote from the manufacturers themselves. They go on: "As of August 17, 2001 there have been 23 reported cases: 22 in adults and one in pediatric patients. It is generally recognized that post-marketing data are subject to substantial under-reporting."

BETA-BLOCKERS

Beta-blockers, such as **Inderal** (propranolol); **Lorpressor** or **Torprol** (metoprolol); and **Tenormin** (atenolol) are used for long-term management of angina (chest pain), mitral valve prolapse (MVP), irregular heartbeat, and high blood pressure. I'm always amazed at how many of my patients are taking these drugs for MVP, even with their very serious side effects.

These drugs slow the heart rate, which reduces cardiac output and leads to low blood pressure and fatigue. The brain and muscles then aren't getting enough blood and oxygen, and this can lead to fuzzy thinking, poor memory, depression, anxiety, and fatigue.

Potential side effects of beta-blockers: According to Mark Houston, MD, associate clinical professor of medicine at Vanderbilt School of Medicine, side effects associated with beta-blockers include congestive heart failure, reduced cardiac output, fatigue, heart block, dizziness, depression, decreased heartbeat and function, cold extremities, paresthesia (a feeling of "pins and needles"), shortness of breath, drowsiness, lethargy, insomnia, headaches, poor memory, nausea, diarrhea, constipation, colitis, wheezing, bronchospasm, Raynaud's syndrome (burning, tingling, pain, numbness, or poor circulation in the hands and feet), claudication, muscle cramps, muscle fatigue, lowered libido, impotence, postural hypotension, raised triglycerides, lowered HDL, raised LDL, and high blood sugar.

Natural alternatives: Dr. Houston recommends Hawthorne berry as a natural beta-blocker alternative.[31] Hawthorne berry is an ACE inhibitor; it works by blocking the angiotensin-converting enzyme. This enzyme is what causes the constriction of arteries, which raises blood pressure and heart rate. Recommended dose of Hawthorne berry is 160–900 mg. of standardized extract daily.

In my experience, the best way to stop the symptoms associated with heart irregularities, including MVP, is to correct magnesium deficiency. Magnesium is a natural sedative that relaxes muscles, and the heart is, of course, mostly muscle. The smooth muscle contained in the blood vessel lining is also dependent on magnesium.

Magnesium acts like a beta-blocker by inhibiting stimulatory hormones including norepinephrine and epinephrine (hormones that increase heart rate). Fortunately, magnesium doesn't cause fatigue or the other symptoms associated with prescription beta-blockers. Certainly, 500–700 mg. of magnesium daily is a lot safer than a beta-blocker![32,33,34,35]

I have found that most people can wean off beta-blockers and other high-blood-pressure medications by increasing their omega 3 and magnesium. Some individuals will also need niacin (vitamin B3) at rather high doses. For more information about cardiovascular disease, including MVP, please see my book *Heart Disease: What Your Doctor Won't Tell You.*

STIMULANTS

Stimulants such as **Adderall** (amphetamine); **Concerta, Metadate,** or **Ritalin** (methylphenidate); **Cylert** (pemoline); **Dexedrine** (dextroamphetamine); and **Focalin** (dexmethylphenidate HCl) are used to increase adrenaline. They can be helpful in increasing a person's energy. But remember the saying "speed kills." These medications are nothing more than various forms of amphetamines ("speed") and are incredibly hard on the adrenal glands. Long-term use can cause adrenal burnout at least and full blown Addison's Disease at worst.

Provigil (modafinil) is a different kind of stimulant than those listed above and is being recommend by some for the fatigue associated with FMS and CFS. It can help wake you up in the morning and make you more alert. However, the reason you're tired is that you're not going into deep restorative sleep each night. This is the problem that needs to be solved. This medication, rather than help you sleep well, will interfere with your normal circadian rhythm (sleep-wake cycle).

Potential side effects of stimulants: Insomnia, Tourette's syndrome (a movement disorder), nervousness, anxiety, mania, depression, irritability, aggression, rapid heartbeat, high blood pressure, abnormal muscle movements, psychosis, headaches, seizures, visual disturbances, unwanted weight loss, aplastic anemia (arrested development of bone marrow), liver dysfunction, and blood disease.

When you (working with your doctor) wean off these stimulants, you'll probably feel lethargic and even depressed for awhile. So wean off slowly, over a four-week period.

You can counter the withdrawal symptoms by taking 4,000–10,000 mg. of the amino acid L-phenylalanine twice daily on an empty stomach (but not later than 4 p.m.). Or you can use SAMe (S-adenosylmethionine), 600–1,000 mg. daily, taken on an empty stomach. SAMe and L-phenylalanine both boost norepinephrine, which quickly increases adrenaline levels and results in more mental and physical energy (without all the side effects).

STATIN DRUGS

Statin drugs are used to lower cholesterol. They include **Lipitor** (atorvastatin calcium), **Lescol** (fluvastatin sodium), **Altocor** or **Mevacor** (lovastatin), **Pravachol** (pravastatin sodium), **Zocor** (simvastatin), and **Crestor** (rosuvastatin). Most conventional medical doctors are convinced that statin drugs are harmless and should be routinely prescribed for anyone with cholesterol levels above 200. These doctors cite a number of studies in which statin use has lowered the number of coronary deaths compared to controls. But if we look a little deeper into these studies, we see that statin medications don't *significantly* reduce the risk of death associated with heart disease.

Potential side effects of statin drugs: In fact, statins increase the risk of death overall. *The British Journal of Clinical Pharmacology* reported on an analysis of all the major controlled trials before the year 2000 and found that long-term use of statins for primary prevention of heart disease produced a 1% greater risk of death over 10 years, compared to placebo.

The New Lipitor Ads

Pfizer is now running full-page Lipitor ads in numerous papers, including the *New York Times* and *USA Today.* The ads feature Dr. Robert Jarvik, inventor of the artificial heart, and read, "In patients with multiple risk factors for heart disease, Lipitor reduces risk of heart attack by 36%*." The noteworthy part of this ad is the asterisk. It leads to a little note that discloses, "That means in a large clinical study, 3% of patients taking a sugar pill or placebo had a heart attack compared to 2% of patients taking Lipitor." Not quite as impressive when you put it that way.

Another Jarvik Lipitor ad in the Times proclaims, "In patients with type-2 diabetes, Lipitor reduces risk of stroke by 48%* if you also have at least one other risk factor for heart disease." The asterisk explanation here reads, "That means in a large clinical study, 2.8% of patients taking a sugar pill or placebo had a stroke compared to 1.5% of patients taking Lipitor."

We're spending $26 billion a year for a 1%–2% decreased risk for heart attack or stroke? That's what all the fuss is about? It almost seems like snake oil. Yet some doctors are recommending we put statins in the drinking water. Others are even suggesting that infants with a family history of heart disease take statins as a preventative measure.

And perhaps your doctor, convinced that statin drugs are harmless, routinely prescribes them for anyone with a cholesterol level above 200. He might even cite a number of studies in which statin use has lowered the number of heart attack deaths compared to controls. But if we look a little deeper into these studies, we see that statin medications do not *significantly* reduce the risk, and some studies have shown no improvement at all. A meta-analysis of 26 controlled cholesterol-lowering trials found an *equal number* of cardiovascular deaths in the treatment and control groups.[36] And by reducing your cholesterol, statins can actually *increase* your risk of death overall.[37]

So the question isn't, "Do statin drugs reduce the incidence of certain kinds of deaths for certain kinds of people?" The real question is this: "Do statin drugs reduce deaths?" That would be my definition of life-saving. Whether it's from heart attack or side effects, death is death, friend. And we want to avoid it.

(From *Heart Disease: What Your Doctor Won't Tell You,* by the author)

Statins, beta-blockers, tricyclic antidepressants, and benzodiazepine drugs can all suppress the body's formation of coenzyme Q10 (CoQ10). CoQ10 is an enzyme that works with other enzymes to keep the body's metabolic functions working at optimal levels. Small amounts of CoQ10 are found in food, but blood levels of CoQ10 decrease with age, high blood pressure, statin use, diabetes, and atherosclerosis. CoQ10's main purpose is to increase the function of the mitochondria, the "power plants" in each cell. A CoQ10 deficiency can lead to diffuse muscle pain and weakness similar to that seen in FMS and CFS, fatigue, angina, hypertension, accelerated aging, mental confusion, poor memory, tingling or pain in the hands and feet, and heart disease.

A growing body of research shows that CoQ10 may benefit those suffering from any number of unwanted health conditions, including fibromyalgia, achy muscle pain, type-2 diabetes, periodontal disease, chronic fatigue, migraine headaches, skin cancers, infertility, cardiovascular disease, immune dysfunction, asthma, muscular dystrophy—even Alzheimer's and Parkinson's! And though there is some CoQ10 found in foods, getting enough in our diets is a challenge. We find it in meat, dairy, and certain vegetables. But it would take, for instance, one pound of sardines or two-and-a-half pounds of peanuts to provide just 30 mg. of CoQ10 And, especially if you're taking a medication that depletes CoQ10, you'll need much more.

Dr. Karl Folkers, who has been honored with the Priestly Medal—the highest award bestowed by the American Chemical Society—for his work with CoQ10, believes that suboptimal nutrient intake in people is nearly universal and that these tendencies prevent the biosynthesis of CoQ10 He suggests that the average or "normal" levels of CoQ10 are really suboptimal, and that the very low levels observed in advanced disease states are only the tip of the deficiency iceberg. Unless we are supplementing with CoQ10, we may be in fact suffering from a CoQ10 deficiency, especially considering the added stress posed in today's society and the need for an ever-increasing amount of antioxidants. Could it be that many (if not all) of our chronic illnesses are indirectly linked to a CoQ10 deficiency?

This biosynthesis of CoQ10 from the amino acid tyrosine is a complex, highly vulnerable, 17-step process. It requires at least seven vitamins (B2, B3, B6, folic acid, B12, C, and B5), and a number of drugs used to treat fibromyalgia are known to deplete the body of some of these vitamins.

We also tend to absorb and utilize less CoQ10 as we age. It doesn't take much of a decrease in absorption for our health to suffer. Researchers estimate the as little as a 25% decline in bodily CoQ10 will initiate several disease states, including high blood pressure, heart disease, fatigue, cancer, and immune dysfunction. My book *Heart Disease: What Your Doctor Won't Tell You* goes into greater detail about CoQ10 and its use in treating high blood pressure, congestive heart failure, mitral valve prolapse, and other heart-related conditions. You can also visit www.treatingandbeating.com for more information on CoQ10.

To end the use of any of these drugs, always consult your doctor first. Stopping medications can trigger a host of withdrawal symptoms. First, start your jump-start program (chapter 13), build up your stress-coping system, and allow your body to start healing itself. After you start feeling stronger (it may be a few months)—and only with the help of your doctor—slowly start weaning off the medications. Most of the medications can be weaned off and never missed. Some will have to be restarted until you become stronger or find other less toxic options.

SOME MEDICATIONS THAT CAN CAUSE NUTRITIONAL DEFICIENCIES

- **ACE inhibitors** (Accupril, Aceon, Altace, Capoten, Lexxel, Lotensin, Mavik, Monopril, Lisinopril, Prinivil, Tarka, Univasc) deplete zinc.
- **Acid reducers** (Prevacid, Prilosec, Nexium, Aciplex) deplete B12 and calcium.
- **Antibiotics** deplete *Lactobacillus acidophilus, Bifidobacteria bifidum,* and other good bacteria; vitamins B1, B2, B3, B6, B12, and K; biotin; and inositol.
- **Aspirin** depletes folic acid, iron, potassium, and vitamin C.
- **Benzodiazepines** (Klonopin, Valium, Ativan, Xanax, BuSpar) deplete vitamin B12 and CoQ10.

- **Beta-blockers** (Atenolol, Tenormin, Lopressor, Toprol, Inderal) deplete CoQ10.
- **Bile acid sequestrants** (Questran, Lopid, Atromid) deplete beta carotene, folic acid, calcium, magnesium, zinc, and vitamins B12, A, D, E, and K.
- **Carbamazepine** (Tegretol) depletes biotin, folic acid, and vitamin D.
- **Centrally acting antihypertensives** (Catapres, Tenex) deplete CoQ10.
- **Corticosteroids** (cortisone, dexamethasone, hydrocortisone, prednisone) deplete calcium, folic acid, magnesium, potassium, selenium, vitamin C, vitamin D, and zinc.
- **Digoxin** (Lanoxin) depletes calcium, magnesium, phosphorus, and vitamin B1.
- **Estrogens** (Estrace, Premarin) deplete magnesium, omega-3 fatty acids, vitamin B1, and zinc.
- **Famotidine and other H2-blocking drugs** (Pepcid, Pepcid AC, Axid, Tagamet, Zantac) deplete calcium, folic acid, iron, vitamin B12, vitamin D, and zinc.
- **Glucophage** (Metformin) depletes vitamin B12.
- **Hydrochlorothiazide** (Dyazide, Maxzide, Microzide) depletes calcium, folic acid, and vitamin B6.
- **Lamictal** depletes vitamin B12 and CoQ10.
- **Loop diuretics** (Lasix, Bumex) deplete calcium, magnesium, potassium, zinc, and vitamins B1 and B6.
- **NSAIDS** (Celebrex, Mobic, Advil, Motrin, Aleve, Relafen) deplete folic acid.
- **Omeprazole** (Prilosec) depletes vitamin B12.
- **Oral contraceptives** deplete vitamin C, vitamin B2, folic acid, magnesium, vitamin B6, vitamin B12, and zinc.
- **Pravastatin** (Pravachol) depletes CoQ10.
- **Ranitidine** (Zantac) depletes calcium, folic acid, iron, vitamin B12, vitamin D, and zinc.
- **Statin drugs** (Lipitor, Zocor, Crestor, Vytorin, etc.) deplete CoQ10.

- **Sulfonylureas** (Diabeta, Micronase, GluCovance) deplete CoQ10.
- **Tetracycline,** since it's an antibiotic, depletes *Lactobacillus acidophilus, Bifidobacteria bifidum,* and other good bacteria; vitamins B1, B2, B3, B6, B12, and K; biotin; and inositol. It also depletes calcium, magnesium, and iron.
- **Thiazide diuretics** (Enduron, Microzide) deplete magnesium, potassium, zinc, and CoQ10.
- **Triamterene** (Dyrenium) depletes calcium, folic acid, and zinc. This could cause fatigue, depression, anxiety, and poor immunity.
- **Tricyclic antidepressants** (Elavil, Pamelor, Doxepin, Trazodone, Sinequan, Tofranil, Remeron) deplete CoQ10 and vitamin B2.
- **Trileptal** depletes vitamin B12 and CoQ10.
- **Valproic acid** (Depacote) depletes carnitine and folic acid.

For more information, see Ross Pelton et al., *Drug-Induced Nutrient Depletion Handbook, 1999–2000* (Hudson, Ohio: Lexi Comp, 1999).

TREATING WITH NATURAL MEDICINE

Natural medicine uses naturally occurring foods, vitamins, minerals, amino acids, essential fatty acids, and herbal supplements to augment the nutritional status, and therefore the health, of the body.

Herbs have always been integral to the practice of medicine. The word "drug" comes from the old Dutch word *drogge* meaning "to dry," as pharmacists, physicians, and ancient healers often dried plants for use as medicines.

Today approximately 25% of all prescription medications are derived from trees, shrubs, or herbs. The World Health Organization notes that of the 119 plant-derived pharmaceutical medicines, about 74% are used in modern medicine in ways that correlate directly with their traditional uses as plant-based medicines by native cultures. Yet, for the most part, modern medicine has ignored the potential benefits of using pure herbs in treating disease. One of the reasons for this is due to the political and economic factors involved in the pharmaceutical industry. Herbs are naturally available, and drug companies can't patent their use. Without exclusive patents, these companies are not able to reap profits from the millions it may take to bring the product to market.

According to James Duke, PhD, a scientist and USDA specialist in the area of herbal medicine, "one of the reasons that research into the field of herbal medicine has been lacking is the enormous financial cost of the testing required to prove a new drug safe." This price is more than 200 million dollars. "What commercial drug company is going to want to prove that saw palmetto is better than this multimillion dollar drug, when you and I can go to Florida and harvest our own saw palmetto?" This paradigm seems to be changing as our country is starting to mirror the European model of treatment with herbals and natural therapeutics. In Germany, the Ministry of Health has a separate commission that deals exclusively with herbal medicine. German doctors study herbal medicine in medical school, and since 1993, all physicians in Germany must pass a section on these medicines in their board exams. European physicians, health professionals, and researchers have formed the European Scientific Cooperative for Phytotherapy (ESCOP). This organization has published (and continues to do so) monographs on individual herbs used in clinical medicine. These monographs, representing the culmination of all the scientific information known on each herb, are published in the *European Pharmacopoeia.*

In general, herbal medicines work in much the same way as do conventional pharmaceutical drugs, via their chemical makeup. Herbs contain a large number of naturally occurring chemicals, and those chemicals have biological activity. In the past 150 years, chemists and pharmacists have been isolating and purifying active compounds from plants in an attempt to produce reliable pharmaceutical drugs. Examples include digoxin (marketed Lanoxin) from the foxglove plant, resperine (marketed Serpasil) from Indian snakeroot, and morphine from the opium poppy.

According to Andrew Weil, MD, of Tucson Arizona Medical School, because herbs and plants use an indirect route to the bloodstream and to target organs, their effects are slower and less dramatic than those of purified drugs administered more directly.

"Doctors and patients accustomed to the rapid, intense effects of synthetic medicines may become impatient with botanicals for this reason." However, the common assumption that herbs are slow to act and therefore free of side effects is not true. Herbal medicines should be prescribed by a professional who is familiar with the actions and interactions of herbals and prescription medications. Still, herbals have an extremely large window of safety, especially when compared to synthetic prescription drugs.

Most U.S. medical schools are still woefully deficient in training physicians in nutrition and herbals. But it's estimated that over 80% of the population takes at least one nutritional supplement a day, and sales of nutritional supplements have contributed greatly to the $27-billion natural-health industry. With this much money involved, it is no wonder that many of the large pharmaceutical companies that were previously opposed to nutritional supplements have started marketing their own line of vitamins, minerals, and herbals.

MY EXPERIENCE WITH NATURAL MEDICINE

I've been a chiropractor for years and strongly believe in the benefits of chiropractic, but when I began to add diet and nutritional advice into my practice, I started seeing significant changes in my patients. They were little things at first, like recommending magnesium to a patient and finding that he didn't need to see me for chiropractic every week after all. I found that patients who took a good multivitamin and mineral supplement had less pain, more energy, and better health overall. Then I was hooked. I read dozens of medical, nutritional, and biochemistry books. I traveled around the country and trained with some of the masters of nutritional and integrative medicine. I took all the post-graduate classes I could on nutrition and biochemistry and then went back and relearned all the biochemistry I had forgotten from chiropractic school.

Slowly my practice changed from 70–80 musculoskeletal patients a day to 15–25 "medical misfits" a day. These complicated and challenging patients had either fallen through the conventional medical cracks by not responding to treatment, or they were seeking a more natural way to restore their health. I have learned a great deal about integrating conventional and alternative methods, and I've found that correcting a person's biochemistry is the key to restoring her inborn healing mechanisms. Prescription medications can, in some cases, be helpful, but they can never take the place of our own self-regulating, God-given healing mechanisms. This doesn't mean I don't refer to medical doctors; I often do. But now that I've been on both sides of the fence (conventional medicine and nutritional medicine—see my story in chapter 1), I know that the type of nutritional medicine I practice works! Even if conventional medicine insists otherwise.

> "Each progressive spirit is opposed by a thousand mediocre minds appointed to guard the past."
>
> —Maurice Maeterlinck

Today, patients call, email, or travel from all over the world to consult with me. These "medical misfits" have usually been to dozens of medical doctors, sometimes including those at Mayo and Johns Hopkins. Yet, conventional medicine has failed them. But some little chiropractic nutritionist in Birmingham, Alabama is able to help them.

And I'm not the only doctor getting these results; more and more doctors are turning to nutritional medicine. The tide is turning, and conventional medicine is beginning to lose some of its luster. It has so many positive things to offer; if only it would remove its head from the sand and acknowledge that the path it has led us down is, in fact, the wrong one.

I will offend those who can't change paradigms quickly enough to realize that every science, no matter how loftily held, must be open to scrutiny. In the spirit of the children's fable, someone has to stand up and declare that the emperor has no clothes.

In the following chapters, we'll examine how my nutritionally based protocols—refined over the past 10 years—can help you feel good again.

NOTES

1. Public Citizen, "2002 Drug Industry Profits: Hefty Pharmaceutical Company Margins Dwarf Other Industries," Congress Watch (June 2003), www.citizen.org/congress/reform/drug_industry/corporate/articles.cfm?ID=9923.
2. Families USA, "Profiting from Pain: Where Prescription Drug Dollars Go," Publication 02-105 (July 2002), www.familiesusa.org/assets/pdfs/PPreport89a5.pdf.
3. Marcia Angell, *The Truth About the Drug Companies* (New York: Random House, 2004).
4. ibid.
5. Tyler Chin, "Drug Firms Score by Paying Doctors for Time," *American Medical News* (May 6, 2001).
6. Arnold S. Relman, "Defending Professional Independence: ACCME's Proposed New Guidelines for Commercial Support of CME," *Journal of the American Medical Association* 89 (2003): 2418–2420.
7. Jerome P. Kassirer, "How Drug Lobbyists Influence Doctors," editorial, *Boston Globe* (February 13, 2006).
8. Spear et al., "Clinical Application of Pharmacogenetics," *Trends in Molecular Medicine* (May 2001).
9. Steve Connor, "Glaxo Chief: Our Drugs Do Not Work on Most People," *The Independent* (December 8, 2003).
10. Public Citizen, "The Other Drug War II: Drug Companies Deploy an Army of 623 Lobbyists to Keep Profits Up," Congress Watch (June 2002), www.citizen.org/congress/reform/drug_industry/contribution/articles.cfm?ID=7908.
11. Jerome P. Kassirer, "How Drug Lobbyists Influence Doctors."
12. Melody Petersen, *Our Daily Meds: How the Pharmaceutical Companies Transformed Themselves into Slick Marketing Machines and Hooked the Nation on Prescription Drugs* (New York: Sarah Crichton, 2008): 19.
13. Vince Parry, "The Art of Branding a Condition," *Medical Marketing and Media* (May 2003).
14. Rachel Christensen Sethl and the Employee Research Institute, "Prescription Drugs: Recent Trends in Utilization," *Expenditures and Coverage* 265 (January 2004).
15. Pennsylvania Health Care Cost Containment Council, "Prescription Drug Safety," PHC4 FYI (May, 2004), www.phc4.org/reports/fyi/fyi25.htm.
16. "World Health Organization Assesses the World's Health System," press release of the World Health Organization (June 21, 2000).
17. Daniel Haley, "The Other Drug War," *Alternative Medicine* 43 (September 2001).
18. Categories included are deaths from adverse drug reactions, medical errors, bedsores, infection, malnutrition, outpatient treatment, unnecessary procedures, and complications related to surgery.
19. Gary Null et al., "Death by Medicine," *Life Extension,* web special (March 2004), www.lef.org/magazine/mag2004/mar2004_awsi_death_01.htm.

20. D.W. Bates, "Drugs and Adverse Reactions: How Worried Should We Be?" *Journal of the American Medical Association* 279(15) (1998): 1216–7.
21. Kaiser Family Foundation, from calculations using data from IMS Health, www.imshealth.com.
22. Gary Null et al., "Death by Medicine," *Life Extension,* web special (March 2004), www.lef.org/magazine/mag2004/mar2004_awsi_death_01.htm.
23. Melody Peterson, *Our Daily Meds.*
24. Curt Furberg and Bruce Psaty, Epidemiology and Prevention Council of the American Heart Association, meeting notes, San Antonio (March 10, 1995).
25. Letter to doctors from Janssen Pharmacuetica, June 26, 1998, www.fda.gov/medwatch/safety/1998/propul.htm.
26. Carrie Louise Daenell, "Drug Induced Nutrient Deficiencies," www.natural-healthsolution.com/nutrientdeficiencies.htm.
27. I.H Kahn et al., "Seizures Reported with Tramadol," *Journal of the American Medical Association* 278 (1997): 1661 (letter).
28. Melody Petersen, *Our Daily Meds.*
29. Alicia Mack, "Examination of the Evidence for the Off-label use of Gabapentin," *Journal of Managed Care Pharmacy* (Nov–Dec 2003).
30. Keith Winstein, "Suit Alleges Pfizer Spun Unfavorable Drug Studies," *Wall Street Journal* (Oct 8, 2008).
31. James A. Duke, *The Green Pharmacy* (Emmaus, PA: Rodale, 1997).
32. L.M. Klevay and D.B. Milne, "Low Dietary Magnesium Increases Supraventricular Ectopy," *American Journal of Clinical Nutrition* 75(3) (2002): 550–4.
33. B. Gonzalez-Flecha, *Research Interests and Select Publications,* 2002.
34. F.J. Simoes et al., "Therapeutic Effect of a Magnesium Salt in Patients Suffering from Mitral Valvular Prolapse and Latent Tetany," *Magnesium* 4(5–6) (1985): 283–90.
35. M. Shechter et al., "Oral Magnesium Therapy Improves Endothelial Function in Patients with Coronary Artery Disease," *Circulation* 102(19) (2000): 2353–8.
36. U. Ravnskov, "Cholesterol Lowering Trials in Coronary Heart Disease: Frequency of Citation and Outcome," *British Medical Journal* 305 (1992): 15–19.
37. I.J. Schatz et al., "Cholesterol and All Cause Mortality in Elderly People in the Honolulu Heart Program: A Cohort Study," *Lancet* 358 (2001): 351–355.

FOR FURTHER READING AND RESEARCH
• P.M. Brooks et al., "NSAID and Osteoarthritis: Help or Hindrance," *Science* April 19, 2002.
• P.M. Brooks and R.O. Day, *New England Journal of Medicine* 324(24) (1991): 1716–25.
• "Carcinogenicity of Lipid-Lowering Drugs," *JAMA* January 1996.
• G. Farrell, "Pfizer Settles Fraud Case for $430 Million," *USA TODAY*

- N.R. Farnsworth et al., "Medicinal Plants in Therapy," *Bulletin of the World Health Organization* 65(6) (1985): 965–81.
- P.R. Jackson, *British Journal of Clinical Pharmacology* 52 (2001): 439–46.
- I. Kirsch et al., "The Emperor's New Drugs: An Analysis of Antidepressant Medication Data Submitted to the U.S. Food and Drug Administration," *Prevention and Treatment,* American Psychology Association (5)23 (July 15, 2002).
- Public Citizen Congress Watch, "2002 Drug Industry Profits: Hefty Pharmaceutical Company Margins Dwarf Other Industries," June 2003 (www.citizen.org).
- Robert W. Simms, MD: Associate Professor of Medicine, Clinical Director, Rheumatology Section, Boston University Arthritis Center, Boston, Massachusetts. Posted to ACR website Oct. 8, 2004 (www.rheumatology.org).
- M. Shechter et al., "Oral Magnesium Therapy Improves Endothelial Function in Patients with Coronary Artery Disease," *Circulation* 102(19) (2000): 2353–8.
- M.J. Shield, "Anti-inflammatory Drugs and Their Effects on Cartilage Synthesis and Renal Function," *European Journal of Rheumatology and Inflammation* 13 (1993): 7–16.

· 7 ·
TREATING WITH
ORTHOMOLECULAR
MEDICINE

"The doctor of the future will give no medication, but will interest his patients in the care of the human frame, diet, and in the cause and prevention of disease."—Thomas Edison

The proceeding chapters have hopefully laid the groundwork for why I place such an emphasis on the use of nutritional supplementation for treating and beating fibromyalgia and chronic fatigue syndrome. Our body's homeostatic mechanism, the HPA-axis, and in fact, every cellular process, depends on the proper amount of essential nutrients. The raw biochemical material that makes up our physical and mental being first originates from foods. The entire process is amazing: macromolecules of carbohydrates, fats, and proteins are ingeniously used to provide the vitamins, minerals, essential fatty acids, enzymes, and amino acids to the body as it manufactures bone, muscle, organs, cells, hormones, enzymes, antibodies, white blood cells, neurotransmitters, and other life-sustaining elements. We truly are what we eat.

I realize that the idea of treating, and even beating, such complicated illnesses as FMS and CFS with nutrition and supplements might sound unreasonable at first—even simple minded. However, no one suffers from a drug deficiency. **The levels and interactions of vitamins, minerals, amino acids, and essential fatty acids determine our state of health.** You can live without Ambien, Klonopin, Lyrica, and other drugs. But you would be dead in days without these essential nutrients. They help determine every bodily function: sleep, levels of pain, energy, moods, immune function, digestion, elimination, thyroid production, metabolism, and more. Every cell in the body is dependent on having the right amounts and right interaction of these essential nutrients to work correctly.

Amino acids and B vitamins are needed to make the feel-good neurotransmitter, serotonin, and also dopamine, norepinephrine, and gamma amino butyric acid (GABA). Magnesium, along with calcium, regulates every cell by controlling what enters and exits through the outer cell membrane. The amino acid L-tyrosine, along with selenium and iodine, make the thyroid hormone thyroxine. Vitamin B5 is needed for proper adrenal gland function.

(I'll provide an in-depth look at vitamins, minerals, amino acids, and essential fatty acids later in this book.)

WHAT IS ORTHOMOLECULAR MEDICINE?

When we establish nutritional deficiencies, our health suffers. Man-made chemicals (synthetic prescription drugs) can't correct these deficiencies, but a nutritional-replacement therapeutic program can. This is the very premise of orthomolecular medicine, which means, "right molecules in the right concentration."

Linus Pauling, two-time winner of the Nobel Prize, is regarded as one of the greatest biochemists of our times. He defines orthomolecular medicine as "the preservation of good health and the treatment of disease by varying the concentrations in the human body of substances that are normally present in the body." This concept involves a medical approach based on the physiological and enzymatic actions of specific nutrients present in the body, such as vitamins, minerals, and amino acids. The idea that to beat a disease one has simply to "get healthy" may seem trivial to those with such life-robbing illnesses as FMS and CFS. Still, it's hard to argue with the results.

Synthetic drugs may be helpful at times, but they always have an inherent ability to cause harm. Not only are nutrients such as vitamins, minerals, amino acids, and essential fatty acids unharmful, the body depends on them for survival. The body knows what to do with—and depends on—vitamin B6. The same certainly can't be said for Elavil. The World Health Organization's definition of health is "a state of complete physical, mental, and social well-being and not merely the absence of disease or infirmity." These words advocate to us the need to correct the biochemical causes of disease rather than merely covering up the symptoms with drugs.

The Centers for Medicare and Medicaid stated in a recent report that the nation spent $140.6 billion in the year 2000 on prescription drugs. And of course this number is rapidly escalating; over one billion prescriptions were written last year. But even though the United States spends more money on health care per capita than any other country in the world, The World Health Organization ranks the overall health of the United States as 15th among the 25 industrialized countries.

Even with this dismal ranking, things in the United States are changing. A new paradigm is emerging, one based on taking responsibility for our own health through abstinence from dangerous habits—like nicotine, trans-fats, sedentary lifestyles, and excessive stress—and through proactive behavior like regular exercise, healthy diet decisions, and optimal nutritional supplementation.

VITAMIN AND MINERAL SUPPLEMENTS

Dr. Janet Travell, White House physician for Presidents John F. Kennedy and Lyndon B. Johnson, and Professor Emeritus of Internal Medicine at George Washington University, co-wrote *Myofascial Pain and Dysfunction: The Trigger Point Manual,* which is acknowledged as the authoritative work on muscle pain. In one chapter alone, 317 studies are referenced showing that problems such as hormonal, vitamin, and mineral deficiencies can contribute to muscle pain and soreness.

We'll see in later chapters how vitamins, minerals, amino acids, essential fatty acids, and certain enzymes, when properly supplemented, can provide profoundly beneficial results for those suffering from poor health. Below is a sample listing of essential nutrients and their contributions to the treatment of FMS and CFS.

• **Vitamin E** helps to relieve pain in CFS patients. It can also improve nighttime leg cramps, which interfere with sleep.

• **Vitamin C** boosts the immune system by increasing natural-killer (NK) cells, B cells, and T cells.

• **Magnesium and malic acid** have been found by controlled studies to be effective in relieving the symptoms of FMS. Magnesium is essential to healthy muscle function, and, working with malic acid, it increases cellular energy, reduces pain, and enhances immune function by increasing NK cells. Magnesium is also a natural muscle relaxant and critical for the relief of muscle pain.

- **Inositol** enhances the immune system by increasing NK cells.
- **Selenium** supports the immune system by enhancing antibody production.
- **Vitamin D** regulates many immune functions.
- **Amino acids,** such as glycine, serine, taurine, and tyrosine, are essential for the production of energy in the body and for brain function.
- **Zinc** supports the immune system by enhancing white-blood-cell activity and supporting healthy antigen-antibody binding.

These nutrients are amazing, aren't they? Sadly, though, many of them are deficient in our society. And it's no secret; numerous published studies demonstrate the need for vitamin and mineral supplementation. Our food supply is tainted with poisonous chemicals and laden with preservatives that rob the body of needed nutrients. We simply can no longer get all the nutrients we need from the foods we eat.

Many so-called experts will tell you not to worry about taking vitamins if you are eating a balanced diet. If you ever encounter a doctor who says this, simply smile and head for the nearest exit! By making such a statement, this physician has demonstrated herself to be 20 years behind in the research. How could someone who is supposed to be looking after our health be so ignorant to think that eating bleached bread; toxic meats; allergy-producing dairy products; and nutritionally void, simple carbohydrates could provide the necessary vitamins and minerals the body requires to be healthy? Remember, most medical doctors receive only three classroom hours of nutritional education! This isn't their fault, but they have no excuse for not staying abreast of latest findings that appear in their very own medical journals.

The facts are that most of our foods are processed, and therefore the nutrients have been leeched out of them. As a result, 70% of the population is deficient in magnesium, 65% is deficient in zinc, 48% is deficient in calcium, and 56% is deficient in vitamin C.

It's clear that everyone can benefit from taking a good multivitamin and mineral formula, and there are thousands of studies that demonstrate its benefits. This daily habit reduces the incidence of heart disease, heart attack, stroke, glaucoma, macular degeneration, type-2 diabetes, senile dementia, and various cancers.

BUT I ALREADY TAKE A VITAMIN

You might be thinking, *I've taken a vitamins for years, and I haven't noticed a difference.* You probably haven't been taking enough to even make a dent in your deficiencies. If you compare Centrum or One-A-Day vitamins to our Essential Therapeutics multivitamin and mineral formulas, you'll notice that our specially designed vitamins have 50 times—and in some cases, 100 times—the recommended daily allowance (RDA). This is because the RDA is an outdated system that does not take into account the depletion of our nutrient-rich top soil, environmental pollutants, chemical food processing, the addition of artificial ingredients, and the increased demands placed on an individual's homeostatic system in the 21st century.

So nearly as criminal as not recommending vitamin and mineral supplements is the recommendation of them based on the RDA. It was never intended to advance health, only to prevent deficiency diseases like scurvy and rickets. Taking the minimum amount of a nutrient to prevent gross deficiency doesn't help those people who want to be truly healthy and not just free of severe symptoms. And optimal health should be the goal for all of us.

Years ago, our ancestors ate locally grown food harvested from mineral-rich soil that was free of pesticides and toxic fertilizers. Their meats had no added hormones and antibiotics, and they didn't eat processed foods robbed of their nutrients, and their foods weren't loaded with preservatives and simple sugars. Their diets consisted mainly of grains and vegetables with a little dairy and organic meats. They didn't need supplements to shore up their diets.

Life is different for us. We're also living a lot longer, and as we age, our nutrient needs can increase dramatically.

See below a selection of nutrient levels as recommended by the RDA and the more prudent ODA (optimal daily allowance).

Nutrient	RDA	ODA
Vitamin A	1,000 mcg.	10,000 mg.
Vitamin D	200 IU	100 IU
Vitamin E	15 IU	400 IU
Vitamin K	80 mcg.	60–80 mcg.
Vitamin B1	1.5 mg.	50–100 mg.
Vitamin B2	1.7 mg.	50 mg.
Vitamin B3	19 mg.	50 mg.
Vitamin B5	7 mg.	200–400 mg.
Vitamin B6	2 mg.	50–200 mg.
Folic Acid	200 mcg.	400–800 mcg.
Vitamin C	60 mg.	1,000–2,000 mg.
Calcium	800 mg.	500–1,200 mg.
Chloride	750 mg.	Not usually recommended
Chromium	50–200 mcg.	200–400 mcg.
Copper	1.5–3.0 mg.	1 mg.
Fluoride	1.5–4.0 mg.	Not usually recommended
Iodine	150 mcg.	Not usually recommended
Iron	10 mg.	Not unless needed
Magnesium	350 mg.	500–1,000 mg.
Manganese	2.5–5.0 mg.	10–20 mg.
Molybdenum	75–250 mcg.	Same (unless deficient)
Phosphorus	800 mg.	Not usually recommended
Potassium	2,000 mg.	100 mg.
Selenium	70 mcg.	200 mcg.
Sodium	500 mg.	Not usually recommended
Zinc	15 mg.	25 mg.

ARE THESE HIGHER DOSES SAFE?

One of the arguments against megavitamin treatment is that a high dose of certain vitamins are toxic and may cause certain adverse reactions. Let me present some statistics to you and let you decide for yourself.

The American Medical Association reports that death from medical errors is now the third leading cause of death in the United States, behind only heart disease and cancer. As reported in *JAMA*, over 250,000 Americans die each year from medical therapies, including at least 113,000 from the negative effects of prescription medications.

The total number of deaths from vitamin/mineral therapy during the years of 1983 to 1990 was zero. Nevertheless, problems can occur with megavitamin or herbal therapy. But if symptoms arise, reducing or stopping the therapy will almost always put an end to any side effects. Working with a physician who specializes in vitamin, mineral, or herbal therapies will usually help you avoid any negative effects in the first place. In the 10 years I've been using orthomolecular doses of vitamins, minerals, and amino acids, both intravenously and orally, there has not been a single major side effect observed in my patients.

SHARON

I'd say along with the adrenal supplements, the CFS/FMS Formula has made the biggest difference in how well I feel. If I miss a few days of either supplement, I start to feel sluggish and run down. I've taken dozens of different supplements over the last few years, but none have seemed to have helped like the ones Dr. Murphree recommended. I like the convenience of taking a pack in the morning and one in the afternoon. Before, I had to carry pills around in my pockets or purse. Sometimes I'd lose them, sometimes they would melt and stain my clothes. And I was buying bottles of all different things. So usually I would just lose interest and give up.

Don't *you* give up. There is a "wonder cure" out there, after all...and it's your own body!

FOR FURTHER READING AND RESEARCH
- B.M. Altura and B.T. Altura, "Role of magnesium in patho-physiological processes and the clinical utility of magnesium ion selective electrodes," *Scand J Clin Lab Invest Suppl* 224 (1996): 211–34.
- M. T. Cantorna et al., "In vivo up regulation of interleukin-4 is one mechanism underlying the immunoregulatory effects of 1,25-dihydroxyvitamin

D(3)," *Arch Biochem Biophys* 377 (2000): 135–8.

• M. de la Fuente et al., "Immune function in aged women is improved by ingestion of vitamins C and E," *Can J Physiol Pharmacol* 76 (1998): 373–80.

• L. Doan et al., "Metal ion catalysis of RNA cleavage by the influenza virus endonuclease," *Biochemistry* 38 (1999): 5612–9.

• G.W. Dyke et al., "Effect of vitamin C supplementation on gastric mucosal DNA damage," *Carcinogenesis* 15 (1994): 291–5.

• M.D. Fernandez et al., "Effects in vitro of several antioxidants on the natural killer func- tion of aging mice," *Exp Gerontol* 34 (1999): 675–85.

• F. Girodon et al., "Impact of trace elements and vitamin supplementation on immunity and infections in insti- tutionalized elderly patients: a randomized controlled trial," *Arch Intern Med* 159 (1999): 748–54.

• H. Hasegawa et al., "Effects of zinc on the reactive oxygen species generating capacity of human neutrophils and the serum opsonic activity in vitro," *Luminescence* 15 (2000): 321–7.

• G. Heuser and Vojdani, "Enhancement of natural killer cell activity and T and B cell function by buffered vitamin C in patients exposed to toxic chemicals: the role of protein kinase-C," *Immunopharmacol Immunotoxicol* 19 (1997): 291–312.

• *Myofascial Pain and Dysfunction: The Trigger Point Manual* by Dr. Janet Travell and Dr. David Simons.

• C.F. Nockels, "The role of vitamins in modulating disease resistance," *Vet Clin North Am Food Anim Pract* 4 (1988): 531–42.

• A. Saini et al.,"Regulation of macrophage growth responses to colony-stimulating factor-1 by 1,25-dihydroxyvitamin D3," *J Am Soc Nephrol* 5 9 1995): 2091–3.

• V. Tuovinen et al., "Oral mucosal changes related to plasma ascorbic acid levels," *Proc Finn Dent Soc* 88 (1992): 117–122.

• N. Wellinghausen et al., "Zinc serum levels in immunodeficiency virus-infected patients in relation to immunologic status," *Biol Trace Elem Res* 73 (2000): 139–49.

· 8 ·
YOUR STRESS-COPING SAVINGS ACCOUNT

We're all born with a stress-coping "savings account" filled with chemicals—such as hormones, amino acids, and nutrients—that can be deposited and then withdrawn when needed. Depending on our genes, some of us have large accounts, and some of us have smaller ones. The more stress we're under, the more withdrawals we make. If we make more withdrawals than deposits, we get overdrawn, and poor health quickly follows. Individuals with fibromyalgia and/or CFS have bankrupted their stress-coping savings account.

Although some patients bankrupt their accounts with one overwhelming event, most experience a series of stressful events over the years. These events typically involve stressful jobs, marriages, family dynamics, surgeries, illnesses, loss of a loved one, divorce, financial failure, etc.

Many of my patients can remember the day when their account went belly-up. It might have been after a surgery or following the loss of a parent. Whatever happened, the person was never the same from that point on; she just couldn't get well. My CFS patients often relate how they came down with a bad case of flu and just never completely got over it. Once these individuals get enough rest and stop making withdrawals, they may attempt to do something as mundane as sweep the kitchen floor only to be wiped out once again. And forget about grocery shopping! That could put them in bed for weeks.

FMS and CFS are the result of internal biochemical (hormonal, enzymatic, neuronal, and chemical) imbalances that manifest themselves as physical symptoms (pain, weakness, and mental impairment). So in order to right the homeostatic system, you must correct the underlying biochemical problems. Just like an onion, you peel away one layer at a time until you get to the core. But we'll discuss these practical steps soon. For now, let's make sure that you understand all of these "layers of the onion." One of these is dysautonomia.

DYSAUTONOMIA AND THE HPA AXIS

Dysautonomia is defined by *Taber's Cyclopedic Medical Dictionary* as "a rare hereditary disease involving the autonomic nervous system with mental retardation, motor in coordination, vomiting, frequent infections, and convulsions." But dysautonomia symptoms are usually nowhere near this severe. Dysautonomia patients are more likely to be suffering from mitral valve prolapse and neurally mediated hypotension (dizziness upon standing) than mental retardation and vomiting.

A better description, then, of dysautonomia would be a malfunction in the body's master regulating (homeostasis) system, which—as you may recall from earlier chapters—is known as the autonomic nervous system or the HPA axis. The HPA axis (comprised of the hypothalamus, the pituitary gland, and the adrenal glands) controls millions of involuntary actions such as breathing, releasing of endocrine hormones, blood flow, smooth muscle tone, immune response, heartbeat, detoxification, and elimination. We don't have to think about breathing; we just do it. We don't try to pump blood through the heart and into the muscles; it is initiated and monitored by our HPA axis.

Normally all the systems in the body speak to and coordinate with one another. This is the essence of homeostasis. But when a person depletes her savings account of stress-coping chemicals, her HPA axis begins to self-destruct. This is dysautonomia. It's as if the immune system starts to speak in Spanish, the endocrine system in German, the musculoskeletal system in Greek, and the digestive system in French! And when no one can communicate, chaos results!

To check for dysautonomia, you don't need a doctor's tilt-table test. Instead, follow these simple instructions (or ask a health-care professional for help) to check for adrenal dysfunction: take your blood pressure while lying down. Then stand up. After 30 seconds has past, take your blood pressure again. Normally the systolic (top number) pressure will go up 10 or more points. A decrease in the systolic number indicates adrenal dysfunction. If a person has mitral valve prolapse, NMH, and a positive adrenal dysfunction test, it's pretty clear she has dysautonomia.

HYPOTHALAMUS GLAND DYSFUNCTION

The actions of the autonomic nervous system are coordinated by the hypothalamus gland (The "H" of the HPA axis). This gland helps maintain water balance, sugar and fat metabolism, blood sugar levels, blood volume, body temperature, endocrine hormones, and a phenomenal portion of the body's activity. The hypothalamus also releases several different chemicals, including epinephrine, norepinephrine, and corticosteroids. Plus, the hypothalamus has immunologic functions. It's one amazing gland.

Improper functioning of the hypothalamus can cause a variety of problems, including neurally mediated hypotension (NMH). This occurs when the blood pressure drops suddenly after standing, causing dizziness and weakness. And since the hypothalamus also plays an immune role, any dysfunction can interfere with your ability to stay well. Let's investigate other conditions that can result from a dysfunctioning hypothalamus.

DEHYDRATION

Dysfunction of the hypothalamus leads to low levels of vasopressin, which is an antidiuretic hormone. This causes decreased ability to hold on to fluid and results in frequent urination and increased thirst. Dehydration then occurs, despite increased water intake. And believe it or not, something as "simple" as dehydration can cause many of the chronic symptoms seen in FMS and CFS, including NMH, depression, excess body weight, high blood pressure, fatigue, low back and neck pain, and headaches. Dehydration also depletes the neurotransmitter tryptophan, and a reduction in tryptophan is associated with insomnia, increased pain, and depression. Feeling thirsty yet?

LOW LEVELS OF HUMAN GROWTH HORMONE

When the hypothalamus is dysfunctioning, human growth hormone (HGH) levels drop. HGH helps increase energy, repair damaged muscles, stimulate immune function, reduce body fat, improve sleep, and enhance mental acuity (especially short-term memory). Does this sound like anyone you know? Long-term studies have revealed even more, as psychological well-being continues to go downhill for those short of HGH. The best way to increase HGH levels is by getting eight hours of deep, restorative sleep each night, but there are also over-the-counter supplements that can help. HGH-replacement injection therapy is available by prescription. Exercise also helps build HGH levels.

LOW LEVELS OF DHEA

DHEA (dehydroepiandrosterone) is used by the body to make other hormones, including estrogen and testosterone. It's important in creating appropriate energy levels and maintaining feelings of well-being, but a dysfunctioning hypothalamus can cause the adrenal glands to produce less DHEA than is needed.

LOW LEVELS OF CORTISOL

Decreased levels of this adrenal stress hormone cause immune dysfunction, increased inflammation, hypoglycemia (low blood sugar), and hypotension (low blood pressure).

LOW OVARIAN AND TESTICULAR FUNCTION

We've talked about how a dysfunctional hypothalamus can lead to low estrogen levels. But did you know that low estrogen can contribute to decreased blood flow to specific areas of the brain? This may explain some of the "fibro-fog" that occurs in some CFS and FMS patients. And low testosterone, both in males and females, can cause immune dysfunction. (Research is now showing that males with low testosterone have an increased risk of heart disease.)

HYPOTHYROIDISM

The symptoms of FMS and CFS are consistent with those associated with hypothyroidism (low thyroid function): low body temperature, cold hands and feet, tingling in the extremities, fatigue, and depressed mental acuity.

Recent studies show that over 43% of FMS patients have low thyroid function, and it's estimated that those with FMS are 10 to 250,000 times more likely than those without to suffer from thyroid dysfunction. For more information on thyroid disorders, see chapter 14.

THE OTHER LAYERS OF THE ONION
Intestinal Permeability (Leaky Gut Syndrome): Most of the individuals I evaluate are plagued by poor digestion. Much of this is caused by intestinal permeability, which occurs when the lining of the small intestine becomes irritated and leaks undigested proteins across the cellular membrane. This is like turning on a damaged garden hose and watching helplessly as water leaks from hole after hole.

In your body, this "leaking" creates a potentially hazardous situation as the food proteins become allergic irritants. The irritants initiate an immune reaction, and chronic inflammation results.

Malabsorption Syndrome: A close cousin of intestinal permeability, malabsorption is when many vital nutrients are simply not absorbed. Deficiencies of these nutrients lead to depression, insomnia, fatigue, pain, decreased immunity, poor memory, and other ill effects. For more information on intestinal permeability and malabsorption syndrome, see chapter 12.

The Liver and Detoxification: The body's ability to eliminate toxins largely determines its health, and detoxification is an ongoing, never-ending process. A number of toxins—including heavy metals, pesticides, solvents, and microbes—are known to cause significant health problems.

The body eliminates toxins either by directly neutralizing them or by excreting them by way of the urine, feces, lungs (breathing), and skin (sweat). Toxins that the body is unable to eliminate build up in the tissues, typically in our fat cells. Most individuals with FMS/CFS are suffering from an overburden of various toxins because of a dysfunctioning liver. To learn more about detoxification, see chapter 19.

Nutritional Deficiencies: "If you eat a balanced diet you'll get all the nutrients you need." The "health experts" who continue to cling to this draconian idea must not have read the research studies written on nutrition over the past 20 years. The standard American diet (even if you eat fruits and vegetables every day) is overloaded with toxic, artificial chemicals. And modern processing methods remove 25–75% of the original nutrients.

An FDA study analyzing 234 foods over two years found that the average American diet contains less than 80% of the RDA of one or more of the following: calcium, magnesium, iron, zinc, copper, and manganese. **Other studies have demonstrated magnesium deficiency in well over 50% of the population.** A magnesium deficiency can contribute to arterიolosclerosis, fatigue, tight muscles, leg cramps, insomnia, constipation, cardiac arrhythmia, and heart disease. More junk food, anyone?

Let's look at what a deficiency in just one common vitamin can mean to your body. Vitamin B6 deficiencies are common in women of childbearing age, as estrogen and progesterone tend to consume B6 during its metabolism in the liver. So how much harm could one deficiency cause?

Well, optimal levels of the neurotransmitter serotonin are dependent on adequate quantities of B6 Some cases of PMS

> Women who have had multiple pregnancies or long-term use of birth-control pills are at special risk of developing a B6 deficiency.

have also been attributed to B6 deficiency. A deficiency of B6 results in the loss of cell-mediated immunity and a reduction in the size and weight of the thymus gland, an important part of the immune system. Numbers of lymphocytes decrease, and the body is compromised in its fight against infection and disease.

In short, there is no such thing as a superfluous nutrient! And this doesn't only include vitamins and minerals. Well intentioned health professionals have been recommending low fat diets for the past 10–15 years, and this has been disastrous for our nation's health. Americans are now the most overweight country in the world, and we're still low in the fats that we really need. While on this so-called health diet, the average American has gained over 10 pounds. And cases of heart disease, cancer, type-2 diabetes, and other chronic conditions have actually increased.

A low-fat diet is also usually a low-protein diet, and protein deficiency contributes to depression, fatigue, poor concentration, poor detoxification, and many other illnesses. This is because our bodies need the essential amino acids that make up a protein. They regulate our neurotransmitters, sex hormones, immune system, glucose-insulin levels, wound healing, and thousands of essential bodily functions. See more about fats in chapter 29, protein in chapter 28, and vitamins and minerals in chapters 26 and 27.

Parasites: Based on medical records and disease patterns, public health experts estimate that 60% of Americans will experience parasitic infections in their lifetime. Over 1 million Americans are infected with roundworm *(Ascaris lumbricoides),* and 20–30 million are infected with pinworm *(Enterobius vermicularis). Giardia lamblia* infects 8–10 million and has been implicated, along with *Entamoeba histolytica* and roundworm, as a contributing factor to CFS. See more about parasites in chapter 20.

Food Allergies and Hypersensitivities: Albert Rowe, MD, past president of the American Association for the Study of Allergy, has described a syndrome known as "allergic toxemia" that included the symptoms of fatigue, muscle and joint pain, drowsiness, difficulty concentrating, nervousness, and depression. This syndrome was known as the "allergic tension-fatigue syndrome" in the 1950s, and it sounds to me a lot like CFS or FMS!

Hypersensitivity to environmental chemicals is a growing public concern, afflicting an estimated 15% of the American public. The offenders include odors from cosmetics, perfumes, new carpet, paint, smog, cigarettes, newsprint, copier machines, fabrics, vinyl, household cleaners, and other man-made products. Chapter 18 explains all about identifying and handling food allergies.

Candida **Yeast Syndrome/Intestinal Dysbiosis:** *Candida albicans*
is a yeast that lives in your intestinal tract. It cohabits in a symbiotic relationship with over 400 forms of healthy intestinal bacteria,
which help produce many nutrients and also keep the *Candida*
in check. When these good bacteria die (from antibiotics) or are
suppressed (by steroids), *Candida* is allowed to grow to unhealthy
levels, causing intestinal dysbiosis. *Candida* can also increase during
times of stress.

Trauma, Especially Neck Injuries: Many FMS patients can trace
the beginning of their illness to some type of trauma. And recent
findings reveal that people with neck injuries are more likely to develop fibromyalgia than are those with other types of injuries. One
study published by *Arthritis & Rheumatism* in 1997 focused on
102 subjects with a neck injury and 59 who had had a leg fracture,
assessing them all one year later. Of those with neck injury, 22%
developed fibromyalgia, compared to 2% of those with lower-
extremity fractures.

Depression: Some physicians would like us to believe that FMS is
nothing more than depression. Studies show, however, that FMS
is not caused by depression. But FMS can be a cause of reactive
depression (depression due to circumstances). Who wouldn't be depressed with such an illness? Individuals with FMS have lost their
lives to an illness they can't control and largely don't understand.
Some level of depression is natural.

Infections: Although viral infections are more closely associated
with CFS than FMS, remember that these two syndromes are two
sides of the same coin. Viral, bacterial, fungal, and mycoplasmal infections are common in both types of patients that I treat, through
viral infections like Epstein-Barr have received the most attention.

Poor Sleep: Nonrestorative sleep reduces the production of serotonin and HGH, lowers the pain threshold, and—of course—
causes fatigue and mental decline. Read all about this in chapter 10.

All of these "layers of the onion," as I call them, can force you to
make continuous withdrawals on your stress-coping savings account until you simply don't have a dime left to your name.

FOR FURTHER READING AND RESEARCH

- P.F. Basch, "Enterobias," in: J.M Last (ed) *Public Health ND Preventative Medicine* 11th edition, (New York: Appleton-Century-Crofts, 1980).
- I. Cox et al., "Red Blood Cell Magnesium and Chronic Fatigue Syndrome," *Lancet* 227 (1991): 757–60.
- R.C.W. Hall and J.R. Joffe, "Hypomagnesemia: Physical and Psychiatric Symptoms," *JAMA* 224(31) (1973):1749–51.
- J.F. Jones et al., "Evidence for Active Epstein-Barr Virus Infection in Patients with Persistent, Unexplained Illnesses: Elevated Anti-early Antigen Antibodies," *Annals of Internal Medicine* 102(1) 1985):1–6.
- G.F. Kroger, "Chronic Candidiasis and Allergy," in: J. Brostoff and S.J. Challacombe (eds) *Food Allergy and Intolerance* (Saunders, 1987): 850-72.
- J.C. Lowe et al., "Effectiveness and Safety of T3 (triiothyroxine) Therapy for Euthyroid Fibromyalgia: a double-blind placebo-controlled response-driven crossover study," *Clinical Bulletin of Myofascial Therapy* 2(2/3) (1997a): 31–58.
- H. Moldofsky, "Fibromyalgia, Sleep Disorder and Chronic Fatigue Syndrome," in: G. Bock and J. Whelan (eds) *CIBA Foundation Symposium* 1731993: 262–79.
- J.A. Pennington and B.E. Young, "The selected Minerals in Foods Surveyed from 1982 to 1984," *Journal of the American Dietetic Association* 86 (1986): 7,876.
- J.J. Plorde, "Intestinal Nematodes," in: G.W. Thorne et al. (eds) *Harrison's Principles of Internal Medicine* (New York: McGraw-Hill, 1977).
- A.H. Rowe and A. Rowe Jr., *Food Allergy: its manifestations and control and the elimination diets: A compendium* (Springfield: Charles C. Thomas, 1972).
- M.S. Seelg, *Magnesium Deficiency in the Pathogenesis of Disease: early root of cardiovascular, skeletal, and renal abnormalities,* (New York: Plenum Med. Book Co., 1980).
- M. Tobi et al., "Prolonged Atypical Illness Associated with Serological Evidence of Persistent Epstein-Barr Virus Infection," *Lancet* 1 (1982): 61.

· 9 ·
STRESS AS A
CATALYST FOR ILLNESS

"Stress" is experienced when a person perceives that the demands made upon her exceed the mental, physical, personal, or social resources she is able to mobilize.

Most of us can handle the ups and downs of our daily lives, even the occasional catastrophe. We dig in our heels, persevere, and eventually learn to cope. However, some individuals have an altered stress-coping system, which prevents them from managing daily stress. Human studies suggest that for some folks, the cumulative effects of physical, mental, chemical, or emotional burdens in early childhood may increase the affects of stress later in life. (It's possible that the reason for his effect is an overstimulation or dysfunction of the HPA-axis). Retrospective studies show that the stress of emotional, physical, or sexual abuse during childhood also increases the future risk of developing certain symptoms, including many associated with FMS and CFS.

Apparently, for some children and adolescents, too many traumatic or stressful events decondition their normal homeostatic stress-coping abilities. Thus stress, particularly traumatic stress, early in life may alter the set point of their stress-response system. As they get older, have more responsibilities, and experience an increase in their daily stress, they often find their health beginning to suffer. They may start to have bouts of anxiety and depression, or perhaps they're just tired all the time. They become extremely vulnerable to major stressors: the death of a loved one, chronic illness, invasive surgery, physical trauma, etc. Like a ticking time bomb, it's only a matter of time before they explode.

This is especially true for those who have a genetic predisposition that makes them more susceptible to the ill effects of daily stress, including reduced serotonin levels. Some research has suggested that FMS/CFS patients may in fact by afflicted by this genetic abnormality.

Sadly, I find that many of my FMS and CFS patients have experienced physical, emotional, or sexual abuse as a child. Some patients report abuse from their spouse (sometimes physical but more often emotional). This stressful situation, though begun in adulthood, can still eventually deplete their stress-coping chemicals and lead to a state of disease.

The symptoms of fatigue, pain, poor sleep, poor digestion, irregular bowel movements, mental confusion, poor memory, anxiety, and depression are all warning signs that certain stress-coping chemicals (including vitamins, minerals, amino acids, essential fatty acids, and hormones) have become deficient. These deficiencies then complicate one another until the body's homeostatic mechanism and HPA-axis become dysfunctional.

The final tick of the time bomb may be just another part of chronic daily stress, or it may be a sudden traumatic event like the birth of a new baby. I know I didn't think I'd survive the first colic-plagued six months of my daughter's life. And I'm extremely healthy! I pulled my weight and spent every other night walking and rocking my crying daughter into the early morning, and this is main reason it took another nine years before my wife could convince me to have another child!

It's no wonder that many of my patients report that their fibromyalgia began after the birth of a child, often a firstborn. Anyone with children can relate to sleeping (if you can call it that) with one eye and two ears open, making sure the baby is breathing. Or how about trying to sleep without moving so that you don't wake the baby up? Then there's the endless nights of breast and bottle feedings, diaper changes at two in the morning, and the early morning piercing cry: "I'm awake, folks!" It's enough to bankrupt anyone's stress-coping savings account! Whew! Let's move on.

I want you to read about some people who really understand what you're going through. These are edited accounts from real people, though their names have been changed. (You can read more testimonials in chapter 2.) See if you can find yourself in their stories. I pray that you will also soon find yourself in their recoveries.

TYPE A: THE DRIVER

I've found that most of my FMS and CFS patients fall into one of two personality types: A or B. A's are the driven perfectionists; they do, do, do, until they're done out. Bs are the caregivers; they give, give, give, until they're given out.

Type A's have a schedule filled with activities, which may include a full-time job (which could be staying at home with kids), household duties, family responsibilities, soccer practices, PTA meetings, volunteer work, church duties, and more. They push themselves harder and harder trying to do more, be more, have more. They don't want to settle for second best. These perfectionist can't stand to be idle. They must be busy doing something, and they love to multitask. They'll be talking on the phone counseling a co-worker, cooking dinner, emptying the dishwasher, feeding the baby, and looking over the day's mail all at the same time. They're used to pushing themselves and often feel guilty asking for extra pay or time off, even though they perform above and beyond their call. If asked to volunteer for a good cause, they nearly always accept. If the boss calls and asks them to head an additional committee, they accept once again. "No" is a rare word in their vocabulary.

Unfortunately, these type A's can get so caught up in "doing" that they never take time to be human "beings." They don't know what true downtime feels like. Finally, the years of constant stress catch up to them, and they literally burn themselves out.

JEAN

I'm 59 years old, and I work as an insurance agent. Until 12 years ago, I had been very active in sports. I've raised three boys, mostly on my own, and I've always been involved in the community.

I had to have surgery, and from there went downhill. Very sick, no energy, lots of pain. Over the next three years, I went through eight doctors and finally found one who put a name to it: fibromyalgia. I read every book that I could find on the subject, trying to find out what caused it and what to do for it. I saw two rheumatologists who told me there was nothing to do for it and it was just something that I was going to have to live with. I had decided that they were right.

There were times that I'd go for weeks and feel really bad and then a period of time where I wouldn't feel so bad. Then about three years ago I got real sick and stayed in bed for several weeks. I couldn't get out of bed, put on my own clothes, cook, or anything. I had always done everything for my sons. And now I was needing them to help take care of me! It was terrible. I was very frustrated.

My doc had put me on antidepressants, pain meds, anything to give me some relief. I know that he was trying to help, but I had reached a point to where I was not sleeping. Two hours a night maybe. Sometimes two or three days with no sleep. I was weak and tired, but my brain was racing 90 miles an hour. I started realizing that the worse I felt, I could not remember things, even things that had just happened. My fibro-fog was bad.

Then I found out about Dr. Murphree by accident from my Sunday school teacher who had seen an article in the paper about a seminar, but at that point, I was too sick to attend. But I looked up his office and got in to see them the very next day. When I read his book, I knew that this was my life story. Everything that he was talking about was me and all that I had gone through. I had been on vitamins off-and-on for a long time and just finally gave up because they did not seem to be doing any good. In reading his book and taking the supplements that he recommended, it made all the difference in the world.

I am now sleeping six to eight hours or more a night; the pain is so much better. I do occasionally have a flare-up, especially if I have a cold, but it doesn't last nearly as long as it used to. Since I have been on the supplements, I mentally, physically, and emotionally, feel so much better. I would highly recommend that anyone read his book. It has so much information as to what you need to do with your health. My coming to the clinic has been very beneficial. The heat therapy and re-alignment has helped me so much.

I also think that Dr. Murphree's approach is the most important thing. He tries to get to the root of the problem and doesn't just give you drugs, or try a lot of different therapies, or try to cover it up. Each body is different and needs different supplements, and he's willing to work with you to get the right ones. I would say on a scale from 0 to 10 that my pain is at a 2. Compared to where I was, that's great improvement.

MAUDY

I've finally learned that I don't have to be the best at everything. My parents always wanted me to be the best that I could be, which is good in a way, but it can really get out of hand. So I graduated from college in three years with honors and immediately began my dream job in advertising. My first year out of college I met my husband, got married, and we wanted to have children right away. We have three children now—two boys and a girl. Mathew, Michael, and Rachal are all about two years apart. I worked up until delivery and took only a month off for each child. I worked full-time, and really more than full-time.

Matt's work requires him to travel several days a month, which can be tough on us. But for the first 10 years, we were doing well. I know that Matt likes his job, and I had had several pay increases, and we both liked to serve on community volunteer boards. Our kids are into soccer, baseball, and basketball, and we tried to make all their games. We also were having a lot of dinner parties for clients. And I was taking some Spanish classes for work. And Matt was working towards his master's.

I would be lying if I said that I didn't love the success we were enjoying. We had a large home we loved, two luxury cars, a lakehouse, happy kids in private school, and I was definitely on track to make VP at the firm.

But one day the bottom just sort of fell out, and my life became un-manageable. My husband starting spending more and more time away on business, Michael was diagnosed with a learning disability, my mother died of a long illness with emphysema, I really had more work than I could handle at the firm, and my health started to suffer. At first it was colds that hung around and wouldn't easily go away. Then I started chronic headaches. Some days I had to drag myself through the day living on coffee. My boss even mentioned that I was yawning all the time. I was so embarrassed.

At first I thought I was just tired and needed a rest, so my husband and I took our first extended vacation—four days—away from our children. I felt a little better when we returned and jumped right back into my old routine. There was always so much do when I got home from work. Some nights I didn't get in bed until early the next morning. Then I'd be blasted by my alarm clock at 5:30 a.m. I'd get up and immediately start getting breakfast ready for the kids.

One day I just couldn't get out of bed. The alarm clock went off but I couldn't even make myself get out of bed to turn it off. Instead it continued to buzz until finally, half an hour later, my son Mathew came into my room and turned it off.

I made an appointment with our family doctor who ran a bunch of tests. He said they didn't show anything was wrong, but maybe I was depressed from the death of my mother and recommended I take an antidepressant. I knew something must be wrong so I started taking the medicine and thought it would get me back on track again. It didn't. I went to doctor after doctor trying to find someone to help me. I continued to get worse with headaches, irritable bowel problems, insomnia, sinus infections that wouldn't go away. I felt like I had the worst case of the flu, 24 hours a day.

I hated taking sick days from work. I was always the one who never did. But I started missing several days of work each month. And I felt like I lived at the doctor's office. I honestly saw 12 doctors about this, but I continued to get worse. My mind seemed to turn to mush. Even the simplest decisions became a big ordeal. I couldn't remember where I put my car keys; had I taken my medicine; what was I supposed to pick up at the store?

My friends were sweet, but I just stopped communicating with them. And the thought of a dinner party just made me want to cry. So I really had no social life anymore. I didn't have the energy to walk the dog. And I couldn't stand sitting in the bleachers at games. They were just too hard on my back. When I was still working, I'd be in bed by nine, sometimes as early as 7:30. Of course I couldn't sleep but dozed off only to wake up in pain.

I had to take an early retirement from my job. I had run out of sick days, and it was getting pretty pathetic at work. I was losing every-thing I had worked for. My marriage was becoming strained, and our finances were dwindling due to all the doctor bills, prescriptions, tests, and the huge increase in health insurance once I retired.

I read an article about Dr. Murphree and his fibromyalgia program. I had run out of options and felt that he was my last hope and told him so. I started the program and faithfully did all the therapies recom-mended by the doctors at the clinic. The first thing that improved was my sleep. I finally began to sleep through the night or least get five hours of what Dr. Murphree called "restorative" sleep. I was able to discontinue my sleep medicines. I was glad to be off these drugs, which left me feeling hung over the next morning. I started to feel better. I had more energy. The pain slowly but steadily became tolerable and continues to be manageable unless I overdo it.

I think the vitamin formulas have made a huge difference. If I forget to take them for a few days, the pain and fatigue start to return. I'm not 100% better, but I'm getting my life back. I now have a social life again. I'm even thinking about going back to work part-time. But I won't try to be the best at everything!

JULIE

I played tennis and golf and was a cheerleader in college. After college, I got married and started my career. I remember coming down with the most terrible case of the flu and not being able to shake it.

I was prescribed antibiotics and bed rest. I stayed home for three sick days, but I was just exhausted, and every muscle in my body hurt. I managed to go back to work, but I still felt terrible and would have to go right to bed when I got home after work. I would just walk in the door and walk straight to my room. Sometimes I'd climb in bed with my shoes on! I went back to my family doctor, and he did dozens of tests over a period of two months. Nothing showed up on my lab work. No matter what I tried—drugs, vitamins, exercise, rest—nothing helped for long. I just couldn't shake it. My family doctor said he thought I was exhausted and needed a vacation. He asked me if my husband was abusing me. That was definitely not the case, but it got me thinking that maybe I was very stressed out.

I took some time off, went to the beach, and lay on the beach for a week. I still felt exhausted and couldn't shake the nagging muscle pains. I couldn't sleep because of the pain. I returned to my doctor who said he thought I should try a new antidepressant and come back in a month. The antidepressant didn't seem to help and I was now starting to get tingling in my right arm and hand. I was referred to a neurologist who said I may have some nerve damage in my arm. The neurologist prescribed Neurontin and recommended I see an orthopedic surgeon. The orthopedic surgeon said my MRI was negative and recommended more drugs.

I was getting worse and started to miss a good deal of work. My social life had gotten pretty awkward. My marriage was being strained from the stress of almost a year of poor health. I mean I couldn't even take the trash out to the curb without becoming totally exhausted. I couldn't sleep, no matter what medicines were prescribed: muscle relaxers, tran-quilizers, antidepressants, whatever. They made me tired, but I didn't really sleep. It seemed like my family doctor resented that I was not any better. He referred me to a rheumatologist and told me that there was really nothing more that he could do for me.

The rheumatologist ordered dozens more tests, all of which came back normal. He then told me I had fibromyalgia. I had never heard of it. He explained what it was. He said they weren't sure what caused it and that there was very little that could be done for it. Most of what he recommended I'd either tried or was already on. He did recommend exercise, which was new, but I just couldn't bring myself to even start. Just putting on my sports bra was actually exhausting. I did feel re-lieved to know I wasn't crazy or just making these things up. Someone had finally found out what was the matter with me.

The rheumatologist prescribed lots of drugs and also physical therapy. At first I seemed to be a little better. After a couple of weeks I started get-ting terrible stomach pains. The doctor said it was probably due to the Celebrex, so I stopped taking it. Then I started having more and more trouble just waking up in the morning. And so I stopped Zanaflex and started Ambien. This definitely helped, and I didn't feel so hung over in the morning. My pain continued to be as bad, though, and I was given trigger-point injections. These didn't help and sometimes made me hurt like crazy. After a couple of months, the Ambien stopped working and I couldn't get to sleep once again. I stopped going to the physical therapist, because some of that also seemed to make me worse. I think it was just too intense.

I read book after book on fibromyalgia and decided that I needed to try a more natural approach. So I started taking various supplements and watching my diet a little closer. I stopped all caffeine, sodas, and alcohol. This was hard to do, but it seemed to help. Massage therapy worked some. And I started seeing a chiropractor and an acupuncturist: two things I never would have even thought of doing before. The relief was short-term, and I had to go a lot. I just couldn't afford it after a while. And it was hard to tell what exactly was working, because I was trying all this alternative stuff at the same time.

One day I was watching the news when they started talking about a local clinic that specialized in fibromyalgia. I went to a talk and realized everything Dr. Murphree said about my illness was true. I just wanted to cry. I felt hope inside me rising up again.

I began the program in October, and by January I was back at work. I still don't have the stamina I once did, but I don't pass out from exhaustion and pain at the end of the day. I know I'll always need to monitor my stress, eat right, and take the supplements Dr. Murphree recommends. When I try to do too much, I'm reminded that I have fibromyalgia. Otherwise I feel good most all the time.

TYPE B: THE CAREGIVER

Type Bs may or may not be as driven as type A's, but they are just as taxed. They spend considerable time and energy taking care of spouses, children, extended family, and friends. Their lives revolve around the ups and downs and daily challenges of those they look after. They may have an invalid living in their home. They may be continuously running back and forth between the hospital and nursing home. Or they may just see it as their duty to especially care for those around them, even those who don't ask for help. And since they don't have enough time in the day to take care of the needy and themselves, they often struggle late into the night to get everything done.

They like to be needed (don't we all?) and feel a sense of duty that makes them continue to give more. They can spend years giving and giving while getting little in return and leaving no time for themselves. This constant emotional strain can certainly take its toll on a marriage. They are often too tired to simply enjoy time with their spouse, who usually gets pushed to the bottom of the priority list (right above them- selves, that is). Finally—and it's inevitable— these individuals either change dramatically, or they crash.

VICKY

I heard about the clinic from a friend of the family. I figured I had nothing to lose at this point. I called and got the first available appointment, and three weeks later I drove seven hours to be seen. The best thing about my visit was knowing I wasn't crazy. There were other patients from all over the country who had the same symptoms as I did. We couldn't all be crazy. The doctors took my history, examined me, and then explained why I felt as I did. They said they'd need to do some more tests but were pretty certain I had chronic fatigue syndrome. I'd never heard of it, but after they began to explain it, everything started to add up.

They asked, When have you last really felt good? It was probably about six years ago. That's when I had started getting chronic sinus infections. I was treated with cortisone shots and antibiotics. I'd have four or five infections a year. No matter how many shots or pills I'd take, they'd hang on for weeks at a time. Each time I'd take antibiotics, I'd get a raging yeast infection. I'd started having lots of stomach problems, bloating, gas, and pain. Two years ago, I developed pneumonia and was hospitalized.

The doctor at the clinic also asked what happened about six years ago. I hadn't really thought about, it but I'd been under a tremendous amount of stress. My mother had died and then my father had a stroke. He came to live with us and needed around-the-clock attention. I couldn't leave him but for a few hours at a time. My husband tried to get me to hire full- time sitters, but I just couldn't bring myself to do that. I know that's not what mom would have wanted for dad. We were in and out of the hospital many times, but dad always managed to pull through. My teenage daughter had a bad car accident, so she too was in and out of doctors offices for over a year.

I never seemed to get better from then on, and I was totally exhausted. I couldn't even go to the grocery store without being wiped out for days. I never got up earlier than 11 o'clock. I drank a pot a coffee and several Diet Cokes just to make it through the day. I had a CAT scan, MRIs, nerve tests, and tons of blood tests. All my tests came back pretty normal, though they did discover some heart irregularities. I was beginning to think I was just crazy; I know my family already thought so.

I tried to be a good wife, mother, and daughter. I kept the house clean, took care of my husband, father, and children. I would have to get up several times a night to check on dad. Sometimes, I was just too tired to go back to sleep. I'd stay awake and enjoy what little free time I could. I'd make sure everyone got their break- fast and was off to school or work on time.

Some days I felt like I was a hundred years old. My father died, and then there was the funeral and the estate to look after. I got through this and was actually looking forward to getting my life back when I my chronic sinus infections turned into pneumonia. I was never the same after that. I've been sick every day now for at least five years.

Dr. Murphree told me I had chronic fatigue syndrome. He explained how my autonomic nervous system had been overwhelmed by the years of chronic stress. My immune system had stopped working like it should. I was placed on an elimination diet, supplements, and some prescription medications.

I didn't notice much improvement, and after two weeks, I started be coming discouraged once again. Then something seemed to change. One day I woke up with more energy than I'd had in years. I felt almost normal. Unfortunately it didn't last but for one or two days. Each week, though, I seem to be getting stronger, feeling better.

JEANETTE

I've been a nurse for over 20 years. I'm the head nurse for the critical care unit at a large hospital. I'm responsible for overseeing dozens of nurses, nursing aids, and medical technologists. We have the sickest *of the sick patients, but I enjoy my work. It's demanding, stressful, but rewarding. Many of our patients don't make it out of CCU. The constant threat of death is too much for some nurses who rotate through the department. Sometimes you'll get close to a patient and their family only to watch them die.*

Until last year, I thought I'd be happy to stay in this position for another 20 years. But now I can't seem to muster up the energy needed to sustain me through the day. It seems I've lost something; I don't know what. I'm sick a lot. I feel like I've got some infection just underneath the surface that just won't go away. None of the doctors I've seen can tell me what's wrong with me. I'm on several medications but don't feel any better. I wonder if I'll ever be healthy again. But I'm willing to try your plan, Dr. Murphree. What can I lose?

FOR FURTHER READING AND RESEARCH

- K.L. Brunson et al., "Neurobiology of the Stress Response Early in Life: evolution of a concept and the role of corticotropin-releasing hormone," *Molocular Psychiatry* 6 (2001): 647–56.
- E. Charmandrari et al., "Pediatric Stress: hormonal mediators and human development," *Hormone Research* 59 (2003): 161–79.
- V.J. Felitti et al., "Relationship of childhood abuse and household dysfunction to many of the leading causes of death in adults," The Adverse Childhood Experience (ACE) study *American Journal of Preventive Medicine* 14 (1998): 245–58.
- C. Heim et al., "Pituitary-adrenal and autonomic responses to stress in women after sexual and physical abuse in childhood," *JAMA* 284 (2000): 592–7.
- P. Hrycaj et al., "Platelet 3H-imipramine uptake receptor density and serum serotonin levels in patients with fibromyalgia/fibrositis syndrome," *Journal of Rheumatology* (1993):1986–8.
- K. Imbierowitcz and U.T. Egle, "Childhood adversities in patients with fibromyalgia and somatoform pain disorder," *European Journal of Pain* 7 (2003): 113–9.
- M. Offenbaecher et al., "Possible associations of fibromyalgia with a polymorphism in the serotonin transport gene regulatory region," *Arthritis and Rheumatism* 42 (1999): 2482–8.
- D.S. Pine and D.S. Charney, "Children, stress, and sensitization: an integration of basic and clinical research on emotion?" *Biological Pschiatry* 52 (2002): 773–5.

- S. Romans et al., "Childhood abuse and later medical disorders in women. An epidemiological study," *Psychotherapy and Psychosomatics* 71 (2002): 141–150.
- B. Va Houdenhove et al., "Victimization in chronic fatigue syndrome and fibromyalgia in tertiary care: A controlled study on prevalence and characteristics," *Psychosomatics* 42 (2001): 228.

· 10 ·
THE IMPORTANCE OF A GOOD NIGHT'S SLEEP

The first question I ask new patients is, "How are you sleeping at night?" If they don't get a good night's sleep, they're not going to get well. It really is that simple.

Most people with FMS/CFS haven't slept well in years. Many of our patients take tranquilizers, muscle relaxants, or over-the-counter sleep aides to get them to sleep. But most of them never go into deep, restorative sleep. It is in this delta-wave sleep that the body repairs itself by making human growth hormone (HGH) and other hormones that help repair damaged muscles, tissues, and organs. Deep sleep also builds and rejuvenates the immune system.

GET GOOD SLEEP FOR GOOD HEALTH

We've all heard that we need eight hours of restful sleep each night. The amount of sleep an individual actually needs will vary from person to person. A five-year-old might need 11–12 hours of sleep; an adult, 7–9 hours. Poor sleep has been linked to various health problems including depression, fatigue, CFS, FMS, and headaches. This is not news to those who suffer from FMS and CFS. They already know that their symptoms get worse when they don't get a good night's sleep.

One study showed that college students who were prevented from going into deep (REM) sleep for a week developed the same symptoms as those with FMS and CFS: diffuse pain, fatigue, depression, anxiety, irritability, stomach disturbances, and headache.

Another study, conducted by the University of Connecticut School of Medicine, compared the sleep patterns and associated symptoms of 50 women with FMS. The study showed that a poor night's sleep was followed by an increase in symptoms, including body pain. This increase in symptoms then went on to prevent the subject from getting a good night's sleep the next night, even though the person was exhausted. For FMS/CFS patients, this cycle continues and creates a pattern of declining health.

Research presented in June 2002 at the Endocrine Society in San Francisco showed that sleep deprivation markedly increased inflammatory cytokines (pain-causing chemicals)—by a whopping 40%.

Poor sleep also affects your human growth hormone (HGH) levels, and low HGH causes further fatigue, reduced capacity for exercise, muscle weakness, impaired cognition, depression, pain, and decreased muscle mass. Deep sleep, however, initiates the pituitary to release *more* HGH. Eighty percent of HGH is produced during delta-stage sleep, so the best way to boost HGH levels is to get 8–9 hours of sleep a night.

If you have fibromyalgia, you know all too well that when you don't get a good night's sleep—which is often—you have more pain, fatigue, anxiety, foggy thinking, and depression. Most of my patients haven't slept well in years and have tried one sleep medicine after another. Unfortunately, these medicines may work for a while but usually lose their effectiveness over time. And many actually prevent you from going into the deep, restorative sleep you need to get well. Some even deplete melatonin, your natural sleep-regulating hormone.

> "Our cells pulse in a rhythm whose timekeeper is the universe as a whole. The flow of intelligence that regulates mind and body in us attends to its own cycles and functions best when these cycles are closely heeded."
>
> —Deepak Chopra, MD

Sleep medications that don't promote deep, restorative sleep include **Gabitril** (tiagabine) and **Neurontin** (gabapentin). These are sedating but rarely yield any pain relief in FMS or CFS patients. In addition, they are loaded with potential side effects. **Zanaflex** (tizanidine) is a dangerous muscle relaxant. **Xanax** (alprazolam), **Ativan** (lorazepam), **Valium** (diazepam), **Tranxene** (clorazepate dipotassium), **Serax** (oxazepam), **Librium** (chlordiazepoxide), **Klonopin**

(clonazepam) and **Restoril** (temazepam) are addictive benzodiazepines with numerous potential side effects. **Soma** (carisprodol) is a muscle relaxant that can be very sedating. **Unisom** (doxylamine) is an over-the-counter antihistamine.

Sleep medications that do promote deep, restorative sleep include Ambien, Elavil, Flexeril, Trazadone, and Lunesta. However, these medications still have potential side effects (see chapter 6) and usually start to lose their effectiveness over time. It's not uncommon to hear stories like the one below:

MARGARET

I'd taken every sleep medicine there is. My doctor said I couldn't sleep because I was depressed. I didn't know why I wasn't sleeping, but I knew I was exhausted. So, even though I didn't think that all of my problems were due to depression, I was willing to try Prozac. It seemed to help for a while, but after about six months, I was worse than when I started the medicine. I then started Celexa, but it wore off after a few months. I used Elavil for a while. It helped me get to sleep, but I usually felt hungover the next day. I was in a downward spiral that I couldn't escape.

I consulted a rheumatologist for my pain, and he diagnosed me with fibromyalgia. He prescribed Ambien for my insomnia and Zanaflex for my pain. I felt better for a while—maybe a couple of weeks. But the medicines made me feel drugged out. The Ambien worked for several months, but then I started needing a higher and higher dose. Finally it also stopped working. I then tried Sonata, but it would only work for four hours. I'd wake up at 3:00 in the morning—wide awake—and wouldn't be able to go back to sleep.

I walked around for four years totally exhausted and in so much pain. I was losing all hope until I tried 5-HTP. It, along with the other supplements Dr. Murphree recommended, allowed me to consistently fall asleep and wake feeling rested. After about a month, I noticed my constant pain was getting better. It was less of an issue. I actually had energy to go shopping and fix dinner. I used to have so much anxiety about going to sleep. The closer it got to bedtime the more worried I got that I wouldn't be able to get to sleep. Now I simply take my 5-HTP, and in 30 minutes, I'm asleep.

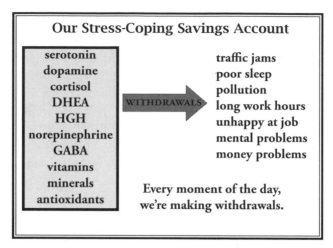

Our Stress-Coping Savings Account

| serotonin dopamine cortisol DHEA HGH norepinephrine GABA vitamins minerals antioxidants | WITHDRAWALS → | traffic jams poor sleep pollution long work hours unhappy at job mental problems money problems |

Every moment of the day, we're making withdrawals.

STRESS LEADS TO POOR SLEEP

As mentioned earlier, we are all born with a stress-coping savings account filled up with chemicals we need for the body to work properly. These chemicals—serotonin, dopamine, norepinephrine, cortisol, DHEA, HGH, and others—help us deal with stress.

Every time we are exposed to stress (chemically, emotionally, mentally, or physically), we make withdrawals from our stress-coping savings account. These withdrawals can be triggered by any stimulus, including sounds (especially loud or irritating noise), odors, and bright light. You may have noticed that the longer you've had your illness, the less tolerant you are to certain odors, chemicals, or noises.

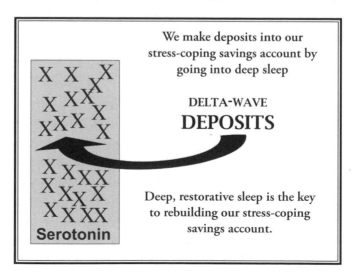

We make deposits into our stress-coping savings account by going into deep sleep

DELTA-WAVE
DEPOSITS

Deep, restorative sleep is the key to rebuilding our stress-coping savings account.

Serotonin

Emotionally stressful situations cause the body to release adrenaline, cortisol, and insulin, and these stress hormones stimulate the brain to secrete serotonin. Long-term stress and poor dietary habits can therefore deplete the body's serotonin stores. If we aren't careful we'll find that we are making more withdrawals than deposits, bankrupting our own account. And when we do, FMS and CFS are often the result.

But when a person enters deep, restorative sleep, she makes more serotonin, which then gets deposited into her stress-coping savings account. The more stress a person is under, the more serotonin she'll need to replenish. It's a vicious cycle. If she doesn't have enough serotonin, she won't be able to go into the stage of sleep in which she is able to make more serotonin!

SEROTONIN AND TRYPTOPHAN

The neurotransmitter (brain chemical) serotonin helps regulate sleep, digestion, pain, mood, and mental clarity.

- It raises your pain threshold by blocking substance P,
- helps you fall asleep and stay asleep through the night,
- regulates your moods, reducing anxiety and depression,
- reduces sugar cravings and overeating,
- increases mental abilities,
- regulates normal gut motility (transportation of food-stuff),
- and reverses irritable bowel syndrome (IBS) (surveys have shown that as many as 73% of FMS patients suffer from IBS).

One source of serotonin is **tryptophan**, an essential amino acid. Ninety percent of tryptophan is used for protein synthesis, 1% is converted to serotonin, and the balance is used to make niacin.

Replacing optimal serotonin stores by supplementing amino acids—such as tryptophan—is the first step toward a better night's sleep for you. Once this has occurred, and it may take months, your body starts to normalize, and you start to feel a whole lot better. But tryptophan is hard to come by, to say the least. It was taken off the market and labeled a prescription drug in 1989. So what do you do?

I've got good news for you. It's called 5-HTP, and it's what tryptophan becomes on its way to becoming serotonin. It's perfectly natural, perfectly legal, and inexpensive. And it's a better way to "get" your serotonin for other reasons:

First, whereas tryptophan needs to be helped by a transport molecule to cross the blood-brain barrier, 5-HTP moves easily into the brain, so it does not compete with other amino acids for passage. And unlike tryptophan, which is made from bacterial fermentation and is hence subject to contamination, 5-HTP is plant-derived *(Griffonia simplicifolia.)* Lastly, 5-HTP is converted directly into serotonin, unlike tryptophan, which must first be broken down.

The Brain Function Questionnaire in chapter 16 will help you determine if you are low in serotonin. However, if you have fibromyalgia, it's a safe bet that you are. Whether it's a cause or an effect of the illness, individuals with fibromyalgia tend to display low levels of tryptophan, serotonin, and 5-HTP.

WHY YOUR SEROTONIN LEVELS ARE LOW

Stress often plays a role in serotonin deficiency. Emotionally stressful situations cause the body to release adrenaline, cortisol, and insulin, and these stress hormones stimulate the brain to secrete serotonin. In this way, long-term stress and poor dietary habits can deplete the body's serotonin stores.

Stimulates like caffeine, nicotine, chocolate, diet pills, sugar, and nicotine also cause a rapid rise in blood insulin levels, which is followed by serotonin release. That's why you feel better and think clearer after using them. The feeling is only temporary, though, as a stimulate high is always followed by an unpleasant low. This low leads to stimulant cravings and eventually to addictions, as people become dependent on stimulates to raise serotonin levels. Sadly, this addictive process causes further depletion of serotonin. Eventually, no stimulant will help.

Normally we get plenty of tryptophan and thus 5-HTP from the protein foods we eat. However, those with FMS have physiological or biochemical glitches that prevent dietary tryptophan from converting into serotonin. We know this because studies have found FMS patients to have higher levels of metabolites in the kynurenine pathway, and this situation diverts tryptophan away from serotonin production.

SOLVING YOUR SEROTONIN PROBLEM

The first reaction of many physicians to a patient's serotonin deficiency is to recommend a selective serotonin reuptake inhibitor (SSRI) drug. But while prescription antidepressants can be helpful, they have some serious potential side effects (see chapter 6). In addition, they tend not to work for FMS patients. And here's why: SSRIs can help a patient hang onto and use their naturally occurring stores of serotonin. They work like a gasoline additive would work in your car, helping to increase the efficiency of "fuel." But most of the patients I see with fibromyalgia are running on fumes! A gasoline additive is not likely to help. If you don't have any serotonin to re-uptake, then using a serotonin re-uptake inhibitor drug is pointless.

And by pointless, I mean exactly that. It's money thrown away. In fact, depending on which study you quote, from 19% to 70% of those taking antidepressant medications would do just as well on a placebo. This is precisely why I recommend that my fibromyalgia patients boost their serotonin levels by taking 5-HTP, not an antidepressant. Why put an additive in your gas tank...when you can just fill it up with what it's really thirsty for?

Q: If tryptophan is a natural amino acid, why can't I buy it at a health food store?

A: Because the sloppy processing practices of Showa Denko—the Japanese company that used to supply most of the tryptophan in the United States—caused some patients to become ill, and a few died as a result. But tryptophan is a very safe supplement! Many foods contain tryptophan as an additive, including baby formulas.

Clearly, the FDA overreacted in banning tryptophan supplements—a natural, effective treatment for depression and insomnia—while at the same time advocating the use of harmful antidepressants. I can't help but wonder: is it mere coincidence that tryptophan was banned shortly before Prozac and other antidepressants hit the market?

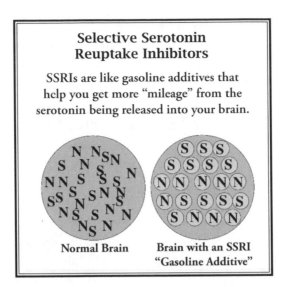

Selective Serotonin Reuptake Inhibitors

SSRIs are like gasoline additives that help you get more "mileage" from the serotonin being released into your brain.

Normal Brain

Brain with an SSRI "Gasoline Additive"

THE MYRIAD BENEFITS OF 5-HTP

5-HTP treats **insomnia** beautifully, improving sleep quality by increasing REM sleep and increasing the body's production of melatonin by 200%.

It's also common for the symptoms of **irritable bowel syndrome** (diarrhea and constipation) to disappear in 1–2 weeks once essential nutrients, especially serotonin levels, are normalized. In fact, there are more serotonin receptors in the intestinal tract than in

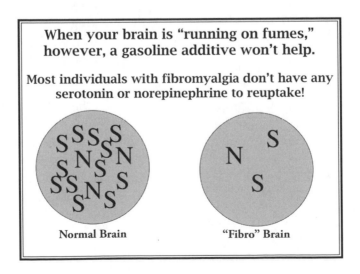

When your brain is "running on fumes," however, a gasoline additive won't help.

Most individuals with fibromyalgia don't have any serotonin or norepinephrine to reuptake!

Normal Brain

"Fibro" Brain

the brain. The brain and gut are connected through neuroreceptors that regulate the perception of visceral pain and gastrointestinal motility (the speed at which food moves through the intestinal tract). These receptors are one reason that people get butterflies in their stomach when they're nervous.

Double-blind placebo-controlled trials have shown that patients with FMS were able to see the following benefits from taking 5-HTP:

- decreased pain,
- improved sleep,
- fewer tender points,
- less morning stiffness,
- less anxiety,
- increased energy,
- and improved moods in general, including in those with clinical depression. See chapter 16 for more about 5-HTP's amazing usefulness—superior to many antidepressant drugs—in this area.

SUPPLEMENT 5-HTP TO RESTORE SLEEP

All my FMS patients start their therapy by taking 50 mg. of 5-HTP 30 minutes before bed, on an empty stomach (90 minutes after or 30 minutes before eating), with four ounces of grape juice. The juice causes the body to release a little insulin, which, though not necessary for 5-HTP to pass the blood-brain barrier, seems to heighten the supplement's effect. (If you have problems with your blood sugar levels, try taking your 5-HTP with water or milk.) Patients continue to increase their dose over time, and I've typically found 300 mg. to be the optimal therapeutic amount.

Q: I'm taking a prescription sleep medication and sleeping fine. Why should I mess with something else?

A: If you're taking a drug that promotes deep restorative sleep, falling asleep within 30 minutes, dreaming, and sleeping 7–8 hours, then good for you! Still, you should add 5-HTP (50 mg.) three times daily with food. If no problems arise after three days, increase to 100 mg. with each meal. Why? Remember that the reason you're taking these prescription drugs is because you have a serotonin deficiency, not a drug deficiency. Even if you are building up some serotonin stores in the night through deep sleep, you'll quickly use them up in one very stressful day. The key is to build up your serotonin levels for good, and nothing does that better than 5-HTP and its cofactors.

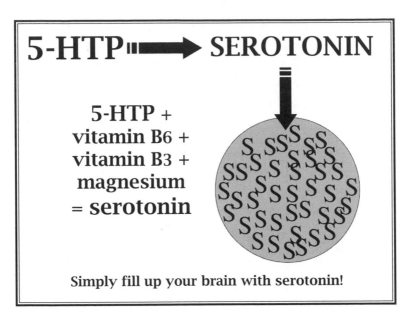

5-HTP ⇒ SEROTONIN

5-HTP +
vitamin B6 +
vitamin B3 +
magnesium
= serotonin

Simply fill up your brain with serotonin!

One of three things will happen when you start by taking 50 mg. of 5-HTP:

1. You fall asleep within 30 minutes and sleep through the night. If so, you should stay on this bedtime dose and add an additional 250 mg. at dinner (for a total of 300 mg. daily). You may find you sleep even better by taking 100 mg. at bedtime and 200 mg. with dinner.

2. Nothing happens. This is a typical response to such a low dose. You should add an additional 50 mg. each night (up to a max of 300 mg.) until you fall asleep within 30 minutes and sleep through the night. Once you've discovered your bedtime dose, subtract that amount from 300 mg. and take the remainder with dinner to keep serotonin levels optimal. If you are taking 300 mg. at bedtime and still can't get to sleep and stay asleep after two days on this dose, then see "Still Can't Sleep?" on p. 167.

3. You have a reaction. Instead of making you sleepy, the dose makes you more alert. This occurs more often in CFS and chemically sensitive patients who have a sluggish liver. If this happens, discontinue 5-HTP at bedtime. Instead take 50 mg. at a mealtime for two days. (Taking 5-HTP with food slows its absorption, allows the liver to process it more effectively, and shouldn't make you too sleepy). After two days on 5-HTP with food, increase to 100 mg. with each meal (300 mg. a day). You may need to play around with your dosing. For instance, you can try taking 100 mg. at breakfast and 200 mg. at lunch. If you are only taking 5-HTP at meals and none at bedtime, then you can increase your dose up to 400 mg. daily if it helps.

If your reaction to serotonin goes beyond alertness to rapid heart rate, increased pulse, elevated blood pressure, and agitation, see your doctor. But don't be alarmed. I have thousands of individuals on 5-HTP, and I assure you that such a reaction is rare. Just be sure to follow the instructions in this chapter carefully.

Increasing serotonin levels is beneficial for 95% of my patients. But there are those—usually at the far CFS end of the spectrum—who have the **serotonin sensitivity reaction** described in number 3 above, and it just can't be helped, even by taking 5-HTP with food. Excessive serotonin levels can cause these patients insomnia, headaches, hyperactivity, and increased heart rate.

Some doctors have theorized that CFS patients actually have too much serotonin already, and this is why they are so tired. So more serotonin just makes them feel worse. I suspect, however, that most patients who have a serotonin reaction do so because of a sluggish liver. These are usually the same patients who have trouble taking most medications. They get depressed on antidepressants and hyperactive on sleeping pills. And they usually need less than the normal dose of any given medicine they take.

I have recommended 5-HTP to thousands of people and have had thousands more order it from my web site and office. In 10 years, I've had *three* individuals who have reported a serotonin sensitivity reaction. Two of them had heard me at a speaking engagement and, in their excitement to enjoy 5-HTP's benefits, had taken 300 mg. at bedtime the *first* night. They then experienced rapid heartbeat, increased pulse rate, and agitation for a few hours. Each one called my office for guidance and eventually built up to 300 mg. a day with food and adjusted great to the supplement. Incidentally, both of these individuals had CFS, a history of funny reactions to medications, and elevated liver enzymes in past blood tests (a sign of a poorly functioning liver). Had they been patients of mine with such obvious signs of sluggish liver, I would have suggested from the beginning that they take 5-HTP only with food and never at bedtime. The third individual is actually a patient of mine. She has extreme sensitivity and just can't take anything without having a reaction.

5-HTP COFACTORS

5-HTP is amazing stuff, but it can't make serotonin alone. It needs help from calcium, magnesium, and some B vitamins. So make sure that you're getting plenty of these along with your 5-HTP.

Your first step is to take a high-dose broad-spectrum multivitamin and mineral formula daily with a minimum of 700 mg. of magnesium (like my CFS/Fibro Formula). If you aren't having a daily

---

Q: *Can 5-HTP be taken with any of my prescription medications?*

A: Yes. Remember, it has a funny name, but it's a perfectly natural brain chemical.

Q: *Can I take 5-HTP along with an antidepressant?*

A: Yes, you can take 5-HTP or any amino acid along with antidepressant medications. In fact, 95% of my patients are already taking antidepressants when they come to see me. Most are on SSRIs—such as Paxil, Prozac, Zoloft, Lexapro, or Celexa—which are trying to work with the serotonin they have. Or in this case, the serotonin they don't have. Once they start filling their brain up with serotonin by taking 5-HTP, the prescription SSRI medications then actually have something to work with!

Q: *Can I take 5-HTP along with sleep medications?*

A: Yes. Start using 5-HTP until you sleep through the night. At some point, you should be able to work with your medical doctor to slowly wean off the prescription sleep medication. Taking 5-HTP along with some prescription sleep medications may cause a morning hangover, though 5-HTP alone never will. Weaning off the sleep medication (again, with your doctor's help) should fix any hangover problem.

Q: *Is there anyone who shouldn't take 5-HTP?*

A: I wouldn't recommend 5-HTP for patients with manic depression or schizophrenia. These conditions are best referred to an orthomolecular psychiatrist who specializes in these complicated disorders.

---

bowel movement, then you're probably still deficient in magnesium.

Increase your magnesium by 140–150 mg. (use magnesium chelate, citrate, or taurate) at dinner each night until you begin to have normal bowel movements each day. If you start to have loose bowel movements, reduce the amount.

If you're not dreaming at night, you're probably deficient in vitamin B6. So make sure there's enough B6 (50–100 mg.) in your multivitamin.

Some folks can't convert vitamin B6 into it's chemically active form, pyridoxal-5-phosphate (P-5-P). This isn't common in my patients, but it does show up occasionally. And in that case, all the supplemented B6 in the world isn't going to help. So when I have a patient who isn't improving on 5-HTP and my CFS/Fibro formula, then I'll try them on a trial of P-5-P. This is sometimes the missing link.

STILL CAN'T SLEEP?

If it turns out that 5-HTP isn't the only answer to your problem, then read on. First, let's make sure you understand the basics of how sleep works:

There are two types of sleep: REM (rapid eye movement) sleep and non-REM sleep. During REM sleep, the eyes—still closed—rapidly move back and forth as dreaming takes place.

Non-REM sleep is divided into four stages. Stages one and two, while important in maintaining the correct sleep cycle, don't provide the restorative efforts of three and four. Stage four is the deepest and is crucial for overall well-being. Non-REM sleep begins when we first fall asleep. Its first two stages have a faster brain-wave pattern (as measured with an electroencephalogram [EEG]) than the final two, and they are considered lighter. As brain activity begins to slow down, we enter into stages three and four of non-REM. This usually occurs about 90 minutes after falling asleep.

The non-REM cycle is then interrupted by ten minutes of REM sleep, which elicits a flurry of brain activity as you dream. These

Q: What if I'm using one of the sleep medications that doesn't promote deep, restorative sleep?

A: Well, it depends. If you're not sleeping well, definitely start taking 5-HTP as directed in this chapter, along with your medication.

If this combination makes you feel hungover the next day, try working with you medical doctor to reduce the dose or frequency of your prescription medication. If you are already sleeping well, start with 50 mg. of 5-HTP with food and, after a couple of days, increase to 100 mg. with each meal. After a couple of weeks, you can try (with the help of your medical doctor) to slowly reduce your sleep medications and switch your 5-HTP dosages from mealtimes to bedtime. Start with moving 50 mg. to bedtime, and increase this amount each night until you fall asleep within 30 minutes and sleep through the night.

cycles occur five to six times night. The time spent in REM continues to grow and may last up to an hour in the final cycle of sleep.

MELATONIN

The pineal gland is located at the base of our brain, and the ancient Greeks considered it the seat of the soul. This thought may not be far off, since the pineal gland is responsible for releasing melatonin, an extremely important hormone that plays a vital role in regulating the body's sleep-wake cycle. Normally, melatonin levels in your body begin to rise in the mid-to-late evening, remain high for most of the night, and then decline in the early morning hours.

But some things can work against your body's production of melatonin. Levels gradually decline with age, and some older adults produce very small amounts or none at all.

Melatonin is also affected by a person's exposure to light. Levels start to rise as the sun goes down and drop off as the sun comes up. The eyes are extremely sensitive to changes in light, and an increase in light striking the retina triggers a decrease in melatonin production. Conversely, limited exposure to light increases melatonin production.[1] Those suffering from insomnia should avoid bright light two to three hours before bed.

Exposure to electromagnetic fields can also deplete melatonin. Do you keep any of these things in your bedroom? Electric clock or radio, electric blanket, sound machine, cell phone, electric telephone, electric fan, television, or computer? In fact, any plugged-in electrical device generates electromagnetic fields. Living near a power station or substation also poses a risk of being affected by electromagnetic fields.

Melatonin levels can also be decreased by NSAIDs. So besides intestinal bleeding, leaky gut, and an increased risk of heart attack, here's another reason to avoid chronic use of NSAIDS. Other drugs that can deplete melatonin include SSRIs and anti-anxiety meds (benzodiazepines). Yes, the very same drugs used to help you with depression may deplete melatonin, preventing you from getting the deep, restorative sleep you need to make serotonin.

Other culprits include anti-hypertensive drugs, steroids, over 3 mg. of vitamin B12 in a day, caffeine, alcohol, tobacco, evening exercise (for up to three hours afterwards), and depression.

Once a curiosity to scientists, melatonin is now known to slow down or perhaps even reverse the effects of aging. It's also a powerful antioxidant that, unlike other antioxidants, can cross the blood-brain barrier and attack any free radicals floating around in the brain. Melatonin protects cell nuclei and thus the DNA blueprint of each cell. This is a major reason why melatonin is able to fend off the adverse affects of cancer.

Says Joan Mathews-Larson, PhD: "Melatonin rejuvenates the thymus gland to protect our immunity....Melatonin will "reset" your immune system when it has been under siege from infections, cancer, stress, and so on. Such attacks disrupt its rhythms and diminish its effectiveness."

It's easy to put two and two together. If you're deficient in melatonin, you can't get to sleep at night. A deficiency of restorative sleep leads to accelerated aging, lowered immune function, and susceptibility to cancer and brain oxidation.

Chronic insomnia leads to a gradual disconnection to our own sleep/wake rhythm, and we begin to lose the ability to right ourselves through homeostasis. This in turn leads to further chemical, physical, and emotional stress. Eventually we lose the ability to sense anything our body is trying to tell us. We begin to lose the very essence of who we are.

SUPPLEMENTING MELATONIN

Remember, start with 5-HTP therapy first. It's serotonin that reduces pain, anxiety, depression, mental fatigue, and IBS. And 5-HTP is not only responsible for making serotonin, it also naturally boosts melatonin levels by 200%. There might be no need for you to supplement melatonin at all.

But for those who need it, melatonin can act as a powerful sleep-regulating agent. Low doses have also been shown effective in treating jet lag. In a recent study, volunteers were given either a .3 mg. dose of melatonin, a 1 mg. dose, or a placebo. Both levels of melatonin were effective at decreasing the time needed to fall asleep.

If, after a full week on 300 mg. of 5-HTP at bedtime, you still aren't able to fall asleep within 30 minutes, try taking 3 mg. of sublingual (dissolves under the tongue) melatonin 30 minutes before bed, followed by your 300 mg. dose of 5-HTP at bedtime. If you're taking the 5-HTP with food to avoid reactions, make sure you're taking 300 mg. a day (or up to 400 mg. if

Q: What are some of the potential side effects of 5-HTP?

A: I hear very few complaints about 5-HTP. The literature says that individuals may have headaches and nausea from taking it, but I have had fewer than half a dozen patients exhibit these side effects, and their symptoms went away after a couple of days. Some patients do complain of fatigue when taking 5-HTP during the day with food. If so, I have them discontinue any 5-HTP at breakfast, take 100 mg. at lunch, and take 200 mg. at dinner. If they continue to have problems with fatigue, I suggest they take all 300 mg. at dinner.

Q: Do I still need to increase my daily dose up to 300 mg. of 5-HTP if I'm sleeping well on less than that?

A: You can most likely stay at your present dose, if you're falling asleep quickly; sleeping through the night; dreaming; enjoying less pain, depression, and anxiety; and noticing improved energy and mental clarity. However, if you continue to have IBS, sugar cravings, low moods, or a lot of pain, continue your night dose, and add additional 5-HTP with food during the day (up to 300 mg. daily).

Q: What do you do when you still can't fall asleep and sleep through the night even when taking 300 mg. of 5-HTP?

A: OK, I said that this could be done; I didn't say that it was going to be easy. There are always those people who won't respond completely—or at all—to 5-HTP therapy. That's when it's time to supplement with melatonin.

Q: I wake up famished in the middle of the night. Why?

A: Some people have bouts of hypoglycemia during the night, and this wakes them up, because low blood sugar stimulates the release of cortisol. Sleep with a banana by your bed. If you wake up during the night, eat half the banana (or some other carbohydrate-rich food) and that should help you go back to sleep.

taking only with food), and add 3 mg. of sublingual melatonin at bedtime.

If you find it hard to fall asleep before the early morning hours and then end up sleeping through the day, you may be suffering from delayed sleep phase insomnia, a disruption of normal circadian rhythms. Studies have shown that 5 mg. of melatonin taken at 11 p.m. helps advance and reset these rhythms.

An alternative to supplementing is to get more melatonin in the foods you eat. Foods high in melatonin include oats, sweet corn, rice, Japanese radishes, tomatoes, barley, and bananas. Some drugs also raise melatonin levels. These include fluvoxamine (marketed as Luvox), desipramine (marketed as Norpramin), most MAOIs, and St. John's wort.

Be especially careful to follow the protocols closely if you are taking a prescription sleep medicine and 5-HTP and melatonin. And take it slow so as to avoid any unpleasant hangovers.

TURN DOWN THE LIGHTS

With the invention of electricity, modern man can be bathed in light 24 hours a day. But I recommend that before bed, you turn off the TV and find a comfortable, quiet room (other than your bedroom) where you can read something pleasant by the light of a soft low-wattage lamp. Relax and read or listen to soothing music for 30 minutes to an hour. Then, take your bedtime supplement or medication and move to your bedroom. Keep the lights low, and avoid any stimulation, especially the TV. (In fact, go take the TV out of your bedroom right now!) In the place of your reading or listening time, you may want to try a warm Epsom salt bath. Simply pour one cup of Epsom salts into a warm bath, and soak.

Again, use low light and no stimuli. Consider introducing the calming herb lavender into your nighttime routine. It can be used as a bath gel, lotion, or soap—or sprinkled along with Epsom salts directly into your warm bath.

Q: I have a heart condition. Is 5-HTP safe for me?

A: Absolutely. I use 5-HTP with individuals with known heart conditions, including MVP and heart disease. I always start with the low 50 mg. dose and warn the patient to stop taking it at bedtime if she has a funny reaction. These people are often on incredibly toxic heart medications that increases their risk for heart failure, stroke, and death. I know that if I don't get them into deep, restorative sleep each night, they'll never get well. So I don't worry about 5-HTP. Once you start reading about the medications and combinations of medications you've been taking, you'll realize just how safe 5-HTP really is.

Q: What if I can fall asleep within 30 minutes but can't stay asleep?

A: Make sure you're taking 300 mg. of 5-HTP at bedtime. Then you can add up to 100 mg. with food during the day, for a total of 400 mg. If you continue to wake up throughout the night, try adding melatonin at bedtime.

Q: I get sleepy after dinner but then catch my second wind right before bedtime, what should I do?

A: It sounds like you have high cortisol levels. Some patients have trouble falling asleep because their cortisol levels are too high at bedtime. Your body might be used to trying to stay awake a little longer to finish household chores, care for children, study for a big test, etc. An adrenal cortex profile can help uncover any abnormal cortisol fluctuations (see chapter 11 for more information). Consider supplementing with L-theanine along with phosphatidylserine. Phosphatidylserine helps block the release of cortisol, and the amino acid L-theanine boosts alpha brain waves as it reduces mind chatter. Take 200–400 mg. of phosphatidylserine at dinner or two hours before bed and 100 mg. of L-theanine before dinner and 100 mg. of L-theanine 1–1/2 hours after dinner (on an empty stomach). Then pick a healthy bedtime and stick to it!

Q: Can you recommend any herbs?

A: Personally, I think that nothing beats 5-HTP. But some of my patients prefer herbal remedies. So I've taken three of the best herbal sleep remedies I've found and combined them into one formula. It includes three standardized botanicals into one capsule intended for nighttime use: hops *(Humulus lupulus),* passion flower *(Passiflora incarnata)* leaf, and chamomile *(Matricaria chamomilla)* flower. To order this remedy, you can visit www.TreatingAndBeating.com or call my office at 1-888-884-9577.

Q: Can I have more information?

A: Sure. Visit www.beatfms.com to see my special report on FMS and sleep.

Q: I've tried everything in this chapter, and I still can't sleep! Would you give up on me?

A: Do I sound like a doctor who gives up? Consider ordering a comprehensive melatonin profile and an adrenal cortex profile to find out why you can't get to or stay asleep at night (see Appendix B for more information).

Also consult your medical doctor for a trial of a prescription sleep medication that promotes deep restorative sleep, such as Trazadone, Ambien, Elavil or Flexeril. Continue your 5-HTP along with the medication. After a few months, you may be able to wean off your sleep medication and just use 5-HTP and—if needed—melatonin.

NOTES

1. This explains some individuals' battles with seasonal affective disorder (SAD), a depression triggered by the onset of winter and the subsequent reduction of sunlight. As these people's melatonin levels increase and their serotonin levels decrease, depression sets in. One in 10 people (including children) suffer from SAD. Symptoms include depression, fatigue, lethargy, anxiety, and carbohydrate cravings. One to two hours of exposure to bright, ultraviolet light will usually decrease melatonin levels to a normal level. Individuals with SAD should use these lights for several hours every day during the winter months.

FOR FURTHER READING AND RESEARCH

- Andrea Alberti1, et al. "Plasma cytokine levels in patients with obstructive sleep apnea syndrome: a preliminary study," *Journal of Sleep Research* 12(4) (2003): 305.
- J. Angst et al., "The treatment of depression with L-5-hydroxytrptophan versus Imipramine: Results of two open and one double blind study," *Archiv fur Psychiatrie und Nervenkrankheiten* 224 (1997): 175–86.
- R.C. Cuneo et al., "The growth hormone deficiency syndrom in adults," *Clin Endoc* 37 (1992): 387–97.
- A.B. Dollins et al., "Effect of inducing nocturnal serum melatonin concentrations in daytime on sleep, mood, body temperature, and performance," *Proc Natl Acad Sci USA* 91 (1994): 1824–8.
- P.A. Goldberg et al., "Modification of visceral sensitivity and pain in irritable bowel syndrome by 5-HT3 antagonism (ondansetron)," *Digestion* 57(6) (1996): 32A–36A.
- S. Harding, "Sleep in fibromyalgia patients: subjective and objective findings," *American Journal of the Medical Sciences Fibromyalgia* 315(6) (1998): 367–76.
- P. Hrycaj et al., "Platelet 3H-imipramine uptake receptor density and serum serotonin levels in patients with fibromyalgia/fibrositis syndrome," letter, *J Rheumatol* 20 (1993): 1986–88.
- J.F. Johanson, "Options for patients with irritable bowel syndrome: contrasting traditional and novel serotonergic therapies," Neurogastroenterol Motil 16(6) (2004): 701–11.
- Karl G. Henriksson, "Is fibromyalgia a central pain state?" *J of Musculoskeletal Pain* 10(1/2) (2002): 45–57.
- J. Laporte and A. Figueras, "Placebo Effects in Psychiatry," *Lancet* 334 (1993): 1206–8.
- A. Lerchl et al., "Marked rapid alterations in nocturnal pineal serotonin metabolism in mice and rats exposed to wheat intermittent magnetic fields," *Metalized Biochemical Biophys. Research Communication* 169 (1990): 102–8.
- P.S. Puttini and I. Caruso, "Primary fibromyalgia syndrome and 5-hydroxy-L-tryptophan: a 90-day open study," Rheumatology Unit, L Sacco Hospital, Milan, Italy, *J Int Med Res* 20(2) (1992): 182–9.
- I.J. Russell, "Neurohormonal abnormal laboratory findings related to pain and fatigue in fibromyalgia," *J Musculoskeletal Pain* 3 (1995): 59–65.

- A.N. Vgontzas, "Modest sleep loss increases/alters normal secretion of IL-6, TNF-alpha, cortisol," 84th Annual Meeting of the Endocrine Society, San Francisco, June, 2002.
- T. Wehr et al., "A circadian signal of change of season in patients with seasonal affective disorder," *Archives of General Psychiatry* 58(12) (2001): 1108–14.
- H.A. Welker et al., "Effects of an artificial magnetic field on serotonin in acetyl transferase activity in melatonin content in the rat pineal gland," *Exp Brain Research* 50 (1983): 426–32.
- S. Winberg et al., "Suppression of aggression in rainbow trout (Oncorhynchus mykiss) by dietary L-tryptophan," *J Exp Biol* 204(Pt 22) (2001): 3867–76.
- M.B. Yunus et al., "Plasma tryptophan and other amino acids in primary fibromyalgia: a controlled study," *J Rheumatol* 19 (1992): 90–4.
- I.V. Zhdanova et al., "Sleep inducing effects of low doses of melatonin ingested in the evening," *Clinical Pharmacological Therapeutics* 57 (1995): 552–8.

· 11 ·
ADRENAL FATIGUE
REPAIRING YOUR STRESS-COPING GLANDS

The proper function of our adrenal glands is second only to a good night's sleep in winning the battle against fibromyalgia and chronic fatigue syndrome.

The importance of restoring optimal adrenal gland function can't be overstated. An individual with FMS or CFS who suffers from adrenal fatigue will find her stress-coping abilities to be severely depleted. Simply put, she "stresses out" easily. Consequently, she has to avoid stressful situations in order to just feel OK (which makes for complicated relationships). Stress causes her physical pain, worsens her other symptoms, and can cause a flare-up that lasts well beyond the time of the stressful incident.

If she has a day when she feel good, she'll usually overdo it. Her reason? "I've got so much to do! And who knows when I'll feel good again." So she cleans the house, stays late at work, re-sods the front yard, goes Christmas shopping, and plays outside with the kids. Then she crashes—hard—the next day. She just doesn't have any resistance to stress. If her sister calls at 9:00 p.m. with some bad news, she can just forget about sleeping. And of course she'll feel terrible the next day, so she can go ahead and cancel that lunch date. "But how can I cancel on my friend again? She already thinks I'm avoiding her!" She just can't make any firm plans, because she never knows if she'll be having a good or bad day. Below are some sample accounts from patients of mine who have suffered from adrenal fatigue. Does any of it sound familiar?

ROBERT

Before my illness, I used to play on the company softball team, run regularly, take long hikes in the woods behind my house, and work 60-hour weeks. I've always been an extremely active person, or at least I was before I got sick six years ago. Now I can barely get out of bed, and I spend a great deal of time on the couch. I'm not able to work. I took an early retirement from my law firm. There are those rare days when I feel better than normal, not like I used to, but I do feel better some days than others. But if I try to do anything useful around the house like cleaning out the basement or sweeping out the garage, I'm so exhausted the next day I can barely move. It takes me days to get over it.

TINA

I just can't handle any stress any more. I turn my phone off at 8:00 each night so that no one disturbs me. I've given up trying to shop, entertain, or even manage the checkbook. Loud noises, crowds, certain smells, even changes in the weather bother me. I've become a recluse. I have to be careful not to overdo it, or I'll really be in trouble. I attended a family reunion three months ago and I'm still trying to recover. I'm sick and tired of being sick and tired.

If you can hear your own voice in the descriptions above, than your invaluable adrenals are probably in need of some serious TLC. The adrenal glands release cortisol and other hormones that allow us to be resilient to day-to-day stress. But the majority of patients I see for chronic illnesses, including FMS and CFS, are suffering from malfunctioning adrenals. (One study showed that underactive adrenal glands are evident in about two-thirds of CFS patients.)

The adrenals are a pair of pea-sized glands located atop each kidney. They consist of two sections: the medulla (inner portion) and the cortex (outer portion).

The medulla produces norepinephrine and epinephrine (also called noradrenaline and adrenaline). These hormones are primarily involved in *acute,* immediate responses to stress. Among other tasks, epinephrine increases the speed and force of the heartbeat, raises blood pressure, releases sugar into the bloodstream, and opens the airways to improve breathing. It also inhibits the muscle tone of the stomach, and that is why you may feel a "knot" in your stomach during times of stress.

The adrenal cortex is primarily associated with response to *chronic,* prolonged stress, such as infections or extended mental, emotional, chemical, or physical stress. The hormones released by the cortex are steroids, and the main steroid is cortisol.

Restoring proper adrenal function is a crucial step in peeling away the layers of dysfunction associated with FMS or CFS. Most likely, underactive adrenals are a major contributory factor to your symptoms. In fact, an altered or dysfunctional cortisol-control system may even be the principal cause of your illness. Adrenal fatigue is already known to cause many of the same problems associated with CFS/FMS, such as muscle or joint pain, dizziness, fatigue, decreased mental acuity, low body temperature, a compromised immune system, depression, constipation, diarrhea, and abdominal pain.

So why exactly are your adrenals letting you down? One reason may be that your hypothalamus does not make enough corticotrophin-releasing hormone (CRH), which is the brain's way of telling the adrenals that more cortisol is needed. HPA-axis dysfunction is a prime culprit for why CRH is deficient.

But I suspect that most of my patients are simply suffering from adrenal burnout. Amid years of poor sleep, unrelenting fatigue, chronic pain, excessive stimulants, poor diet, and relying on a plethora of prescription medications, the adrenal glands and the hormones they release have been used up. And once adrenal exhaustion sets in, it's not long before the body begins to break down. Adrenal fatigue then becomes a fact of life—and the beginning of chronic illness—for most, if not all, of my FMS and CFS patients.

YOUR SLEEP-WAKE CYCLE

Sleeplessness is such an integral part of FMS and CFS, and it is directly linked to cortisol levels. Cortisol secretions rise sharply in the morning, peak at approximately 8:00 a.m., and then starts to taper off until they reach a low point at 1:00 a.m. In this way, cortisol helps to regulate the sleep-wake cycle known as your **circadian rhythm.**

Fluctuations in cortisol levels can occur whenever normal circadian rhythm is altered, whether by air travel, a change in work shifts, or stress-induced sleeplessness. Some patients report that their symptoms started when they began working at night. Some will begin to have symptoms after staying up several nights in a row to take care of invalid family members or newborn babies. This is why it is essential for you to try to go to bed (preferably before 11:00 p.m.) and wake up at the same time each day. Establishing normal sleep and wake times is crucial in restoring normal circadian rhythms.

GENERAL ADAPTATION SYNDROME

In today's society, we process more information in one day than our great-grandfathers processed in three months. We experience stress reactions every few minutes, as we are bombarded by stimuli from TVs, radios, traffic, cell phones, pagers, etc. We even start out our days stressfully, waking up to a beeping alarm! All this stress can lead to what's known as the **general adaptation syndrome** (GAS).

Three phases lead up to a person developing GAS. The first is known as the **fight-or-flight response.** This alarm reaction is triggered by messages in the brain that cause the pituitary gland to release adrenocorticotrophic hormone (ACTH). This hormone then causes the adrenal glands to secrete adrenaline, cortisol, and other stress hormones, putting the body on "red alert" and ready for physical and mental activity. The heart beats faster, the breath rate increases, and digestion and other functions not essential for the moment are halted. The liver releases glucose into the blood stream. The body is now ready for any real or imagined danger.

The next phase is known as the **resistance reaction.** While the fight-or-flight response is usually short-lived, the resistance phase can last for quite some time. The major player in this phase is the hormone cortisol, which continues to be released by the adrenal glands. The resistance reaction allows the body to endure ongoing stress such as pain, fatigue, or injury. However, this mechanism doesn't come without a price. Long-term stress can generate a host of health problems, including the third phase, known as **adrenal exhaustion.** When the adrenals are overworked and underpaid, if you will, they simply give out. Exhaustion then leads to chronic poor health.

As an example: it was common for my fellow chiropractic students and me to come down with a bad cold or other illness after taking our finals each quarter. Most of us worked as well as went to school. We'd go to classes in the morning, wait tables at night, and then stay up until dawn studying. We'd survive on pure adrenaline for weeks. Then once our finals were over, we'd all be exhausted and sick. A similar situation may be in effect for your FMS or CFS. When you're adrenal glands became exhausted—whether from chronic illness or stress, surgery, or a traumatic event—you then become susceptible to illnesses. Many of my patients describe just such a scenario to me upon their first visit. They had just tackled some big illness, event, or struggle, and then they'd crashed, became ill, and just couldn't shake it. Once adrenal exhaustion sets in, it's not long before the body begins to break down, rendered defenseless against the continuous chemical, emotional, and physical challenges of daily stress. This is the beginning of chronic illness.

DIAGNOSING ADRENAL FATIGUE

Beyond adrenal fatigue is **Addison's disease.** This severe disorder results in total adrenal insufficiency. The situation is usually permanent and can be identified by a simple blood test. But the adrenal weakness brought on by chronic stress is a marginal and temporary insufficiency. It's much more difficult to diagnose. An exhausted adrenal gland may enlarge a bit, but otherwise it appears structurally sound and usually produces normal blood levels of cortisol. A **saliva adrenal hormone profile** is much more reliable in this case. See Appendix B for more information about this test.

TESTING FOR ADRENAL FATIGUE

There are also some simple tests that you can do at home—or with a doctor's help—to help you determine the state of your adrenals:

Ragland's sign is an abnormal drop in systolic blood pressure when a person arises from a lying to a standing position. Normally, there should be a rise of 8–10 mm. in this number. A drop or a failure to rise indicates adrenal fatigue.

Example: Someone takes your blood pressure while you're lying on your back. The systolic number is 120 and the diastolic number is 60 (120 over 60). Then he takes your blood pressure again immediately after you stand up. The systolic number should increase to 128–130. If it doesn't, you have adrenal fatigue.

Another way to test for adrenal dysfunction is the **pupil dilation exam.** To perform this on yourself, you'll need a flashlight and a mirror. Face the mirror, and shine the light in one eye. If after 30 seconds, your pupil (black center) starts to dilate (enlarge), adrenal deficiency should be suspected.

Why does this happen? During adrenal insufficiency, there is a deficiency of sodium and an abundance of potassium, and this imbalance causes an inhibition of the eye's sphincter muscles. These muscles would normally initiate pupil *constriction* in bright light. However, with adrenal fatigue, the pupils actually dilate when exposed to light.

Adrenal fatigue can be mistaken for a variety of other illnesses. From Dr. David Walther's book, *Applied Kinesiology*, comes this discussion on hypoadrenia (low adrenal function):

"Hypoadrenia displays itself in a variety of ways, such as severe depression, suicidal tendencies, asthma, chronic upper respiratory infections, hay fever, skin rashes, colitis, gastric duodenal ulcers, rheumatoid arthritis, insomnia, headaches, fatigue, fainting spells, obesity, heart palpitations, edema in the extremities, learning difficulties—the list goes on and on....

"The tragedy is that thousands of persons today are suffering from some manifestation of hypoadrenia. They may have sought help for their problems, and been given tranquilizers and psychotherapy for the emotional depression; analgesics for rheumatoid arthritic pain; sedatives for insomnia; amphetamines and diuretics for obesity; anti-cholinergic and a bland diet for colitis; antihistamines and bronchial dilators for asthma....

"They may have had extensive examination, with no pathology found. Therefore, these victims of hypoadrenia are given treatment to diminish the symptoms rather than eliminate the cause."

Rogoff's sign is a definite tenderness in the lower thoracic spine where the ribs attach. It can be an indicator of adrenal exhaustion. Lastly, **salt craving** is another possible sign. And if you've ever experienced it, you know what I'm talking about. In hypoadrenia, more sodium is lost than usual, and more potassium is retained. The kidneys reabsorb less water than is needed, and blood pressure may drop, leading to fatigue.

Those with low adrenal function usually have low blood pressure and fatigue. Increasing water and salt intake may help boost adrenal function and eliminate fatigue.

However, if you suffer from high blood pressure, increasing your salt intake may pose a problem. If you do increase your salt intake in this case, monitor your blood pressure a few times a day. You can purchase a blood pressure cuff at most pharmacies. If your blood pressure begins to go up while increasing salt to your diet, simply reduce your salt intake once again.

THE SIGNIFICANCE OF CORTISOL

You've probably already heard of cortisol and know that it's important. You might have even been prescribed cortisol at one point or another. Since its discovery some 50 years ago, this steroid has gained increasing prominence in treatment of autoimmune diseases, allergies, asthma, and athletic injuries. Over the years, researchers have developed powerful synthetic forms with stronger anti-inflammatory effects. Unfortunately, in continued high doses, cortisol can cause adverse side effects including depression, fluid retention, high blood pressure, bone loss, stomach ulcers, cataracts, and breathing disorders.

THE DHEA CONNECTION

When the adrenals are chronically overworked and straining to maintain high cortisol levels, they lose the capacity to produce sufficient DHEA. DHEA (the full name is dehydroepiandrosterone) is a precursor hormone to estrogen, progesterone, and testosterone and is necessary for moderating the balance of hormones in your body. Insufficient DHEA contributes to fatigue, bone loss, loss of muscle mass, depression, aching joints, decreased sex drive, and impaired immune function.

DHEA is notoriously low in FMS and CFS patients. This is because as chronic stress demands more and more cortisol from the adrenals, they get to where they can't keep up with the demand. As the cortisol levels fall, the body attempts to counter this by releasing more DHEA. Eventually the DHEA also is depleted. And aging makes holding on to DHEA even tougher. Even in healthy individuals, DHEA levels begin to drop after the age of 30. By age 70, they are at about 20% of their peak levels.

And DHEA, like cortisol, is valuable to your body. It helps prevent the destruction of 5-HTP, which increases the production of serotonin, buffering the effects of chronic stress. Studies continue to show low DHEA to be a biological indicator of many different serious illnesses, including cancer and arthritis. It protects the thymus gland, a major player in immune function, and in this way protects your overall well-being.

10—OR FEWER—STEPS TO ADRENAL HEALTH

The best time to have helped your adrenals, of course, was before they were exhausted. But take heart. Many of my patients have seen amazing results by restoring their adrenals through the following protocol:

1. **Sleep.** And make sure your sleep is consistent, deep, and restorative. See chapter 10 for help.

2. **Take a comprehensive optimal daily allowance multivitamin and mineral formula.** I've developed a special CFS/Fibro Formula that my patients use. Visit www.TreatingAndBeating.com or call 1-205-879-2383 for more information.

3. **Take adrenal cortical extracts.** These help repair and restore normal adrenal function. Adrenal cortical extracts are used to replenish and eventually normalize adrenal function. And they have an advantage over prescription cortisol hormone replacement (Cortef) in that they can be instantly discontinued once they have done their job of repairing adrenal function.

Adrenal extracts have been successfully used to treat many conditions related to adrenal fatigue, including many symptoms of FMS and CFS. They can increase energy and speed recovery from illness. Adrenal extracts are not a new treatment. In the 1930s, they were very popular, used by tens of thousands of physicians. They were still being produced by leading drug companies as recently as 1968. Today, these extracts are available without a prescription as adrenal cortical glandular supplements.

Start with 500 mg. of adrenal cortex glandular twice a day with food. You should notice an improvement—including a difference on the orthostatic blood pressure test and or pupil test—within two weeks. If not, double your dose of adrenal cortex, and retest in another two weeks.

Important: *Don't* use whole gland adrenal or adrenal medulla glandular, which are designed to increase adrenaline levels. These can put more stress on your already delicate stress-coping system and cause anxiety, rapid heart rate, and elevated blood pressure.

4. **If your blood pressure runs low (99/60 or below), then increase your salt consumption.** Yes, it's OK to use salt. By increasing your salt intake you'll help reduce inflammatory chemicals. Salt is a natural antihistamine, and histamine—along with its regulators, the hormones known as prostaglandins and kinins—can cause pain. (Salt's antihistamine properties is one reason why saline nasal rinses help prevent sinus congestion.) However, patients with congestive heart failure, pulmonary edema, or high blood pressure should avoid additional salt intake.

5. **Drink water.** I recommend at least 70 ounces daily.

6. **Always eat breakfast, and never skip meals.** If you have low adrenal function, then you are probably not hungry when you wake up. You might have gotten used to using chemical stimulants—such as coffee, sodas, or cigarettes—to get you going. These stimulants do raise blood sugar and serotonin levels, but they also increase adrenaline and cortisol levels, which curbs the appetite even further. In the morning, your body needs to break the eight-hour fast it has been under. Your brain especially needs

to be fed; forty percent of all food fuel goes to maintain proper brain function.

7. **Limit your consumption of adrenal-hormone robbers.** Start to eliminate—or at least drastically reduce—caffeine, nicotine, sugar, and alcohol in your diet. I know this can be tough, but if you want to get well, this is really not an option. Take two–three weeks to wean off caffeine in order to avoid headaches.

If you continue to experience adrenal fatigue symptoms even after taking the steps above, then continue on....

8. **Try supplementing with DHEA.** CFS patients are generally more likely than FMS patients to benefit from DHEA supplementation. But if you have FMS and truly aren't responding to adrenal cortical extract therapy, then taking DHEA is the next step. It's best to have your DHEA levels tested before supplementing DHEA, especially if you take a dose above 50 mg. (See Appendix C for ordering a home test). Most females with FMS or CFS who benefit from DHEA therapy need 10–25 mg. daily. The males generally need 50–100 mg. daily. I've found sublingual (dissolving under the tongue) to be the best form of DHEA, but micronized forms of DHEA are also a good choice. When needed, supplementing with DHEA boosts your energy, sex drive, resistance to stress, immune system, mood, strength and stamina, and overall health.

9. **Increase vitamin C intake if necessary.** It is perhaps the most important nutrient in facilitating adrenal function and repair. In fact, until it was possible for scientists to measure adrenal steroid hormones, vitamin C levels were used to judge adrenal health in animal studies. If you're taking my CFS/Fibro Formula, then you are taking in 1,800 mg. of vitamin C already, and I don't usually find that a patient needs to increase her intake beyond that. However, if nothing else is working, it won't hurt to add even more. If you do, begin with 1,800–2,000 mg. the first day.

Then increase by an additional 1,000–2,000 mg. each day, up to a maximum of 10,000 mg. or until you have a loose bowel movement. If you have such a bowel movement, reduce your dose by

1,000 mg. the next day. Keep reducing the dose by 500–1,000 mg. daily until you no longer have loose stools. This is your ideal dose of vitamin C.

10. **Treat any remaining low blood pressure.** If your blood pressure remains low even after supplementing salt in your diet, start taking licorice root extract *(Glycyrrhiza glabra)* to raise blood pressure. It has been used for over 5,000 years and is one of China's most popular herbal medicines. Licorice root extract acts like the adrenal hormone aldosterone, which is involved in salt and water metabolism.

Large amounts of licorice root can cause water retention, potassium deficiency, and elevated blood pressure, so take it slow. But if you need it, raising the blood pressure with licorice root extract can have dramatic effects on your symptoms. Your nausea, dizziness, and fatigue may simply disappear. I recommend licorice root extract when blood pressure is at or below 95/60 even after supplementing with adrenal cortical extract. But since the adrenal cortical extract contains aldosterone, as well as cortisol and DHEA, it will often normalize low blood pressure on its own.

FOR FURTHER READING AND RESEARCH
- *Adrenal Fatigue: The 21st Century Stress Syndrome* by James L. Wilson, ND, DC, PhD.
- *Applied Kinesiology: The Advanced Approach in Chiropractic* by David S. Walther, DC.
- M.A. Demitrack, "Chronic fatigue syndrome: a disease of the hypothalamic-pituitary-adrenal axis?" *Ann Med* 26(1) (1994): 1–5.
- N.N. Lizko et al., "Events in the development of dysbacteriosis of the intestines in man under extreme conditions," *Nahrung* 28 (1984): 599–605. As reported in *Alternative Medicine Review* 4(4) (1999): 249–62.
- S. Melamed and S. Bruhis, "The effects of chronic industrial noise exposure on urinary cortisol, fatigue and irritability: a controlled field experiment," *J Occup Environ Med*; 38(3) (1996): 252–6.
- *Practical Organotherapy* by HR Harrower, MD.
- J. Teitelbaum and B. Bird, "Effective treatment of severe chronic fatigue: a report of a series of 64 patients," *Journal of Musculoskeletal Pain* 3(4) (1995): 91–110.
- *Textbook on Physiology* by Arthur Guyton, MD.

· 12 ·
THE DIGESTIVE SYSTEM: OUR FRAGILE ALLY

**The state of our health is largely determined by not only
what we eat but how well we digest and absorb it.
Nutrients are worthless if they can't
be broken down and utilized by the body.**

In the proceeding chapters, I've reported on the importance of re-establishing deep restorative sleep, building-up your stress-coping savings account, restoring optimal nutrient levels, and rejuvenating your adrenal glands with nutritional therapy. In this chapter, we'll look at the importance of proper digestion and elimination.

Think of your gastrointestinal (GI) tract as your window to the world. It breaks down, absorbs, and assimilates the foods you eat. These carbohydrates, proteins, and fats yield sugars, amino acids, essential fatty acids, and other life-sustaining nutrients. Our food and the nutritional supplements we take provide the building blocks for manufacturing, repairing, and coordinating the vital biochemical components of each bodily function.

But as we'll see in this chapter, the GI tract can become compromised from various biochemical malfunctions: poor diet, bacteria, age, and prescription medications. **Unfortunately, even if you eat a healthy diet and take nutritional supplements, your health will suffer if you have malabsorption syndrome, achlorhydria, intestinal permeability, or pancreatic enzyme deficiencies.** Establishing optimal digestion allows you get the most from the foods you eat and the supplements you take.

You probably don't know it, but your GI tract is one of your most important immune and detoxification systems. But it's assaulted on a daily basis by bacteria, yeast, viruses, and toxins contained in the foods we eat. So the first place to start in establishing a healthy GI tract is your diet. A poor diet leads to poor health, but the right food choices can make all the difference in how you feel.

YOU ARE WHAT YOU EAT

A typical American breakfast might include nitrate-laden bacon cooked in hydrogenated oils, sugary cereal made with bleached enriched flour, and a glass of orange juice (a simple carbohydrate). Lunch might be a fast-food hamburger loaded with saturated and trans-fatty acids, pasteurized preservative-rich cheese (containing aluminum), french fries cooked in hydrogenated oils and loaded with fat, and a Diet Coke ("I'm watching my weight").

Well, this menu does contain all the "recommended" food groups: meat, dairy, grains, and fruits and vegetables. But does this sound healthy to you? Of course not! Cooking in hydrogenated oils, preserving by bleaching, and adding artificial flavors and colors removes essential vitamins and minerals and adds toxins. Is it any wonder that nearly 65% of our population are overweight?

Since 50 years ago, Americans are consuming an additional 31% fat and 50% sugar while decreasing complex carbohydrate consumption by 43%. Much of our food has been processed, bleached, altered with preservatives, and tarnished with toxic pesticides. We are literally eating ourselves into the grave. Over 40 million Americans have been diagnosed with irritable bowel syndrome, and surveys have shown that as many as 73% of FMS patients have it. In chapter 23, we'll look at how to incorporate healthy eating habits into your busy lifestyle. For now, I want to investigate the inner workings of the GI system and how it can affect our health.

HOW THE DIGESTIVE SYSTEM WORKS

The digestive system includes the mouth, salivary glands, esophagus, stomach, pancreas, liver, gall bladder, small intestine, and large intestine. Digestion involves the breakdown of food; its movement through the digestive tract; the chemical breakdown of large molecules into smaller, more readily absorbed ones; and the elimination of waste.

Digestion begins before you even take a bite. Just thinking about or smelling food can trigger certain chemicals, including the hormone gastrin, which stimulates the stomach cells. The process of chewing also initiates chemical reactions that prepare the stomach, gallbladder, and pancreas for proper digestion. Foodstuff is delivered from the **mouth** to the **stomach** by way of the **esophagus,** a 10-inch-long hollow organ. The esophageal sphincter works like a gate, opening to receive food and then closing to prevent stomach acid or food from returning to the throat.

Food is then pushed into the stomach, where digestive enzymes and gastric juices reduce it to a liquid substance known as chyme. The gastric juices contain hydrochloric acid and the enzyme pepsin. Hydrochloric acid breaks down the predigested food, and pepsin breaks down proteins into polypeptides (chains of amino acids). This acidic environment acts as one of the body's first lines of defense, destroying viruses, parasites, yeast, and bacteria.

After four-six hours, chyme passes into the **small intestine,** which is about 22 feet of hollow tubing. The **gallbladder** secretes **bile** to help break down fats in the small intestine, and digestive juices continue to do their work. At the end of the small intestine, the broken-down food is absorbed into the bloodstream and finally routed to the liver.

The **colon** (part of the **large intestine**) receives the leftover unusable chyme and begins to solidify it for evacuation. This semisolid material—known as feces—should produce a bowel movement and be excreted within 36 hours.

All of this, by the way, would not be possible without your amazing **pancreas.** It releases **proteolytic enzymes,** which the stomach uses to break down the food. Then it later releases **sodium bicarbonate** (think nature's Alka-Seltzer) to create the necessary alkaline environment in the small intestine.

HOW POOR DIGESTION AGGRAVATES YOUR SYMPTOMS

• **You might not be secreting enough gastric acid.** If you are age

60 or over, listen up. Numerous studies have shown that acid secretion declines with advancing age. And the resultant rise in stomach pH (to more alkaline) can cause many of symptoms associated with FMS and CFS. It's been estimated that 50% of Americans over the age of 60 suffer from a deficiency in hydro-chloric acid.

FMS and CFS symptoms can certainly suggest that you're not acidic enough. One group of researchers found that 80% of those with achlorhydria (low stomach acid) had soreness, burning, and dryness in the mouth, including a low tolerance for dentures. Thirty-four percent complained of indigestion and excessive gas. Forty percent complained of fatigue.

Gastric-acid secretion is a funda-mental process in assuring proper digestion and absorption, as these secretions are responsible for stimu-lating the release of pancreatic enzymes. But you don't have to be a senior citizen to suffer from low lev-els of acid. If you have symptoms of FMS, I recommend you take digestive enzymes. If your acid levels are already sufficient before you supplement with enzymes, your body will adjust fine. But if your levels are low, you should notice a dramatic improvement in your symptoms with continued use.

> I recommend that you begin taking digestive enzymes, even if you believe you're not currently suffering from a digestive illness. Your pain may be the symptom, even if your stomach feels fine.

Symptoms associated with achlorhydria (low stomach acid levels) include bloating, gas, heartburn, diarrhea, constipation, hair loss in women, rectal itching, nausea (especially after taking supplements), restless legs, sore or burning tongue, dry mouth, post-adolescent acne, undigested food in the stool, and weak, peeling, or cracked fingernails.

- **Your pancreas might not be making enough proteolytic enzymes because it doesn't have enough amino acids to build with.** Proteolytic enzymes help break down food during diges-tion, and they also help block painful inflammatory reactions. Proteolytic enzymes are built from amino acids, so a deficiency in amino acids means a deficiency in the inflammation- and pain-blocking proteolytic enzymes.

Amino acids come from protein. So, if you're not getting enough protein (as is the case on many low-fat diets), you won't have enough amino acids to build these valuable enzymes. And if you already suffer from malabsorption, you might not be digesting the protein you take in anyway. But supplementing with digestive enzyme will help you absorb your proteins. (Did I mention that I highly recommend them?)

- **You may be suffering from a food allergy, intolerance, or addiction.** If so, your pancreas is the first organ to suffer. It can become deficient in bicarbonate, and the proteolytic enzymes can be compromised or even destroyed. Without proteolytic enzymes, protein goes undigested. And if it's leaked across the intestinal cellular membrane, it can trigger inflammatory reactions, resulting in more gastrointestinal stress.

Food reactions, probably of frequently eaten foods, can contribute to many of the symptoms of FMS and CFS. And continuous exposure to allergic foods can trigger a cascade of reactions that can interfere with the absorption of essential nutrients. It's not new news that if you're not getting enough nutrients, you just feel terrible. See chapter 18 to learn more about food allergies.

Nutritional deficiencies, especially amino acid deficiencies, create a burden on the body's regulatory system. Further deficiencies are created as the regulatory system tries to right itself by using up nutritional reserves. It's no wonder FMS and CFS patients must supplement with vitamins and minerals in order to get well. *No one* could eat enough healthy food to keep up with the needs of a FMS/CFS patient's body when her illness is in full swing.

- **You might have a poorly functioning colon.** Healthy individuals should be having two or more bowel movements a day. Anything less than this increases the risk of fecal toxins being reabsorbed and leaking back into the bloodstream. A poorly functioning colon can cause autoimmune disorders, arthritis, skin disorders including eczema and psoriasis, muscles aches, bad breath, offensive body odor, headaches, nausea, and even mood disorders.

HEARTBURN, REFLUX, AND GERD

One estimate is that 40% of the US population has some degree of **esophageal reflux,** with 20% of adults complaining of weekly episodes of heartburn and 7–10% complaining of daily symptoms. Esophageal reflux occurs when the lower esophageal sphincter malfunctions, allowing the backward flow of acid, bile, and other contents from the stomach into the esophagus. Reflux can result from gastritis (inflammation of the stomach itself), peptic or duodenal ulcers, a hiatal hernia, or even the chronic use of NSAIDs.

> The most obvious symptom of esophageal reflux is heartburn. It occurs after eating and can last from a few minutes to a few hours. It feels like a burning sensation in the pit of the stomach and can move up into the chest and throat.

GERD (gastroesophageal reflux disease) can cause esophageal scarring or Barrett's syndrome, a chronic esophageal irritation that causes normal cells to be replaced by precancerous ones. An endoscopy test is used to diagnose GERD. Conventional treatment usually involves H2 antagonists (such as Tagamet, Pepcid, Zantac, or Axid) and antacids (such as Tums or Maalox) as the first line of treatment. Proton-pump inhibitor drugs (such as Nexium, Prevacid, or Prilosec) might also be initiated.

ARE ANTACIDS THE ANSWER?

No! These medications block the absorption of nutrients like zinc, folic acid, B12, calcium, and iron. This can lead to fatigue, anemia, and depression. And long-term use of these medications can block all stomach acid. But your body *needs* acid! Here's why:

- **The esophageal sphincter is stimulated to close by the release of stomach acids.** Picture the esophageal sphincter as being a door that separates our esophagus (throat) from our stomachs. The door is opened by the food we take in and closed when the naturally occurring stomach acid is released. When there's not enough acid present—because antacids have neutralized them—the esophageal sphincter may not close properly, allowing acid to travel back up into the esophagus and cause heartburn. Ironic, isn't it? Antacids can actually make heartburn *worse*.

- **The stomach needs acid to break down proteins for digestion.** No protein digestion means no amino acids. No amino acids means no neurotransmitters (serotonin, dopamine, norepinephrine, etc.). This can lead to all sorts of problems: including intestinal permeability, anemia, fatigue, increased allergy disorders, depression, anxiety, and bacterial and yeast overgrowth.

- **An acidic environment is one of the body's first lines of defense,** destroying viruses, parasites, yeast, and bacteria.

PROTOCOL FOR LOW STOMACH ACID

If you're suffering from heartburn and you have FMS or CFS, low stomach acid is most likely the problem. Try these solutions rather than antacids:

- **Take a digestive enzyme with each meal.** If you've been taking Nexium, Prevacid, Pepcid, Prevpac, Prilosec, Propulsid, Reglan, or Zantac for over three months, then you may have to stay on the medication as you begin the digestive enzyme. But many of my patients have found that they don't need these prescription medications once they start taking a good high-potency digestive enzyme. Still, don't discontinue any prescription medication without consulting your medical doctor first.

I recommend my patients use a potent 8X (double the strength of most) pancreatic digestive enzyme formula that utilizes USP porcine-derived high-potency pancreatin for reliable and consistent enzyme activity.

- **Consider supplementing with hydrochloric acid if the problem persists** (see the next page). If this makes your heartburn worse, then you probably have enough stomach acid. Stop supplementing the HCl, and continue using digestive enzymes.

- **Avoid foods that can relax the esophageal sphincter and make**

heartburn, reflux, and GERD worse. These include fried, spicy, or fatty foods; carbonated drinks; citrus fruits; peppermint; chocolate; coffee; tea; alcohol; tomatoes; garlic; and onions.

Q: I have bloating and gas that seems to be worse when I eat certain foods. Will taking digestive enzymes help?

A: Digestive enzymes help you digest and utilize proteins, fats, and carbohydrates. You should notice that your bloating and gas are eliminated once you start taking digestive enzymes. If after one week, you continue to have bloating, gas, or indigestion, add three capsules of high dose probiotics (good bacteria) on an empty stomach. Usually one to two months of probiotic therapy is enough.

• **Avoid lying down for at least three hours after you finish eating.** When you do lie down, try elevating the head of your bed about six inches (to facilitate keeping the gastric contents in the stomach). You can also try sleeping on your side, which would remove pressure from the esophageal sphincter, helping to keep gastric contents from backing up into your esophagus.

• **Try to eat smaller meals, and more frequently** (perhaps four or five in a day).

SUPPLEMENTING WITH HYDROCHLORIC ACID

Adequate protein intake, digestive enzyme supplementation, and a relaxed emotional state can help increase stomach acidity, but supplementation might also be necessary. Follow the guidelines below.

Don't take HCl if you've been diagnosed with a peptic ulcer. And since HCl can irritate sensitive tissue and corrode teeth, take it in capsule form only, and don't empty capsules into food or beverages. I recommend that you take pancreatic enzymes along with the HCl.

1. **Take one "betaine HCl with pepsin" capsule,** containing 600–650 mg. of hydrochloric acid and 100–200 mg. of pepsin, at the beginning of your meal. Continue taking one capsule with each meal for the next five days.

2. **After five days, increase your dose** to two capsules with each meal. Continue this dose for five days.

3. **If you are experiencing no side effects** (such as warmth, fullness, or other odd sensation in your stomach), **increase your dose** by one capsule each day until you do. Then reduce your dose by one capsule at your next meal.

4. **Establish a comfortable per-meal dose** (five capsules or fewer), and continue at that level. As your stomach regains the ability to produce an adequate concentration of HCl, you will probably require fewer capsules. Listen to your body, and reduce your dose as necessary. You may wish to reduce your number of capsules at smaller meals.

5. **Be consistent.** Individuals with low HCl and pepsin typically don't respond as well to botanicals and supplements, so to maximize the benefits, keep up the supplementation as directed.

> *Q: I've been diagnosed with GERD and have been taking Nexium for several months. Can I stop taking this medication and just take the digestive enzymes?*
>
> A: Try only the digestive enzymes (with each meal) for a week or two, and see if this alone prevents your reflux symptoms. If you continue to have reflux while taking the digestive enzyme, try adding the betaine HCl with pepsin (see "Supplementing with Hydrochloric Acid, p. 196) and probiotics. If you continue to have a problem, then you'll need to go back on the prescription medication. If you do this, discontinue the HCl, but keep taking the digestive enzymes. As always, talk to your medical doctor before discontinuing your prescription medication.

If you continue to have heartburn even after trying these recommendations, get tested for GERD and *H. Pylori*. Ask your doctor for help.

H. PYLORI

Helicobacter pylori bacteria is now thought to be the cause of most stomach ulcers. *H. pylori* is also associated with heartburn and reflux. Blood tests can reveal the presence of the *H. pylori* antibody, and antibiotics can eliminate *H. pylori* from the stomach in a matter of weeks. Then you should be able to discontinue prescription antacids. Be sure to supplement with probiotics 12 hours apart from any antibiotics you may need to take.

IRRITABLE BOWEL SYNDROME

Excuse me, but can we talk about poop? Not necessarily the best topic for a cocktail party, I agree. However, for over 40 million Americans who have been diagnosed with irritable bowel syndrome (IBS), their poop is always on their minds.

Some experts report that IBS affects 10%–20% of the population, though it might go undiagnosed. Over 40 million Americans have been diagnosed with IBS, and surveys have shown that as many as 73% of FMS patients have it.

Research has shown that the cause of IBS is related to a dysfunction in the neuroendocrine (brain and stomach hormones) immune system. The connection between the brain and the stomach is largely mediated by the neurotransmitter serotonin. Serotonin controls how fast or how slow food moves through the intestinal tract. In fact, 90% of serotonin receptors are in the intestinal tract, not the brain! This is one reason people get "butterflies" in their stomach when they get nervous.

So IBS patients might have hypersensitive pain receptors in their GI tracts, which may be related to low levels of serotonin. These decreased serotonin levels might help explain why people with IBS

Diagnosing IBS

Some individuals with this disorder have constipation (IBS-C), and some have diarrhea (IBS-D). Some will swing back and forth between the two extremes (IBS-A). New criteria for diagnosing IBS require that it be present for at least 12 weeks (not necessarily consecutive) in the preceding 12 months. True IBS also includes abdominal discomfort or pain that cannot be explained by a structural or biochemical abnormality. It must also be accompanied by at least two of the following three features:

1. Pain is relieved with defecation.

2. Pain is associated with a change in frequency of bowel movement (diarrhea or constipation).

3. Pain is associated with a change in the form of the stool (to loose, watery, or pellet-like).

---

are likely to be anxious or depressed. Studies show that 54%–94% of IBS patients meet the diagnostic criteria for depression, anxiety, or panic disorder. Consequently, restoring optimal serotonin levels has been the focus of traditional drug therapy.

PRESCRIPTION MEDICATIONS FOR IBS

Some of you are taking prescription medications for your IBS. These might include smooth muscle relaxants (such as Bentyl, Levsin, and Levsinex), antidepressants (such as Prozac or Paxil), anti-diarrhea meds (such as Imodium and Lomotil), bulk-forming laxatives (such as Metamucil). These medications range from innocuous to life endangering!

Zelnorm (tegaserod) was recently hailed as "the drug" for IBS-C. (Did you see the T.V. commercials with the cheerful women and their stomachs?) In a past edition of this book, I warned about the dangers of its side effects. Now it has been pulled off the market for its association with heart attacks and stroke! The percentage of patients taking Zelnorm who had serious, life-threatening side effects was 10 times higher than the percentage of patients taking a placebo.

You should be having at least one bowel movement every 24 hours, and one after each meal is optimal. True, having three or more bowel movements in a day can seem like a lot, when many FMS/CFS patients are used to having one every few days. But taking an optimal daily allowance multivitamin and mineral formula like our CFS/Fibro Formula along with taking digestive enzymes (either HCl or pancreatic enzymes) should result in normal bowel movements with in a couple of weeks. To order, visit www.TreatingAndBeating.com or call 1-888-884-9577.

The FMS/CFS formula will help a lot because it contains magnesium, which naturally relaxes the colon and usually remedies any problems with constipation. However, too much magnesium will cause a loose bowel movement. Obviously you want to find the right balance, and typically this is around 700 mg. daily.

Even before the drug was recalled for cardiovascular risks, many experts were warning about it's other potential side effects, including severe liver impairment, severe kidney impairment, bowel obstruction, diarrhea, constipation, abdominal pain, headaches, abdominal adhesions, gallbladder disease, and back pain.

Lotronex (alosetron) is prescribed for IBS-D. Within eight months of being on the market, reports of ischemic colitis (a life endangering situation in which the blood supply to the intestines is blocked) began to grow each day. Lotronex was responsible for at least four deaths—probably more. Many on the drug reported severe abdominal pain from constipation, and the drug was taken off the market. It is now again approved but with stricter prescribing guidelines.

An editorial in the *British Medical Journal* suggests that as many as 2 million Americans will be eligible for the drug under the new guidelines. According to previous reported side effects, this would result in 2,000 cases of severe constipation, almost 6,000 cases of ischemic colitis, 11,000 surgical interventions, and at least 324 deaths.

Antispasmodics (Levsin, Levsinex, Bentyl) are routinely prescribed for the treatment of IBS symptoms. Potential side effects include bloating; blurred vision; clumsiness; constipation; diarrhea; dizziness; excessive daytime drowsiness ("hungover feeling"); nausea and vomiting; nervousness; rash or hives; difficulty breathing, tightness in the chest, and pounding in the chest; swelling of the mouth, fact, lips, or tongue; fainting; irregular heartbeat; hallucinations; memory loss; muscle pain; trouble sleeping; and weakness.

Why in the world would anyone prescribe this crap? (No pun intended.) This is typical of what is wrong with "cookbook" (symptom-focused) medicine. It is absurd to suggest that high doses of

---

Q: What if I'm taking 300 mg. of 5-HTP daily, the digestive enzymes at every meal, and your CFS/Fibro Formula and still have constipation?

A: The 700 mg. of magnesium (a natural muscle relaxant) in our CFS/Fibro Formula is usually enough to promote normal daily bowel movements. However, some individuals will need to increase their dose of magnesium in order to overcome severe constipation. You should increase your magnesium (use magnesium citrate or chelate) by 140–150 mg. daily at dinner until you begin to have normal daily bowel movements. Then stay on this extra magnesium. You'll find that after a few months of continuing the CFS/Fibro Formula, you'll be able to discontinue the extra magnesium.

---

vitamins and minerals are dangerous while at the same time promoting life-threatening medications that only cover up symptoms.

REVERSING IBS WITH NUTRITIONAL THERAPY

I find that IBS usually disappears rather quickly once my patients follow this protocol:

- **Boost serotonin levels.** I recommend that patients supplement with the very amino acid that's responsible for making serotonin, 5-hydroxytryptophan (5-HTP). Those with IBS should take 300–400 mg. daily with food.

- **Correct poor eating habits.** Increase fiber, and reduce simple sugars, caffeine, and junk food.

- **Uncover any hidden allergies, including gluten intolerance** (Celiac disease).

- **Boost optimal stress-coping chemicals, such as serotonin, magnesium, and B vitamins.** I always recommend people take a good optimal daily allowance multivitamin/mineral formula. Patients with IBS have depleted their stress-coping chemicals and this not only leads to IBS but also prevents them from beating IBS. It is a vicious cycle that can only be broken by taking adequate amounts of essential vitamins and minerals.

Magnesium, involved in over 300 bodily processes, is particularly important for reversing the symptoms of IBS-C. It helps relax the smooth muscle of the colon, acting as a natural laxative and allowing normal bowel movements. While a diet high in nutritious fiber is important, magnesium is even more important. A magnesium deficiency not only causes constipation but can also lead to heart disease, mitral valve prolapse (MVP), depression, anxiety, chronic muscle pain, headaches, migraines, fatigue, and many other health conditions. Those with IBS-C may need up to 1,000 mg. of magnesium each day. Those with IBS-D may need less than 500 mg. I recommend patients begin with 500 mg. of magnesium a day.

- **Restore bowel ecology through probiotics.** This helps to avoid or correct intestinal dysbiosis (see next page).

- **Supplement with digestive enzymes.** Most digestion and absorption takes place in the small intestine and is regulated by pancreatic enzymes and bile. The pancreas aids in digestion by releasing proteolytic enzymes, which help break down proteins into amino acids. Natural digestive enzymes are found in raw fruits and vegetables. Processed foods are usually devoid of digestive enzymes. Overconsumption of these processed foods can lead to enzyme deficiencies, which can lead to malabsorption and/or intestinal permeability syndrome—characterized by bloating, gas, indigestion, diarrhea, constipation, and intestinal inflammation. To ensure proper digestion and absorption, I recommend, then, taking pancreatic enzymes with each meal.

INTESTINAL DYSBIOSIS

A healthy intestinal tract contains some 2–3 lb. of bacteria and other microorganisms, such as yeast, that normally don't cause any health problems. (In fact, you have more bacteria in your body than you do cells...you're outnumbered!) However, when the intestinal tract is repetitively exposed to toxic substances (such as antibiotics, steroids, and NSAIDs), these microorganisms begin to proliferate and create an imbalance in the bowel flora. This is known as **intestinal dysbiosis.** And when this occurs, a person becomes more susceptible to disease. For instance, the infective dose of *Salmonella enteritidis* decreases from 100,000 to approximately 10.

Candida yeast, like bacteria, only causes a problem when it gets out of control. In a normal microflora environment, numerous good bacteria are attached to the inner surface of the intestines. But when they aren't there, *Candida albicans* is able to attach itself, inserting a hook-like tentacle that create increased permeability and allows toxins to leak across the intestinal tract membrane.

These toxins can cause a myriad of health problems, such as *Candida* yeast syndrome, allergies, eczema, vitamin B12 deficiency, autoimmune diseases such as rheumatoid arthritis and lupus, CFS, IBS, colitis, and psoriasis.

To correct this overgrowth and overactivity of *Candida* yeast and bad bacteria, you need to put more good bacteria into your body to tip the scales back over to the "good guys." You do this by taking **pro-biotics.** *Lactobacillus (L. acidophilus, L. casei,* and *L. rhamnosus)* and *Bifidobacterium bifidum* are the two most important. Studies show that probiotics can reduce and even eliminate yeast overgrowth.

INTESTINAL PERMEABILITY: LEAKY GUT

Intestinal permeability occurs when the lining of the digestive tract becomes permeable (leaky) to toxins that cause chronic inflammation. This permeability allows toxins to leak out of the digestive tract and into the bloodstream. This triggers an autoimmune reaction that can create pain and inflammation in any of the body's tissues.

The use of NSAIDs, steroids, antibiotics, antihistamines, caffeine, alcohol, and other prescription and nonprescription drugs can cause intestinal permeability, as they render the intestinal mucosa permeable to toxins and undigested food particles.

Intestinal permeability is associated with many illnesses, but studies

---

Q: What if I continue to have loose bowel movements?

A: Low serotonin will cause loose bowel movements, so make sure you're taking 300 mg. a day of 5-HTP either at bedtime or throughout the day with food (see chapter 10). If you're taking the 5-HTP, digestive enzymes, and the CFS/Fibro Formula for two weeks, and you continue (or start) to have loose bowel movements, then you'll need to decrease the amount of magnesium you're taking.

Stop taking the smallest white tablet in your CFS/Fibro Formula. If after a couple of days you continue to have loose bowel movements, then take only one CFS/Fibro pack a day. If the problem persists, then start probiotics. Stay on the one pack of CFS/Fibro Formula, because the amino acids, vitamins, and especially the fish oil in the formula will help normalize your intestinal tract.

Q: OK, I've done everything you recommend, and I just can't get rid of my IBS! What else can I do?

A: Don't give up! You may need to treat intestinal dysbiosis or permeability. Keep reading.

---

show individuals with CFS are especially plagued with it. A treatment program for patients with CFS that reduced allergic foods and used nutritional supplements to increase liver detoxification pathways yielded an 81.2% reduction in symptoms. You can read more about toxicity issues in chapter 19, but for now, let's continue treating and beating intestinal permeability.

PROTOCOL FOR INTESTINAL PERMEABILITY

Intestinal permeability can be measured by a special functional medicine test available from Genova Diagnostics. To order this test, see Appendix C. But if you suspect that you have intestinal permeability (if the protocols for low stomach acid and for IBS aren't giving you intestinal relief), take the following steps:

1. **Keep supplementing with your digestive enzymes** and HCl if needed.

2. **Start taking probiotics,** three a day on an empty stomach for two months.

3. **Begin the elimination diet** (see next page) to pinpoint any food allergies. Pay particular attention to gluten, a protein found in most grains, because it can be very irritating to the intestinal lining. (For more on food allergies, see chapter 18.)

4. **Keep taking your CFS/Fibro Formula.** If you aren't taking mine, make sure that the supplement you are taking contains **fish oil,** 1,000–2,000 mg. daily. The omega-3 fatty acids in fish oil help repair the intestinal tract, reducing inflammation associated with leaky gut. One study showed that 2.7 grams daily put Crohn's disease patients into remission.

5. **For more and faster relief, add our Leaky Gut Formula** supplement to your regimen. Take six capsules daily in divided doses between meals.

Our Leaky Gut Formula has been developed especially for intestinal permeability and has all the essential nutrients to help correct it: **Large amounts (6,000 mg.) of the amino acid glutamine,** the primary fuel for intestinal cell function, are included to meet the high energy demands of the GI tract, liver, and immune system during periods of physiological stress. Glutamine also transports potentially toxic ammonia concentrations to the kidneys for excretion and restores shortages created by chronic use of NSAIDs or antibiotics. **Acacia** contributes soluble, nonbulking fiber readily fermentable into a supportive environment for growth of beneficial *Lactobacillus* bacteria. It also assists in water absorption and supports colonic cell function. **Nutraflora FOS** supplies nondigestible fructooligosaccharides to further encourage growth of beneficial microorganisms, and **N-acetyl-D-glucosamine** is used as a structural component of intestinal mucous secretions that protect intestinal tissues and help food pass through the GI tract.

THE ELIMINATION DIET

To begin the elimination diet for intestinal permeability, **avoid all known and suspected food allergens.**

For two weeks, also avoid all gluten-containing foods: wheat, barley, oats, millet, spelt, sourdough, and rye. This includes wheat flour, breads, taco shells, muffins, cereals, pastries, cakes, pizza, crackers, pasta, oatmeal, pretzels, and other flour-based products.

Also avoid all dairy products, including milk, ice cream, cream, yogurt, and cheese. Butter and eggs are allowed.

Don't drink any sodas (Coke, Diet Coke, Pepsi, etc.).

Reduce caffeine consumption, including tea (green and herbal tea is allowed), coffee, chocolate, and cocoa. The less caffeine intake, the better. To help prevent withdrawal symptoms (headaches, mood disturbances, and fatigue) slowly wean off caffeine.

Q: I also suspect that I have a yeast overgrowth; chapter 22 describes me perfectly. Can I start your protocol for yeast overgrowth at the same time as I'm treating my digestive system?

A: Yes and no. You can start the yeast overgrowth diet, but don't begin using any supplements or medications to kill off yeast until you have given yourself plenty of time to get your gut healthy and are sleeping through the night on a regular basis.

Start by eliminating one quarter of daily caffeine consumption. For example: each serving of coffee, soda, diet soda, tea, and each chocolate bar equals one caffeine serving. If you consume four cups of coffee in the morning, three glasses of tea at lunch, and a diet Coke before dinner, you consume a total of eight servings of caffeine daily. You should begin by reducing your caffeine servings by one quarter (which is two servings). So drink six servings tomorrow instead. After seven days, reduce your caffeine servings by another quarter. Slowly discontinue caffeine over a manageable period of time. Not every patient must go off all caffeine; you will help yourself if you reduce your intake to no more than one or two caffeine servings a day.

REINTRODUCTION OF ELIMINATED FOOD GROUPS

After one month on the elimination diet, start to reintroduce one eliminated food group at a time. For example, begin by eating a few servings from the gluten group: pasta, crackers, or bread. Then, for three days, eat no gluten-containing foods or any other eliminated food. Keep a journal handy to note any symptoms that occur.

After three days, reintroduce dairy. Have a few glasses of milk or three slices of cheese. Be sure to eat enough servings to let your body experience any negative reactions. If after three days of having challenged a food group, there's no negative reaction (headaches, stomach pain, bloating, runny nose, congestion, muscle/joint pain, low moods, fatigue, etc.), then start to slowly add these items back into your regular diet.

If you do experience a negative reaction to any food group within three days of challenging it, discontinue that group for another month and then repeat the three-day process.

PROTECTING FROM FUTURE DAMAGE

Once you've gotten better, stay better! Try to avoid all NSAIDs, including Advil, Motrin, etc. If you need relief for your chronic pain, try the natural remedies featured in chapter 15.

If you ever need to take antibiotics in the future, always take probiotics as well, 12 hours away from the antibiotics.

> Q: *The protocols from this chapter helped, but my digestion still isn't what it used to be. What else could be wrong with me?*
>
> A: If you don't find the relief that you're looking for through the protocols in this chapter, than you might very well be suffering from a yeast overgrowth or even a parasitic infection. But don't jump immediately to treating this problems unless you're ruled out the other, much more common, possibilities: low stomach acid, IBS, and intestinal permeability. To find out more about yeast overgrowth, see chapter 22. Learn about parasites in chapter 20.

RESOURCES
- **Leaky Gut Formula** is available from my Essential Therapeutics line of supplements.
- **Digestive enzymes** and vegetarian digestive enzymes are also available from my Essential Therapeutics line. Digestive enzymes are also available at your local health food store, but I use a high-potency digestive enzyme that greatly reduces the number of tablets a person needs with each meal.
- **Probiotics** are available at your local health food store or by contacting my office.
- **Testing for leaky gut** is available from my office. To order any of these, visit www.TreatingAndBeating.com or call 1-888-884-9577.

FOR FURTHER READING AND RESEARCH
- A. Belluz et al., "Effects of an enteric-coated fish-oil preparation on relapses in Crohn's disease," *N Engl J Med* 334 (1996): 1557–60.
- L.M. Brown and S.S. Devesa, National Cancer Institute, "Epidemiologic trends in esophageal and gastric cancer in the United States," *Surg Oncol Clin N Am* 11(2) (2002): 235–56.
- S.K. Das et al., "Deglycyrrhizinated liquorice in aphthous ulcers," *J Assoc Physicians India* 37(10) (1989): 647.
- M. Delvaux, "Gastroenterology unit and laboratory of digestive motility," CHU Rangueil, Toulouse, France.
- M. Galland, "Leaky gut syndromes: breaking the vicious cycle," Third International Symposium of Functional Medicine, Vancouver, British Columbia (1996).
- P. Goldberg "Modification of visceral sensitivity and pain in irritable bowel syndrome by 5-HT3 antagonism (ondansetron)," *Digestion* 57(6) (1996): 478–83.
- F. Huwez et al., "Mastic gum kills Helicobacter pylori," *N Engl J Med* 339(26) (1998): 1946.

- G. Ionescu et al., "Abnormal fecal microflora and malabsorption phenomena in atopic eczema patients," *J Advan Med* 3(2)(1990): 71–89.
- J. Marle et al., "Deglycyrrhizinised liquorice (DGL) and the renewal of rat stomach epithelium," *Eur J Pharm* 72 (1981): 219.
- G. Olaison et al., "Abnormal intestinal permeability in Crohn's disease," *Scan J Gastroen* 25 (1990): 321–8.
- F. Pearce et al., "Mucosal mast cells III Effect of Quercetin and other flavonoids on antigen-induced histamine secretion from rat intestinal mast cells," *J Allergy Clin Immunol* 73 (1984): 819–23.
- S. Rigden, "Entero-hepatic resuscitation program for CFIDS," *CFIDS Chron* (Spring 1995): 46–9.
- G.S. Sharp and H.W. Fister, "The diagnosis and treatment of achlorhydria 10 year study," *Journal of American Geriatric Society* 15 (1967): 786–91.
- G.L. Simon and S.L. Gorbach, "The human intestinal flora," *Dig Dis Sci* 31(spl 9) (1986): 147s–62s.
- "Stress and visceral perception," *Can J Gastroenterol* 13(spl A) (1999): 32A–36A.
- A.G. Turpie et al., "Clinical trial of deglydyrrhizinized liquorice in gastric ulcer," *Gut* 10 (1969): 299–302.
- B. Vellas et al., "Effects of aging process on digestive functions," *Comprehensive Therapy* 17(8) (1991): 46–52.
- W.E. Whitehead et al., "Systematic review of comorbidity of irritable bowel syndrome with other disorders: What are the causes and implications?" Division of Digestive Diseases and Center for Functional Gastrointestinal and Motility Disorders, Univ of N. Carolina, Chapel Hill.

· 13 ·
YOUR JUMP-START
PROGRAM

OK, you've learned a lot so far….
I know it can be a bit confusing, especially if you have fibro-fog.
Relax; don't use up your few stress-coping chemicals, because I'm
going to simplify things for you right now.

For the past 14 years, I've successfully treated thousands of patients
with high does of certain vitamins, minerals, amino acids, and
other nutrients—an approach known as orthomolecular medicine
(see ch. 7). It's based solely on biochemistry, using the right chemicals inherently natural to your body's optimal functioning.

In short, by using the natural building blocks that make up your
normal biochemistry, we can correct, drastically improve, or even
reverse the cause of your illness. Nutrients— including vitamins,
minerals, and amino acids—make the hormones that regulate your
body. They compose every essential chemical in the body, including

---

Q: Does this mean that I stop taking all my medication?

A: No. It's too stressful for you to stop then right away. Start the Jump-Start Program first. As your begin to sleep better and have more energy and less pain, you'll become more tolerant to stress. Then follow the suggestions in this book to—working with your doctor—slowly wean off the drugs. Say good-bye to the ones that weren't helping, and restart the ones that were. You might find that even the useful drugs can be reduced in dosage once your body is healthier.

Remember, drugs are foreign to the body, and they have potential side effects. Drug therapy can be useful, however, merely covering up symptoms with drugs often leads to further problems. Learning which drugs to take and which ones to avoid while replenishing your nutrient-depleted body is the foundation of my Jump-Start Program.

---

thyroid hormone, testosterone, estrogen, neurotransmitters (serotonin, norepinephrine, etc.), antibodies, adrenaline, cortisol, and white blood cells.

Unlike with drug therapy, there is never any danger in getting healthy. Once you become familiar with my protocols, you'll realize that they're safer and often more effective than drug therapy alone. And they often work quickly, having a person feel better than she has in years.

I've found that it's best to start with the following core nutrients, which I call the Jump-Start Package. The supplements in this package are essential for reversing fibromyalgia and CFS symptoms, and they don't take a lot of measuring, counting, or reorganizing of your medicine cabinet. Ninety-nine percent of the time, I start my pain-and-fatigue patients on the four pillars of the Jump-Start Program from day one: 5-HTP, adrenal cortex, digestive enzymes, and an optimal daily dose multivitamin and mineral formula.

When my patients begin the jump-start package, they consistently report feeling better within 2–4 weeks. That's because these supplements help address the core issues of fibromyalgia and CFS. I call these the **four pillars,** and we begin them all at the same time.

1. 5-HTP

This builds serotonin and promotes deep restorative sleep, the most important step in beating fibromyalgia and CFS. See chapter 10 to read all about it, including what to do if it doesn't seem to be working for you.

2. ADRENAL CORTEX

Once you get sleeping well and restore you serotonin levels, you should start feeling better than you have in years. However, if you don't repair your sluggish adrenal glands, you'll crash every time you attempt to overdo it. I know you can relate to having a day or two when you feel good and then overtaxing yourself only to "flare up" again and end up in bed for several days. Supplementing with adrenal cortex (500 mg. daily divided into two doses) and/or other supplements that help the adrenal gland repair itself is a crucial step towards avoiding these flare-ups. Check out chapter 11 again if you're not convinced.

3. DIGESTIVE ENZYMES

The majority of my patients are suffering from poor digestion, and most are taking antacids or proton-pump inhibiting medicines to block their stomach acids. As I've already discussed, this can cause further nutritional deficiencies. If you're not breaking down and assimilating the nutrients in your foods or the supplements your taking, you'll be wasting your money and never feel as good as you could. That's why I recommend that all of my patients take an 8X pancreatic digestive enzyme—or betaine HCl with pepsin enzyme—with each meal. Read more in chapter 12.

4. OUR CFS/FIBRO FORMULA

I've already established the important roles vitamins, minerals, essential fatty acids, and amino acids play in reversing many of the most troubling symptoms of fibromyalgia and CFS. After working with fibromyalgia and CFS patients for over a decade, I'm firmly convinced that without taking a good optimal daily allowance multivitamin-and-mineral formula similar to the one I've developed, patients are doomed to a life-long battle with poor health. Chapters 26–29 will give you more details about the ingredients in the CFS/Fibro Formula.

The CFS/Fibro Formula is taken as one pack with food, twice a day. I've designed what I consider to be (and which has proved itself to be) the best on the market, if I do say so myself.

GET JUMPING

This Jump-Start Package is the place to begin in your journey to wellness. Start here, and give yourself some time to improve. As your stress-coping savings account builds up for a couple of weeks, you should definitely feel better. Some of you will show a dramatic improvement. You won't be totally well yet, and you might never

What's in the CFS/Fibro Formula?

- **Vitamin A:** 11,250 I.U. (33% from fish liver oil and 67% from natural carotenes [alpha, beta, cryptoxanthin, zeaxanthin, and lutein])
- **Vitamin C:** 600 mg. as calcium ascorbate and magnesium ascorbate buffered complex.
- **Vitamin D3:** 200 I.U.
- **Vitamin E:** 201 I.U.
- **Vitamin K1:** 30 mcg.
- **Thiamine B1:** 50 mg.
- **Riboflavin B2:** 25 mg.
- **Niacin B3:** 100 mg. (75% as niacinamide)
- **Pyridoxine B6:** 25 mg.
- **Folic Acid:** 400 mcg.
- **Methylcobalamin B12:** 50 mcg.
- **Biotin B7:** 150 mcg.
- **Pantothenic acid B5:** 200 mg.
- **Calcium:** 250 mg. (76% as calcium citrate-malate and 24% as calcium ascorbate)
- **Iodine:** 75 mcg. (from kelp)
- **Magnesium:** 350 mg. (54% as magnesium aspartate and ascorbate complex, 28% magnesium aspartate, and 18% as magnesium amino acid chelate)
- **Zinc:** 10 mg. (as amino acid chelate)
- **Selenium:** 100 mcg. (as amino acid chelate)
- **Copper:** 1 mg. (as amino acid chelate)
- **Manganese:** 5 mg. (as amino acid chelate)
- **Chromium:** 100 mcg. (as chromium polynicotinate)
- **Molybdenum:** 75 mcg. (as amino acid chelate)
- **Potassium:** 148 mg. (as potassium aspartate-citrate)
- **Boron:** 1 mg. (as aspartate-citrate)
- **Vanadium:** 50 mcg. (as bisglycinato oxovanadium) This is a potent blood sugar regulator.
- **Choline:** 75 mg.
- **Inositol:** 25 mg.
- **PABA:** 25 mg.
- **Citrus Bioflavonoids:** 50 mg.
- **Malic Acid:** 500 mg.
- **Amino Acid Blend:** 1,000 mg.
- **Essential Fatty Acids:** omega 3, 6, and 9.
- **Potassium-Magnesium Aspartate Complex:** increases metabolism in the cells and mental and physical energy
- **Marine Lipid Concentrate:** supplying eicosapentaenoic acid (EPA) and docosahexaenoic acid (DHA)
- **Organic High-Lignin Flax Seed Oil:** supplying alpha linolenic acid, linoleic acid, and oleic acid
- **Borage Seed Oil:** 50 mg. supplying gamma linoleic acid (GLA), linoleic acid, and conjugated linoleic acid (CLA)

feel like you did when you were 20. But you shouldn't have to suffer like you have been. Let your body exist in this healthier state for up to a month before attempting any of the additional protocols or taking additional supplements I recommend later in this book.

Achieving optimal health will take time and perhaps additional supplements. You may be like the 40% of my patients who suffer from undiagnosed hypothyroid (low thyroid), or you may be low in the energy-boosting neurotransmitter norepinephrine. (We'll look at how to boost energy levels in ch. 16) Or you may have plenty of energy but still suffer a good deal of pain. (Chapter 15 has more information on pain.) A few of you might even report that nothing has helped yet. In the next several chapters we'll look at some of the other important layers of the FMS/CFS onion that need to be peeled away: hypothyroid, food allergies, immune system dysfunction, yeast overgrowth, etc.

· 14 ·
HYPOTHYROID AND CHRONIC ILLNESS

Over 20 million Americans suffer from thyroid dysfunction, and over 500,000 new cases of thyroid disease occur each year.

Like my patient Allison, many individuals with low (hypo) thyroid simply fall through the cracks. It's estimated that more than 10 million women with **thyroid dysfunction** are untreated. And almost another 8 million people with **hypothyroid** go completely undiagnosed.

ALLISON

I really felt terrible most of the time. I had no energy at all. I'd gained 40 pounds over the last year even though I ate very little and tried to follow my Weight Watcher's program. I kept cutting my calorie intake and even started skipping meals in an attempt to lose weight. The less I ate, the worse I felt.

I had numerous sinus infections, which I had never had before. My hair was falling out, I had tingling pain in my hands and feet, and I always felt cold—even in the summer. I had this constant ringing in my ears. I was depressed or anxious a good deal of the time. Every doctor I consulted said that my blood tests were normal so it must be my fibromyalgia that was causing me to feel so bad. I knew something was wrong with me, but I couldn't find anyone who could help me. One doctor said I had all the symptoms of low thyroid, but the endocrinologist she referred me to said all my tests were normal. How could my thyroid be normal when I have all the symptoms of hypothyroid?

Allison's story is a typical one. I routinely have new fibromyalgia and CFS patients who present with all the symptoms of hypothyroid: fatigue, headaches, dry skin, swelling, weight gain, cold hands and feet, poor memory, hair loss, hoarseness, nervousness, depression, dry skin, constipation, joint and muscle pain, and burning or tingling sensations in the hands or feet. The symptoms associated with hypothyroid are, after all, very similar to those of fibromyalgia and CFS. And in fact, up to 63% of patients with fibromyalgia and/or CFS have been shown to have hypothyroid.

I estimate that as many as 40% of my FMS and CFS patients are suffering from low thyroid function.

YOUR THYROID GLAND

The thyroid gland is shaped like a butterfly and is located in the lower front part of your neck (just above the breastbone). It's responsible for secreting thyroid hormones, which travel through the bloodstream and help cells convert oxygen and calories to energy. Basically, thyroid hormones control a person's metabolism.

Metabolism is defined as the sum of all physical and chemical changes that take place within the body; it's all the energy and

---

Symptoms of Hypo (low) thyroid

- fatigue (the most profound symptom)
- headache
- dry skin
- swelling
- weight gain
- cold hands and feet
- poor memory
- hair loss
- hoarseness
- nervousness
- depression
- joint and muscle pain
- burning or tingling in the hands and/or feet
- yellowing of skin from a build up of carotene (conversion of carotene to vitamin A is slowed by hypothyroidism)
- carpal tunnel syndrome
- problems with balance and equilibrium
- constipation
- myxedema (nonpitting edema due to the deposition of mucin in the skin), especially around the ankles and below the eyes
- high blood pressure
- chest pain
- hardening of the arteries
- high cholesterol
- menstrual irregularities, PMS, and infertility
- fibrocystic breast disease
- polycystic ovary syndrome
- reactive low blood sugars
- psoriasis
- nasal allergies

---

material transformation that occur within living cells. So if your thyroid gland becomes dysfunctional, every cell in the body suffers. This is why thyroid disorders can cause so many problems.

When your thyroid gland *produces too much* thyroid hormone, this is known as hyperthyroid. When your thyroid *doesn't produce enough* thyroid hormone, it's called hypothyroid. Below is a more complete list of symptoms associated with **hypothyroid,** many of which sound like the symptoms of FMS/CFS.

UNDERSTANDING THYROID HORMONES

A healthy thyroid gland produces hormones called thyroxine (T4) and triiodthyronine (T3). T4 can then be converted into T3, which is four times more active than T4. T3 is essential for life. Twenty percent of the T3 circulating in the body comes directly from the thyroid gland, and the remaining 80% comes from the conversion of T4.

WHAT CAN GO WRONG WITH THE THYROID GLAND?

There are three types of hypothyroid: primary, secondary, and tertiary. **Primary hypothyroidism** arises from a deficiency in the thyroid gland. **Secondary hypothyroidism** involves the pituitary gland. In **tertiary hypothyroidism,** the hypothalamus gland shuts down in response to overwhelming stress.

An imbalance in the estrogen-progesterone ratio can also interfere with proper thyroid function. So a vicious cycle may ensue when low thyroid function (from chronic stress) alters the normal estrogen-progesterone balance, which then contributes to further low thyroid. This case may be especially true for autoimmune thyroid disease. (An autoimmune disease occurs when the body's immune system becomes misdirected and attacks the organs, cells, or tissues it was designed to protect. About 75% of autoimmune diseases occur in women, most frequently during their childbearing years.)

Overstimulated Immunity: Hashimoto's thyroiditis is a type of autoimmune thyroid disease in which the immune system attacks and destroys the thyroid gland. Symptoms include those normally seen in hypothyroid disease, including fatigue, depression, sensitivity to cold, weight gain, muscle weakness, coarsening of the skin, dry or brittle hair, constipation, muscle cramps, increased menstrual flow, and goiter (enlargement of the thyroid gland). Hashimoto's thyroiditis is the most common form of hypothyroidism and is generally treated with thyroid hormone replacement therapy.

Low progesterone in women age 30–50 may lead to Hashimoto's disease as elevated estrogen levels cause the immune system to become overstimulated. To compound this potential problem, estrogen-like chemical compounds can also block thyroid function. By binding to the estrogen-receptor sites on cells, they cause an increase in circulating estrogen. Thesechemicals include common environmental pollutants such as PCBs (polychlorinated biphenyls), dioxins, and pesticides. Unfortunately, though no longer produced in the US, these chemicals are routinely found in our food and water supply.

Maintaining an optimal detoxification system helps protect us against these chemicals. Along with increasing antioxidants, which assist the liver's detoxification processes, some doctors also recommend supplementing with natural progesterone cream. We'll look at sex hormones in more detail in chapter 31.

STRESS AND NUTRITIONAL DEFICIENCIES

We've already looked at how the HPA axis is affected by stress. The thyroid gland—which is controlled by the hypothalamus and pituitary—may become compromised by any disruption to the HPA axis. So stress definitely takes a toll on thyroid function. Short-term stress causes an elevation of cortisol, which then blocks the conversion of T4 to T3.

> The conversion of T4 to T3 (or reverse-T3) takes place within the cells by the enzyme 5-deiodinase. This enzyme can be inhibited by prolonged stress, acute and chronic illness, steroids (either natural stress hormones or those taken as a drug), and poor nutrition.

Long-term stress further depletes the nutrients needed to keep thyroid hormones at peak levels. Nutrition is involved in every aspect of T4 production, utilization, and conversion to T3. The minerals zinc and iodine; vitamins A, B2, B3, B6 and C; and the amino acid tyrosine are all needed for the production of T4. Selenium is needed to convert T4 to T3, so a deficiency in this mineral can also cause thyroid dysfunction. High blood levels of fatty acids can also inhibit conversion of T4 to T3. A deficiency in iodine or tyrosine especially can lead to thyroid dysfunction.

Iodine is simply *necessary* to generate thyroid hormones (T4 has four atoms of iodine, and T3 has three). While many experts suggest that iodine deficiencies are rare in this country, our consumption has dropped drastically over the last 20 years. One test for iodine deficiency is the skin-patch test. Using a 2% Lugol's solution (available at any drug store), paint a 2-inch square patch onto your abdomen. Iodine deficiency is indicated if the painted patch disappears within 24 hours. If it lasts longer than 24 hours, your iodine status is normal. If you test low in iodine, add one of any number of kelp supplements to your diet.

A deficiency in just about any of the **B vitamins** will contribute to low thyroid function. Low levels of **copper, magnesium** and **manganese** may also prevent optimal thyroid function.

Prescription Medications: Antidepressant medications alter the HPA axis by making the thyroid-releasing hormone and thyroid-stimulating hormone pathway less efficient. Antidepressants also divert L-tyrosine, the precursor for the neurotransmitters dopamine and norepinephrine, from converting into the thyroid hormone T4. This is a bit ironic, since low thyroid function is a major cause of depression.

Interferon typically interferes with thyroid function, and secondary thyroiditis occurs in up to 14% of those taking interferon. **Methadone, synthetic estrogen, Tamoxifen,** and cholesterol-lowering drugs increase the binding of thyroid hormones to chemicals that inactivate thyroid hormones. **Dilantin** (Phenytoin) and **Carbamazeprine** (Tegretol) decrease T4 and T3 by about 20%.

Certain Foods: Some foods may contribute to goiters and alter thyroid function: broccoli, cauliflower, Brussels sprouts, cabbage, mustard, kale, turnips, canola oil, soy, pine nuts, millet, and peanuts.

THYROID BLOOD TESTS UNRELIABLE

Blood tests for thyroid function measure the amount of thyroid hormones in the bloodstream; but the action takes place in the cells themselves. What good is a blood test that only shows what is racing around the bloodstream one second out of one minute, out of one hour, out of a one day? These tests are only an educated guess based on the bell curve theory. Sixty percent of patients will have thyroid levels between the usual testing parameters, 20% will be above, and 20% will fall below these parameters.

Picture it this way: when I arrive at my office each morning I can take an educated guess that since there are 10 cars in the parking lot, my waiting room will be full. However, I'm only guessing, because some of the car owners may be in the pediatric clinic next door. And if there's a virus going around the elementary school, then all 10 of the carloads are probably in the pediatric clinic, while my patients have had to park elsewhere. The same princi- ple is true in thyroid blood tests. We can make an educated guess, but we can never account for the myriad circumstances that could affect the results.

Of course, conventional medical professionals know that thyroid blood tests are less than perfect. The *Journal of Clinical Psychiatry* has reported that "laboratory blood tests for thyroid may be inac- curate for many who get tested for hypothyroid disorder." In 2004, the president of the American Association of Clinical Endocri- nologists (AACE) said, "there are more people with minor thyroid abnormalities than previously perceived."

Thankfully, the parameters for normal thyroid have recently nar-

> Q: *If my lab tests are normal, does this mean I don't need thyroid medication?*
>
> A: Maybe and maybe not. You may have hypothyroid or euthyroid, even if your blood tests are normal. I recommend you rely instead on the results of temperature testing.

rowed. The new guidelines have reduced the range for acceptable thyroid function and will hopefully result in a proper diagnosis for millions of Americans who suffer from mild thyroid disorder. The AACE estimates that the new guidelines actually double the number of people who have abnormal thyroid function, bringing the total to as many as 27 million, up from 13 million thought to have the condition under the old guidelines.

Unfortunately, I still routinely get test results from labs that use the old numbers, leading many doctors to misdiagnose their patients based on outdated parameters.

SAFETY CONCERNS OF TREATMENT

Patients often relate that they, and sometimes their doctors, have suspected a thyroid problem only to have their blood work return normal. Most physicians, in this case, are reluctant to prescribe thyroid replacement for fear of jeopardizing the health of the patient. And certainly the risks of thyroid-replacement therapy should be considered. Excess thyroid hormone can cause elevated heart rate, rapid pulse, and accelerated bone loss.

Still, millions suffer with symptoms far worse then these when their prescription thyroid therapy is withheld. If you weigh the pro's and con's of administering thyroid-replacement therapy to a patient with normal blood tests but all the symptoms of hypothyroid, it's easy to see why I consider it malpractice to withhold prescription thyroid therapy. This is especially true in light of the fact that most of my fibromyalgia and CFS patients are already taking numerous drugs to cover up the symptoms of hypothyroid: Provigil or Adderall to increase energy, antibiotics for chronic sinus infections, a laxative for constipation, NSAIDs for pain, an SSRI medication for depression, and perhaps a benzodiazepine like Ativan or Xanax for anxiety. Once their thyroid disorder is corrected, many of my patients are able to drastically reduce or eventually wean off these medications, some of which are quite dangerous themselves.

This tragic situation is just one reason while I've always advocated treating the patient and their symptoms, instead of treating the blood work.

Important! Check Your Adrenals First.

A major connection exists between low thyroid and low adrenal function. Adrenal fatigue can actually cause a person's thyroid problem to be much worse than it would be otherwise. That's because normal adrenal function (especially of the hormone cortisol) is *essential* to the body's ability to metabolize thyroid hormones.

Instead of getting better, individuals with adrenal fatigue who start thyroid replacement therapy may experience a racing heart, fatigue, pain, agitation, fuzzy thinking, anxiety, and depression. These side effects can cause them to give up on their thyroid treatment. But it's not that they don't need—or can't tolerate—the thyroid replacement therapy but that their adrenal function is too low to support the increase in their metabolism.

Even the manufacturers of thyroid medication themselves acknowledge in their "contraindications" that patients with "untreated adrenal cortical insufficiency" can experience a worsening of symptoms. Unfortunately, many conventional doctors simply choose to ignore adrenal fatigue unless the patient has true adrenal failure (Addison's Disease) and so don't treat their patients with adrenal support therapy.

The saddest story is when the increase in symptoms is blamed on a worsening of arthritis (more drugs) or even clinical depression (more drugs). And the thyroid treatment, which could have cured both of these symptoms, is completely abandoned.

To ensure success with your thyroid replacement therapy, be sure to read and apply chapter 11 before treating any low thyroid.

SICK EUTHYROID SYNDROME

Another reason that a patient might go undiagnosed for thyroid disorder is that some people show symptoms of thyroid illness and

Dr. Barnes's Thyroid-Testing Method

1. First thing in the morning, while still in bed, shake down and place a thermometer (mercury, not digital) under your arm. Leave it there for 10 minutes.
2. Record your temperature in a daily log.

- Women still having menstrual cycles should take their temperature after the third day of their period.
- Readings below 97.8 degrees strongly suggest **hypothyroid**.
- Readings above 98.2 degrees may indicate an overactive thyroid.

might be making plenty of T4 but are not properly converting it to T3. These patients are said to have sick euthyroid syndrome. The blood tests of these patients may not reveal the syndrome, however, unless their doctor orders a special reverse-T3 study (which will reveal that the T4 is being changed into reverse-T3 rather than the vital T3). This condition can be caused by stress, chronic illness, or even acute illness. Individuals with this syndrome might take a synthetic thyroid hormone like Synthroid, which contains T4 only, but since the T4 is not converting efficiently, they continue the symptoms of low thyroid.

SELF-TEST FOR LOW THYROID

Dr. Broda Barnes was the first to demonstrate that a low basal body temperature was associated with low thyroid. His first study was published in 1942 and appeared in JAMA. It tracked 1,000 college students and showed that monitoring body temperature in order to test thyroid function was a valid, if not superior, alternative to thyroid blood tests.

The body works best at the optimal temperature of 98.6 degrees. Higher temperatures (fevers) speed up the metabolism and allow the body to fight off infection. A temperature of 90 degrees or below qualifies as hypothermia, a medical emergency. But it doesn't have to go that low to affect health, because most of the biochemical reactions that occur in the body are driven by enzymes, and these enzymes are influenced by metabolic temperature.

Dr. Barnes recommends that hypothyroid patients take a glandular prescription medication known as Armour Thyroid, which was used before synthetic medications were introduced. Armour Thyroid and other prescription thyroid glandulars (such as Westhroid) contain both T4 and T3. Synthroid and other synthetic thyroid medications contain T4 only, and since some individuals have a difficult time converting T4, these medications may not work at the cellular level. Consequently, patients may take T4 medications for years and never notice much improvement in their symptoms. Their blood tests will look good, but in the meantime, they'll be falling apart: gaining weight, suffering aches and pains, battling one sinus infection after another, and becoming more and more fatigued, depressed, and withdrawn.

> Q: *My doctor has me on Synthroid. Should I switch to Armour, Nuthroid, or Westhroid?*
>
> A: If you're taking one of the T4-only synthetic prescription drugs and haven't noticed much difference in your symptoms: fatigue, weight gain, hair loss, tingling in your hands or feet, etc., then yes, consider asking your doctor to try you on one of these T3-T4 combinations.

Many patients with hypothyroidism do just fine on T4 only. But others don't, so why should doctors prescribe synthetic T4 medications (such as Synthroid, Levoxyl, Levothroid, Eltroxin, and Unithroid) at all? T4 administered *along with* T3 yields the best clinical outcome for many patients, especially those suffering from mood disorders.

RESULTS OF LOW THYROID

Depression: Several studies demonstrate that a combination of T4 and T3, or T3 therapy alone, may provide welcomed relief from a number of symptoms commonly associated with fibromyalgia and CFS. Depressed patients often benefit by taking T3, with or without their antidepressant medications. And thyroid replacement therapy, especially the addition of T3 therapy, helps increase the effectiveness of tricyclic antidepressant medications. As far as SSRIs go, studies show that T3 therapy is more effective in reducing the symptoms associated with depression.

A study published in the *New England Journal of Medicine* showed that patients who received a combination of T4 and T3 were mentally sharper, less depressed, and feeling better overall than a control group who received T4 only. This is good news for the 40% of my patients who suffer from low thyroid. I suspect that it will be good news for many of you reading this book, too.

Fibromyalgia: Research continues to suggest that thyroid hormone deficiency may be a key feature in FMS etiology. Researchers have observed that FMS patients respond best to treatment with thyroid hormone as part of a comprehensive regimen to optimize the patient's metabolism. They stated in the *Journal of Myofascial Therapy* that "virtually all FMS patients dramatically improve or completely recover from the symptoms with this regimen. As long as the patient does not take excessive amounts of thyroid hormone, there are no adverse side effects." In fact, T4 with T3 has improved or eliminated depression, brain fog, feeling of cold, constipation, chronic fatigue, headaches, insomnia, muscle and joint pain, and chronic sinus infections. For some people it has helped them finally lose weight.

> *Q: What if I'm taking one of these combination drugs (Armour, Westhroid, or Nuthroid) but still have a low body temperature and symptoms of low thyroid?*
>
> A: I'd recommend you ask you doctor to consider increasing your prescription medication. If this is not an option or it doesn't help, then start taking GTA-Forte II along with the prescription (see page 228).

You can take T4 with T3 as a desiccated thyroid or a synthetic medication such as Thyrolar. For many patients, synthetic medications are adequate and sometimes preferable; for other patients, synthetic medications don't relieve all their symptoms but desiccated thyroid does.

Pharmaceutical company representatives typically report that synthetic medications for hypothyroidism are superior to desiccated thyroid. They falsely describe desiccated thyroid as unstable or unpredictable. Since these sales reps are the primary source of information about drugs for most doctors, this myth is passed from doctor to patient. However, though the amount of thyroid hormone present in the thyroid gland may vary from animal to animal, Armour Thyroid runs analytical tests—to measure actual T4 and T3 activity—on both their raw thyroid powder and their actual tablets.

In this way, they ensure that their product is consistently potent from tablet to tablet and lot to lot. So Armour Thyroid is an excellent product choice. Still, Thyrolar is available for those who prefer a synthetic.

WILSON'S SYNDROME

E. Denis Wilson, MD, was refining some of the pioneering clinical research of Dr. Barnes, when he discovered that his patients weren't converting T4 to T3.

Dr. Wilson's protocol uses specially compounded timed-release T3 therapy to overcome the buildup of stress-induced reverse T3. Patients start with 7.5 mcg. of timed-release T3, taken every 12 hours. They increase their dose by 7.5 mcg. each day until their temperature reaches 98.2. Once they have "captured" their normal temperature, they then begin to gradually reduce their compounded T3 medication. Dr. Wilson's protocol can be a challenge for doctors and patients alike. However, I've found that for some patients, this complicated therapy has been the final piece of their puzzle. For more information, visit www.WilsonsSyndrome.com.

The symptoms of Wilson's syndrome (failure to convert T4 to T3) include severe fatigue, headache and migraine, PMS, easy weight gain, fluid retention, irritability, anxiety, panic attacks, depression, decreased memory and concentration, hair loss, decreased sex drive, unhealthy nails, constipation, irritable bowel syndrome, dry skin, dry hair, cold and/or heat intolerance, low self-esteem, irregular periods, chronic or repeated infections, and many other complaints. A lot of symptoms for such a little hormone problem, huh?

Perhaps the greatest obstacle Dr. Wilson has had to overcome in his attempts to be recognized by mainstream medicine

> **TESTING FOR WILSON'S SYNDROME**
>
> Like with Dr. Barnes's protocol, patients suspected of Wilson's syndrome monitor their body temperature.
>
> - The temperature is taken 3–4 times daily.
> - Patients shake down and place a (mercury) thermometer under their arm for 10 minutes. An consistently low temperature (less than 97.8) averaged over 5–7 days indicates Wilson's syndrome.

is the vast number of symptoms associated with Wilson's syndrome. Yet all these symptoms can be seen in hypothyroid patients. And *in one study, all the symptoms of FMS were eliminated* by taking high doses (120 mcg.) of T3.

STRESS LEADS TO WILSON'S SYNDROME

The symptoms of Wilson's syndrome tend to come on or become worse after a major stressful event. Childbirth, divorce, death of a loved one, job or family stress, chronic illness, surgery, trauma, excessive dieting, and other stressful events can all lead to hypothyroidism.

Under significant physical, mental, or emotional stress, the body slows down its metabolism by decreasing the amount of T4 that is converted to T3. This is done to conserve energy, and when the stress is over, the metabolism is supposed to speed up and return to normal. This process can become derailed, however, by a buildup of reverse-T3 (rT3) hormone. This rT3 can build to such high levels that it starts using up the enzyme that converts T4 to T3. The more stress, the more likely rT3 can block T4 from converting into T3. The body may then try to correct this by releasing more T4 and its precursor TSH, only to have rT3 levels climb higher. A vicious cycle is created, where T4 is never converted into active T3.

Certain nationalities are more likely to develop Wilson's syndrome: those whose ancestors survived famine, such as the Irish, Scotch, Welsh, Russians, and American Indians. Interestingly, those patients who are part Irish and part American Indian are the most prone of all. Women are also more likely than men to develop Wilson's syndrome.

TREATMENT FOR WILSON'S SYNDROME

To stop the cycle of Wilson's syndrome, reduce your rT3 levels so that T4 can convert to active T3. This is done by taking a specially compounded form of timed-released T3 in gradual increments. T3 is available as the synthetic medication Cytomel in the United States and Canada and Tertroxin in the U.K.

> Q: I'm taking a prescription thyroid medication. Should I start to take GTA-Forte II as well?
>
> A: If you're taking a prescription thyroid medication and your temperature is running 97.8 or below, then yes, you should consider adding GTA-Forte II. I'd recommend one GTA-Forte II in the a.m. and one in the early afternoon. Monitor your temperature (as outlined on p. 223). If it rises above 98.2, then discontinue or reduce the GTA Forte II.

When the body temperature returns to normal, the patient can gradually wean herself off the medicine. This is a big advantage of T3 therapy over other hormone replacement therapies, which are difficult to discontinue.

Wilson's protocol can be inconvenient for patients to follow, but it often yields results when Armour and Westhroid therapies fail, and I've seen dramatic results from it in many of my patients. Some of my patients have been on synthetic thyroid medications for years with very little or no improvement, so I'm often amazed at the turnaround they experience on Cytomel. Many enjoy a newfound energy and metabolism, and it's common for them to lose weight that couldn't be lost, sleep better, rid themselves of chronic infections, and think clearly for the first time in years.

NATURAL GLANDULAR THYROID SUPPLEMENTS

I used to regularly refer my patients to a medical doctor in an attempt to get them on prescription Armour Thyroid medication—It's what I'd prefer they use. However, since many doctors are reluctant to treat a patient for hypothyroid when she has normal thyroid blood tests, I've been forced to find an over-the-counter thyroid glandular replacement therapy. Fortunately, I've discovered a reliable manufacturer of high-quality thyroid glandular that's producing great results.

This over-the-counter treatment, called **GTA-Forte II,** is a natural glandular just like Armour Thyroid. By law, however, they've had the T4 removed, and only T3 is included. Since these raw thyroid tissue concentrates contain the active thyroid hormone T3, they can be used as a first line of treatment for low to moderate hypothyroid dysfunction.

I've been using GTA-Forte II for several years now, and my patients consistently notice improvement in their hypothyroid symptoms. But it's not easy to find. Your naturally oriented physician can order it for you, or you can order it from my office (see "resources," below). Dosing: For low thyroid, start on one tablet twice daily. Monitor your basal temperatures as described above. After two weeks, if your temperature is not going up or you're not feeling better, increase your dose to two tablets in the morning and one in the evening. Continue to monitor your temperatures. If they still don't go up or if you don't feel any better, try adding a thyroid support formula. I use one developed by Dr. Joseph Collins, a leading naturopath. Called Thyro-Mend, this herbal combination helps increase T4's ability to convert into T3. It's available from your naturally oriented doctor or from my office under the name Thyroid Support Formula. For more information on Armour Thyroid, or to obtain a referral to a doctor for Armour Thyroid, go to www. BrodaBarnes.org.

RESOURCES
- www.WilsonsSyndrome.com
- www.BrodaBarnes.org
- GTA-Forte II and Thyro-Mend are available from your nutrition-oriented physician or from my office (to order, visit www.TreatingAndBeating.com or call 1-888-884-9577). You might also find them at your local health-food store.

FOR FURTHER READING AND RESEARCH
- A.J. Halterer et al., "Transthyretin in patients with depression." *Amer J Psychiatry* 150 (1993): 813–5.
- O. Agid and B. Lerer, "Algorithm-based treatment of major depression in an outpatient clinic: clinical correlates of response to a specific serotonin reuptake inhibitor and to triiodothyronine augmentation," *Int J Neuropsychopharmacol* 6(1) (2003): 41–9.
- L.L Altshuler et al., "Does thyroid supplementation accelerate tricyclic antidepressant response? A review and meta-analysis of the literature," *Am J Psychiatry* 158(10) (2001): 1617–22.
- R.G. Cooke et al., "T3 augmentation of antidepressant treatment in T4-replaced thyroid patients," *J Clin Psychiatry* 53(1) (1992): 16–8.

- H.O. Eidenier Jr., "A clinician's view of biotics research products," lecture, July 2003.
- A. Gaby, " 'Sub-laboratory' hypothyroidism and empirical use of Armour Thyroid," *Altern Med Rev* 9(2) (2004): 157–79.
- *J Clin Endocrin and Metab* 88 (1998): 3401–8.
- J.C. Lowe et al., "Triiodothyronine (T3) treatment of euthyroid fibromyalgia: a smaller replication of a double-blind placebo controlled study." *Clin Bulletin Myofas Ther* 2(4) (1997): 71–88.
- K. Kellman, "Thyroid Deficiency," *Life Extension* (Sept 2004): 52–59.
- R.P. Kraus et al., "Exaggerated TSH responses to TRH in depressed patients with 'normal' baseline TSH," *J Clin Psychiatry* 58 (1997): 266–270.
- J.C. Lowe et al., "The process of change during T3 (Triiodthyronine) treatment for euthyroid Fibromyalgia: a double-blind placebo-controlled crossover study," *Clinical Bulletin of Myofascial Therapy* 2(2/3) (1997b): 91–124.
- "Recovery from FMS by hypothyroid patient resistant to T4 and desiccated thyroid," *Journal of Myofascial Therapy* 1(4) (1995): 21–30.
- Y. Suzuki et al., "Plasma free fatty acids, inhibitor of extra thyroid conversion of T4 to T3 and thyroid hormone binding inhibitor in patients with various nonthyroid illnesses," *Endocrinol Jpn* 39(5) (1992): 445–53.

· 15 ·
CHRONIC PAIN *CAN* BE STOPPED!

If you still have a good deal of pain after two to three weeks of sleeping well and implementing the jump-start plan, then you might require additional supplements.

Most individuals with FMS/CFS will show a tremendous improvement in their pain by implementing my jump-start program outlined in chapter 13—adding the hypothyroid protocol (chapter 14) if needed. Follow this plan first; see if it doesn't heal your chronic pain. If not, then read on.

ANDREA

My fibromyalgia began after I had a hysterectomy three years ago. Before then I was in pretty good health. I was a little overweight and often struggled with long, stressful hours as a plaintiff's attorney. But while I sometimes felt tired and run down, I never had pain. At least not the allover pain I now experience. The pain started with my neck and shoulders. Now I have pain in my mid back, low back, legs, knees, chest. I've been to several doctors, including a rheumatologist, orthopedist and neurologist. All my tests are normal, yet I hurt every day. I think some of the doctors thought I was only trying to get pain meds. It really wears me out. I've tried taking various drugs: Advil, Celebrex, Mobic, Skelaxin, Cymbalta, Neurontin, even pain meds. Nothing helped. About two months ago, I started taking 5-HTP and several of the supplements recommended in Dr. Murphree's book. I'm now sleeping through the night—first time in years. I have more energy and less pain.

SAMe

SAMe (S-adenosyl-l-methionine) is a naturally occurring amino-acid compound. My patients often report that it was the missing link in helping them reduce pain, boost energy, improve moods, increase mental clarity, and restore deep restorative sleep. Sounds pretty amazing huh? Unlike some multilevel "latest and greatest" fad supplements, I find that SAMe consistently helps my patients feel better. So I've been recommending it more and more often. If it's what you need, it will work rather quickly, within hours, to reduce many of your pain symptoms and help boost mental and physical energy. It also serves as a potent antidepressant and helps the liver work more effectively.

Before starting on SAMe, take the Brain Function Questionnaire in chapter 16. If it reveals a deficiency in norepinephrine and/or dopamine, then SAMe is likely for you.

SAMe plays a role in the immune system, maintains cell membranes, and helps produce and break down serotonin, melatonin, dopamine, and vitamin B12. Powerful substances in the body called catecholamines (linked with mood and stress response) depend on SAMe in order to function effectively. SAMe is also needed by the pineal gland in the brain to properly synthesize melatonin from 5-HTP.

You can read in chapter 16 about how SAMe boosts the energy-producing neurotransmitters norepinephrine and dopamine; these two brain chemicals also help reduce pain. SAMe also increases the production of endorphins, the bodies natural pain-blocking chemicals, more powerful than morphine. Several studies involving SAMe and fibromyalgia patients yielded substantial improvement in overall pain levels, sleep, and mood.

Until recently, SAMe was exceedingly expensive to produce. Fortunately prices have come down, but high-quality very potent SAMe, which comes from Italy, is still rather expensive: around $50.00 for a month's supply. Cheaper SAMe, most of which comes from China or India, is readily available. But beware, because you get what you pay for. In this case, trying to save a few dollars doesn't make sense. Studies have shown that cheaper SAMe knockoffs may only contain about 50% of the active compound. SAMe is highly unstable and needs to be enteric coated and kept in a moderate-temperature storage facility. The SAMe I use is straight from Italy and pharmaceutical grade. I think this is why I'm getting such good results.

To take SAMe, start with 200 mg. on an empty stomach (30 minutes before or 90 minutes after eating). If you don't see an improvement in your mental and physical energy, increase your dose by 200 mg. each day—up to 1200 mg.—until you do. You can take SAMe in divided doses if needed, but always on an empty stomach. Don't take it past 3:00 p.m. as it may interfere with your sleep.

Potential side effects of SAMe include increased heart rate and blood pressure, dry eyes, and dry mouth. While my patients rarely report problems with taking SAMe, even those with mildly elevated blood pressure should use it cautiously and under the care of a health care professional familiar with SAMe.

DL-PHENYLALANINE

DL-phenylalanine, otherwise known as DLPA, is a combination of the D and L forms of the amino acid phenylalanine. DL-phenylalanine acts as a natural pain reliever by blocking the enzymes responsible for the breakdown of endorphins and enkaphalins, substances within the body that help relieve pain. Endorphins, morphine-like proteins, also act as appetite suppressants and mild stimulants.

Although caution is advised for individuals with high blood pressure, DL-phenylalanine is an effective supplement in treating musculoskeletal pains, including those associated with FMS. Many of my fibromyalgia patients have benefited from DL-phenylalanine. A clinical study shows subjects taking DL-phenylalanine had a remarkable improvement in their condition: improvements were seen in 73% of low-back pain suffers, 67% with migraines, 81% with osteoarthritis, and 81% with rheumatoid arthritis.

For pain control, or as an antidepressant, take 1,000–4,000 mg. of DL-phenylalanine twice daily on an empty stomach. Phenylalanine can elevate blood pressure, and very high doses can cause rapid heart rate. So start with a low dose and increase to a higher one only as needed—and only if no side effects are noticed. I typically recommend DL-phenylalanine when a patient scores high in the opioid ("O") section of the Brain Function Questionnaire, which is included in the next chapter.

TAKING SAMe WITH DL-PHENYLALANINE

I don't combine DL-phenylalanine with SAMe initially, opting instead to start with SAMe and then add DL-phenylalanine if needed. In this case, the dosage is 400–800 mg. of SAMe in the morning and 400–800 mg. of DL-phenylalanine in the afternoon.

TREATING CHRONIC INFLAMMATION

While inflammation hasn't been found to be the cause of fibromyalgia pain, the majority of my patients have one or more types of inflammation that contribute to their chronic pain.

> ### A Vitamin D Connection
>
> Low vitamin D levels have also been associated with chronic pain. For more information, see chapter 26. Everyone with fibromyalgia should supplement vitamin D, but if your pain persists, consider having your vitamin D levels checked. Your doctor can order a blood test for 25-hydroxy vitamin D.

Inflammation may be due to arthritis, elevated substance-P levels, autoimmune reactions, scar tissue, lactic acid buildup, allergic reactions, leaky gut, intestinal dysbiosis, sensitivity to nightshade plants, deficient serotonin, or poor detoxification processes. In these cases, patients may find it difficult to find and successfully treat the sources of their chronic pain, despite employing the jump-start plan. If this is your story, you may have osteoarthritis or rheumatoid arthritis in addition to your fibromyalgia pain; many of my patients do.

HOW THE INFLAMMATORY SYSTEM WORKS

Trauma, infection, reduced blood flow, toxins, poisons, and normal wear-and-tear cause damage and destruction to cells. This damage then triggers an inflammatory response by the body's self-regulating mechanisms. Hormones called inflammatory prostaglandins (PG-2) cause blood vessels to dilate, and the area becomes hot, red, and swollen. The healthy tissue surrounding the damaged area releases anti-inflammatory prostaglandins (PG-1 and PG-3) to combat the inflammatory prostaglandins. White blood cells begin to attack and digest damaged cells, until the proteolytic enzymes tell them that their job is done. As the damaged tissue is removed, less of the pro-inflammatory chemicals and more of the anti-inflammatory chemicals are released. Once the inflammation process is finished, the body begins to repair itself.

The balance between inflammation, destruction, and repair is an ongoing process. Normally, this process is kept in check. When it becomes unbalanced, chronic inflammation is the result.

WHAT IS ARTHRITIS?

Over 50 million Americans suffer from arthritis and its symptoms of pain, stiffness, inflammation, and decreased range of motion.

Rheumatoid arthritis (RA) is an autoimmune disease in which the body actually attacks itself and antibodies develop in joint tissues and cause pain. Women are three times more likely to develop this arthritis than are men. It usually affects the knuckles, wrists, elbows, and shoulders with painful, warm, red swelling.

Osteoarthritis (OA), also known as degenerative joint disease, is the most common of the over 100 forms of arthritis. It occurs when wear and tear of the bony cartilage of the body causes bone spurs or calcium deposits to form on the ligaments surrounding the joint. This leads to inflammation, pain, and decreased joint motion. Over 40 million Americans have OA. Many of my patients can trace the onset of their OA to a car accident, but some don't remember anything that could be causing their neck or low back pain. Some develop it from repetitive motions, poor posture, or from simply carrying more weight than their joints can handle. Heredity also plays a role in osteoarthritis.

OA is characterized by early morning stiffness or pain that eases up as the day goes on, only to return again in the evening. It generally affects the joints of the knees, hands, feet, and spine, and it develops gradually over several years. It usually doesn't cause joint redness, warmth, or swelling like RA does.

Conventional treatments for RA and OA leave much to be desired, to say the least. Short-term use of NSAIDs and analgesics to cover up symptoms is acceptable; long-term use, however, increases the risk of heart attack, stroke, bone destruction, intestinal permeability, yeast overgrowth, ulcers, and internal bleeding. Corticosteroids have serious side effects, including ulcers, osteoporosis, diabetes, glaucoma, and hypertension. The immune-suppressing drug Methotrexate is a toxic therapy that can cause kidney failure and severe liver damage. Gold injections can cause damage to the liver and kidneys, stomach disorders, anemia, headache, neuritis, and ulcerations of the mouth and gums. So how do you find safe relief?

PROTOCOL FOR TREATING RA AND OA

You should be starting with my jump-start program, so some of these steps (1, 5, and 6, specifically) should already be in place.

1. Correct any intestinal permeability. See Appendix C for intestinal-permeability testing, or treat without testing (see chapter 12), especially if you've been on NSAIDs for long periods. Individuals with intestinal permeability are further prone towards developing arthritis, as fragments of intestinal bacteria are allowed to penetrate into the joints. These bacteria fragments may cause the body to release antibodies, which then attack the joint tissue—a typical autoimmune response typical of RA.

RA was absent in prehistory, when cereals and dairy products were not part of a daily diet. In 1992, the *Lancet* reported that "the frequency of gut mucosal lesions and excessive permeability of the intestinal wall found in rheumatoid arthritis patients today suggests that enterocyte enzymes are not adapted for modern food in most patients." Basically, our bodies are not adjusting quickly enough to account for our increasingly junky diet.

2. Strongly consider food allergy testing. Allergies can contribute to a wide range of diseases and certainly have been linked to arthritis. See chapter 18 for more information about allergies.

3. Avoid nightshade foods. These include tobacco, eggplant, bell peppers, tomatoes, and white potatoes. Nightshade (family: *Solana-*

ceae) foods have been linked to an increase in arthritis symptoms. In one study, 70% of those with arthritis reported relief from chronic pain over a period of seven years after eliminating all nightshade foods. Between 20% and 30% of my patients on this regimen experience moderate to dramatic pain relief. They typically report less pain overall but especially in their hands, feet, knees, and ankles.

4. Eat to reduce inflammation. The pro-inflammatory hormone PG-2 is made from arachidonic acid (AA). (See chapter 29 for more about this fatty acid). Since AA is found in corn, and corn products are used as the prominent foodstuff for westernized livestock, red meat, cheese, eggs, and pork products have a high AA content in the United States.

Several research articles have demonstrated that the more animal fats a human eats, the more AA is in his blood and cell membranes and the more likely he is to have inflammation. So reduce your intake of grains, vegetable and seed oils, and corn-fed livestock. If your inflammation is severe, reduce or avoid red meat and dairy as well. Cook with olive oil or canola oil. (Avoid instant coffee, as well. It contains substances that block the receptor sites for endorphins.)

The functional opposite of PG-2, PG-1 and PG-3 are anti-inflammatory hormones. They help reduce and eliminate inflammation and pain. You should increase your intake of these hormones. The best sources of PG-1 and PG-3 are fish oil supplements or a diet high in cold-water fish. This leads us to number 5 in the protocol.

5. Supplement with 3–9 g. of fish oil (EPA/DHA) daily for at least 12 weeks. Some studies have shown that supplementing with fish oils results in a dramatic reduction in a person's leukotrienes (one of the chemicals implicated in asthma and other allergic reactions) by 65%. This correlates with a 75% decrease in their clinical symptoms. Another fish-oil study gave rheumatoid arthritis sufferers 1.8 grams of EPA fish oil daily while reducing their saturated fats (from land animal foods). The subjects showed significant improvement over those who took a placebo. Further, Greenland Eskimos, who naturally consume high amounts of fish oil, rarely develop arthritis. You should already be getting fish oil if you are taking the CFS/Fibro Formula.

6. Supplement with digestive enzymes—HCL or pancreatic enzymes—with each meal. Arthritis patients are typically low in several nutrients, especially zinc. Many are not digesting their food properly due to low stomach-acid levels. See more about digestive enzymes in chapter 12.

7. Take my specially formulated Inflammation Formula (for RA) or Arthro Formula (for OA) twice daily. You should see improvement in three to four weeks. Treatment should continue for a minimum of three months and, since there are little or no side effects, long-term therapy is advisable.

The **Inflammation Formula** contains:

- **Turmeric root extract:** Inhibits enzymes associated with PG-2 inflammatory hormones
- **Rosemary leaf extract:** Helps block synthesis of leukotrienes (a cause of allergic inflammation) and PG-2. Stimulates phase-II liver detoxification
- **Holy basil leaf extract:** Helps boost natural anti-inflammatory chemicals PG-1 and PG-3
- **Green tea leaf extract:** Increases the body's own anti-inflammatory activity and is a potent antioxidant
- **Ginger root extract:** Reduces inflammation and helps regulate inflammatory systems
- **Chinese goldenthread root:** Reduces activity of PG-2 (the bad guy) and boosts function of PG-1 and PG-3 (the good guys)
- **Barberry root extract:** Helps regulate prostaglandins
- **Baikal skullcap root extract:** Reduces inflammatory chemicals, including PG-2
- **Protykin polygonum cuspidatum extract:** Reduces inflammatory chemicals, including PG-2, and is a potent antioxidant

The Arthro Formula contains:
- **Glucosamine and chondroitin:** help eliminate the pain and stiffness of osteoarthritis. A Portugal study involving 1,208 patients and 252 physicians showed it to be quite effective. Studies in

Italy showed that glucosamine reduced arthritis symptoms by one half in 73% of the group, and 20% enjoyed total symptom relief. In one study of patients with OA of the knee, those patients who were administered glucosamine had an 80% reduction in pain. Other studies have demonstrated glucosamine to be more effective than ibuprofen (Motrin, Advil, or Nuprin) in relieving the symptoms of OA—without the side effects. More importantly, **glucosamine and chondroitin sulfate actually slow or even arrest destruction of cartilage.** Glucosamine actually helps repair damaged articular joint tissue. It stimulates cells within the cartilage to produce more proteoglycans, which form a protective netting within the cartilage, helping to prevent its destruction. Chondroitin attracts fluid into the proteoglycan molecules, and this fluid acts as a shock absorber. It also inhibits certain enzymes that can damage cartilage, while stimulating the healthy new cartilage growth. A study conducted in France showed that patients who received three months of chondroitin therapy had actually repaired a significant portion of their degenerated joint tissues.

- **Boswellia:** reduces pain and inflammation. One of the oldest herbs in Indian medicine, it helps shrink inflamed tissue, build cartilage, increase blood supply, and repair damaged blood vessels.

- **Bromelain:** blocks inflammatory chemicals and digests excess fibrin, a chemical implicated in osteoarthritis. Bromelain needs to be taken on an empty stomach.

- **Curcumin/Turmeric:** relieves pain like hydrocortisone does but without the side effects. It is a popular arthritis remedy in India and a powerful pain-relieving anti-inflammatory.

- **Devil's Claw:** acts as a potent anti-inflammatory and pain reliever. A perennial vine native to South Africa, it has been shown very effective in relieving lower back pain and associated sciatica.

8. Exercise to keep the joints moving. Walking on a daily basis helps keep you limber and fit. Many of the back-pain patients that I see are shocked to discover that they can severely reduce or eliminate the back problems they've had for years by simply walking 30–60 minutes a day. If you have ankle, knee, or hip problems, then use a stationary bike or elliptical machine—or better yet, a pool. I would also recommend a beginner's course in yoga or Pilates.

Susan was a very active 50 year-old nurse who often spent hours on her feet while she attended patients. She visited my office with the complaint that her low-back and knee pain had become chronic over the last few years. Her low-back pain had recently become worse and out of desperation, she came to see me as a last resort before agreeing to surgery.

I began weekly chiropractic adjustments to her low back. I also prescribed glucosamine sulfate along with some other nutritional supplements. In three weeks, she reported that she was now completely free of the low-back pain that had plagued her for years. The arthritis pain in her knee, which she had also endured for many years, was nearly gone too.

9. Try your best to lose excess weight. Losing weight can provide dramatic relief to those with OA of the knees and hips. That's because these joints bear loads up to 10 times your weight. For a 200-pound individual, this can translate to one ton of pressure.

10. Consider treating for hypothyroid (see more about this in chapter 14). Patients with hypothyroid have been shown to be at increased risk of developing osteoarthritis.

11. Pursue chiropractic adjustments for OA. Chiropractic has helped millions of Americans with OA every year. Deep tissue massage can also help relieve aching, locked, or immobile joints. When combined together, these two disciplines are extremely successful in reducing and arresting the ravages of OA.

12. Consider these other treatments. Though not as widely successful as glucosamine and chondroitin, these supplements have offered great relief for some.

• **Niacin (vitamin B3)** may decrease the pain associated with OA, especially in the knee. Begin with 100 mg. daily, and slowly increase until one gram can be tolerated three times daily. Use timed-release niacin to avoid flushing. But high doses, even of timed-release niacin can cause nausea, flushing, and elevated liver enzymes. But the elevated enzymes are not really a concern, according to Abram Hoffer, MD, author of numerous books on medicine and the use of niacin therapy.

• **Shark cartilage extracts** may also be beneficial for arthritic symptoms. Several double-blind experiments have shown that individuals who use cartilage extract therapy can see a significant improvement in pain and stiffness. This may be because animal cartilage contains a protein that inhibits tumor growth.

- **D-ribose** helps to increase depleted ATP levels in the body. ATP (adenosine triphosphate) is the body's primary source of energy. It is used by the mitochondria—the body's "cellular power plants," tiny organelles found within each cell—to fuel that cell's energy. **Chronic stress on cells can result in low ATP levels.** When this happens to muscle cells, they can become tight, rigid, and prone to spasm. Studies show that patients with fibromyalgia and CFS have up to 20% less energy in their muscle cells than normal.[1] Without proper energy, the muscles can become tighter and tighter, unable to relax. Muscle fatigue and pain then follow. **B vitamins, magnesium, CoQ10, malic acid, essential fatty acids, and D-ribose all help to boost mitochondrial function and ATP levels.** D-ribose is a five-carbon sugar that all cells need to make ATP. Our bodies make D-ribose from the foods we eat, but the process is slow and laborious. When blood flow and oxygen levels are compromised, as with chronic illness, D-ribose levels become depleted. **D-ribose levels may help restore natural muscle cell energy and function.** A small open study conducted with 41 patients showed that 5 grams of powdered D-ribose three times a day for three weeks and then 5 grams twice daily thereafter led to substantial improvement for 66% of participants.[2] **Personally, I've seen mixed results with patients taking D-ribose.** Some have seen their energy levels increase and pain levels decrease. Others have found little benefit. I recommend trying D-ribose, however, if other therapies have failed to reduce your pain.

- **The Fibromyalgia/CFS Jump-Start Program** certainly can't hurt, even if you are diagnosed only with arthritis. It contains B vitamins, magnesium, and malic acid, all which perform critical roles in the development of ATP. Malic acid helps improve energy production by reversing oxygen depletion of muscle cells. Supplementation of malic acid elevates mitochondrial function and production.

- **CoQ10,** as mentioned, is also essential for proper cellular energy levels. You can supplement with it as directed in chapter 19.

If you are suffering from arthritis, don't let anyone tell you that there is no hope except to cover up your symptoms for the rest of your life. Be proactive, and have the tests done for allergies, intestinal permeability, and hypothyroid. Then clean up your diet, exercise daily, and enjoy the good health you desire and deserve.

NOTES
1. A. Bengtson and K.G. Henriksson, "The Muscle in Fibromyalgia: A Review of Swedish Studies," *Journal of Rheumatology* (supp.) 19 (1989): 144–8.
2. J.E. Teitelbaum et al., "The Use of D-ribose in Chronic Fatigue Syndrome and Fibromyalgia: A Pilot Study," *Journal of Alternative and Complementary Medicine* 12(9) (2006): 857–62.

FOR FURTHER READING AND RESEARCH
- G.E. Abraham and J.D.Flechas, "Hypothesis: management of fibromyalgia: rationale for the use of magnesium and malic acid," *J Nutr Med* 3 (1992): 49–59.
- P. Bendetto et al.,"Clinical evaluation of s-adenosyl-L-methionine versus transcutaneous electrical nerve stimulation in primary fibromyalgia," *Current Ther Res* 53(2) (1993): 22.
- J.H. Bland and S.M. Cooper, "Osteoarthritis: a review of the cell biology involved and evidence for reversibility. Management rationally related to known genesis and pathophysiology," *Sem Arth Rheum* 14 (1984): 106–133.
- T. Bottiglieri, "Folate, vitamin B12, and neuropsychiatric disorders," *Nutr Rev* 54(12) (1996): 382–90.
- T. Bottiglieri et al., "The clinical potential of ademetionine (S-denosylmethionine) in neurological disorders," *Drugs* 48(2) (1994): 137–52.
- L.R. Brady et al., *Pharmacognosy* (8th edn) (Philadelphia; Lea and Febiger, 1981).
- P.M. Brooks PMet al., "NSAID and osteoarthritis: help or hinderence," *J Rheum* 9 (1982): 3–5.
- R.A. Brown and J.B. Weiss, "Shark cartilage reduces joint destruction by inhibiting neovascularization: Neovascularization and its role in the osteoarthritic process," *Ann Rheum Dis* 47(11) (1988): 881–5.
- L.G. Cleland et al., "Clinical and biochemical effects of fish oil supplementation in rheumatoid arthritis," *J Rheumatol* 15 (1988): 1471–5.
- A. Cohen and J. Goldman, "Bromelain therapy in rheumatoid arthritis." *Penn Med J* 67 (1964): 27–30.
- B.M. Cohen et al., "S-adenosyl-L-methionine in the treatment of Alzheimer's disease," *J Clin Psychopharmacol* 8 (1988): 43–7.

- C.A. Cooney et al., "Methylamphetamine treatment affects blood and liver S-adeno-sylmethionine (SAM) in mice: Correlation with dopamine depletion in the striatum," *Ann N Y Acad Sci* 844 (1998): 191–200.
- L.G. Darlington LG. Ramsey NW, and Mansfield JR. "Placebo-controlled, blind study of dietary manipulation therapy in rheumatoid arthritis," *Lancet* (1986): 236–8.
- M. Donowitz, "Arachidonic acid metabolites and their role in inflammatory bowel disease," *Gastroenterology* 88 (1985): 580–7.
- C. di Pavoda, "S-adenosylmethionine in the treatment of osteoarthritis. Review of clinical studies," *Am J Med* 83(suppl 5A) (1987): 60–5.
- M. Fava et al., "Rapidity of onset of the antidepressant effect of parenteral S-adenosyl-L-methionine," *Psych Res* 56(3) (1995): 295–7.
- J. Folkman et al., "Induction of angiogenesis during the transition from hyperplasia to neoplasia," *Nature* 339 (1995): 58–61.
- A. Ford-Hutchison, "Leukotrienes their formation and role as inflammatory mediators," *Re Proc* 44 (1985): 25–9.
- M.D. Galland, "Leaky gut syndromes: breaking the vicious cycle," The Third International Symposium on Functional Medicine, Vancouver, B.C., 1996.
- G. Gatto et al., "Analgesizing effect of a methyl donor (S-adenosylmethionine) in migraine: an open clinical trial," *Int J Clin Pharmacol Res* 6 (1986):15–17.
- S. Glorioso et al., "Double-blind multicentre study of the activity of S-adeno-sylmethionine in hip and knee osteoarthritis," *Int J Clin Pharm Res* 5 (1985): 39–49.
- M. Grasseto and A. Varotto, "Primary fibromyalgia is responsive to S-adensyl-L-methionine," *Curr Ther Res* 55(7) (1994): 797–806.
- W. Grossman and H. Schmidramsyl, *Alt Med Rev* 6(3) (June 2001): 303–10.
- M.F. Harmand et al., "Effects of S-adenosylmethionine on human articular chondrocyte differentiation. An in vitro study," *Am J Med* 83(5A) (1987): 48–54.
- E.F. Hartung and O. Steinbrocker, "Gastric acidity in chronic arthritis," *Ann Intern Med* 9 (1935): 252–7.
- S. Jacobsen et al., "Oral Sadenosylmethionine in primary fibromyalgia. Double-blind clinical evaluation," *Scand J Rheumatol* 20 (1991): 294–302.
- J. Kremer et al., "Effects of manipulation of dietary fatty acids on clinical manifestation of rheumatoid arthritis," *Lancet* i (1985): 184–7.
- R. Langer et al., "Isolations of a cartilage factor that inhibits tumor neovascularization from cartilage," *Science* 193 (1976): 70–2.
- G.M. Laudanno, "Cytoprotective effect of S-adenosylmethionine compared with that of misoprostol against ethanol-, aspirin-, and stress-induced gastric damage," *Am J Med* 83(5A) (1987): 43–7.
- L.J. Leventhal, "Management of fibromyalgia," *Ann Intern Med* 131 (1999): 850–8.
- C.S. Lieber, "Hepatic, metabolic, and nutritional disorders of alcoholism: from pathogenesis to therapy," *Crit Rev Clin Lab Sci* 37(6) (2000): 551–84.

- C.S. Lieber, "Role of oxidative stress and antioxidant therapy in alcoholic and nonalcoholic liver diseases," *Adv Pharmacol* 38 (1997): 601–28.
- C. Loguercio et al., "Effect of S-adenosyl-L-methionine administration on red blood cell cysteine and glutathione levels in alcoholic patients with and without liver disease," *Alcohol* 29(5) (1994): 597–604.
- A. Maccagno et al., "Double-blind controlled clinical trial of oral S-adenosyl-methionine versus piroxicam in knee osteoarthritis," *Am J Med* 83(suppl 5A) (1987): 72–7.
- M. Mandell and A.A. Conte, "The role of allergy in arthritis, rheumatism and polysymptomatic cerebral, visceral and somatic disorders: a double-blind study," *J Int Acad Prev Med* (July 1982): 5–16.
- J.M. Mato et al., "S-adenosylmethionine in alcoholic liver cirrhosis: a randomized, placebo-controlled, double-blind, multicenter clinical trial," *J Hepatol* 30 (1999): 1081–9.
- L.D. Morrison et al., "Brain S-adenosylmethione levels are severely decreased in Alzheimer's disease," *J Neurochem* 67 (1996): 1328–31.
- H. Müller-Fassbender "Double-blind clinical trial of s-adenosylmethionine versus ibuprofen in the treatment of osteoarthritis," *Am J Med* 83(suppl 5A) (1987): 81–3.
- E. Munthe et al.,"Trace elements and rheumatoid arthritis: pathogenetic and therapeutic aspects," *Acta Pharmacol Toxicol* (Copenh) 59 (Suppl 7) (1986): 365–73.
- W. Najm et al., "S-adenosyl methionine (SAMe) versus celecoxib for the treatment of osteoarthritis symptoms: A double-blind cross-over trial," *BMC Musculoskeletal Disorders* 5 (2004): 6.
- D. Palevitch et al., "Feverfew as a prophylactic treatment for migraine: a double-blind placebo controlled study," *Phytotherapy Research* (UK) 11/7 (1997): 508–11.
- S.P. Pandley et al., "Zinc in rheumatoid arthritis," *Indian Jour of Med Res* 81 (1985): 618–20.
- R.S. Panush, "Delayed reactions to foods. Food allergy and rheumatic disease," *Annals of Allergy* 56 (1986): 500–3.
- C.K. Reddy et al., "Studies on the metabolism of glycosaminoglycans under the influence of new herbal anti-inflammatory agents," *Biochemical Pharm* 20 (1989): 3527–34.
- Rozen TD et al.,"Open label trial of CoQ10 as migraine preventative," Thomas Jefferson University Headache Center.
- R. Scimal and B. Dhawan, "Pharmacology of diferuloyl methane (curcumin), a non-steroidal anti-inflammatory agent," *J Pharm Pharmac* 25 (1973): 447–52.
- M.J. Shield, "Anti-inflammatory drugs and their effects on cartilage synthesis and renal function," *Eur J Rheumatol Inflam* 13 (1993): 7–16.
- P.A. Simkin, "Oral zinc sulphate in rheumatoid arthritis," *Lancet* 2 (1976): 539–42.

- G.B. Singh and C.K. Atal, "Pharmacology of abextract of salai guggal ex-Boswellia serrate, a new non-steroidal anti-inflammatory agent," *Agents Action* (1986): 407–12.
- W.F. Stevenson et al., "Dietary supplementation with fish oil in ulcerative colitis," *Ann Int Med* 11 (1992): 609–14.
- M.J. Tapadinhas et al., "Oral glucosamine sulfate in the management of arthrosis. Report on a multi-centre open investigation in Portugal," *Pharmatherapeutica* 3 (1982): 157–68.
- A. Tavoni et al., "Evaluation of S-adenosylmethionine in primary fibromyalgia: A double-blind crossover study," *Am J Med* 83(5A) (1987): 107–10.
- A.L. Vaz, "Double-blind clinical evaluation of the relative efficacy of ibuprofen and glucosamine sulfate in the management of osteoarthritis of the knee in out patients," *Current Medical Research and Opinion* 8 (1982): 145–9.

· 16 ·
DEPRESSION AND OTHER MOOD DISORDERS

Have you been told by doctors that you're depressed?
Well, your symptoms weren't caused by your depression,
but who with your illness wouldn't be depressed?

Mental fatigue, anxiety, depression and "fibro-fog" are common complaints among individuals with FMS or CFS. Although they may in fact be depressed, their depression is not the cause of their FMS/CFS but rather a consequence of having a misunderstood chronic illness.

CONVENTIONAL TREATMENTS

Individuals who consult a family doctor for anxiety or depression usually receive a prescription antidepressant. And while prescription drugs have helped millions of people overcome mental illnesses, their side effects can cause an assortment of health problems. And they often work little better—if better at all—than placebos. Studies show that up to 70% of those taking a placebo fare as well as those on a prescription antidepressant.

Some individuals do experience improvement for a period of time but then notice they need to take higher doses of the drug. Or they are changed to another antidepressant medication altogether. And this dreadful situation should come as no surprise to the scientific community. Studies have revealed that prescription antidepressants actually *reduce* the brain's serotonin receptor cells, and this gets worse the longer a person is on such a medication. Reduced serotonin receptors means reduced ability to take in necessary serotonin. This cycle continues, and once the person's serotonin stores are all used up, she's left to try yet another antidepressant.

THE EVOLUTION OF
MOOD-DISORDER WONDER DRUGS

Prior to the 20th century, mood disorders and mental illnesses were treated with a variety of obscure and often barbaric methods including frontal lobotomies (with no anesthesia), exorcisms, and shamanistic potions.

Dr. Benjamin Rush, the father of American psychiatry, was the first to believe that mental illness is a disease of the mind and not a possession of demons. His classic work, *Observations and Inquiries upon the Diseases of the Mind,* published in 1812, promoted the belief that "madness" was an arterial disease, an inflammation of the brain.

Dr. Rush wrote that as much as "four-fifths of the blood in the body" should be drawn away. Rush bled one patient 47 times, removing four gallons of blood over time. He confined others in his "tranquilizer chair," which completely immobilized every part of their body for long periods and blocked their sight with a bizarre wooden shroud—all while they were doused in ice-cold water.

In the early 1900s, frontal lobotomies and electric-shock therapy were standard fair. Insulin-coma therapy was introduced into psychiatry in 1933. And within a few years, every psychiatric clinic in Germany was practicing insulin-coma therapy, using insulin to induce coma in a patient and then glucose to revive him. The practice received much praise. Unfortunately, it was also associated with a high mortality rate.

In 1954, the first "modern" sedative drug—known as Thorazine and fueled by a huge promotion campaign by Smith, Klein & French—swept the nation. This new medication, along with Haldol, spawned an additional class of drugs known as benzodiazepines (tranquilizers). The effect of taking these drugs was explicitly compared to having a lobotomy, and they were thought to induce "chemical lobotomies." Thorazine became the drug *du jour* during the 1950s; the number of individuals taking it went from 428 in 1952 to over 2,000,000 in 1957.

In the 1960s, Hoffman La Roche were successful in marketing the benzodiazepines (tranquilizers) Librium and Valium. Benzodiazepines became a frequent recommendation for any number of illnesses associated with mental stress. In fact, these drugs became known as "mother's little helper."

To combat the ills of modern-day stress, housewives, college students, and busy executives were encouraged to take these medications. Valium became the best-selling drug at that time. Klonopin, Ativan, and Xanax followed, all hailed as safer and more effective than the anti-anxiety drugs that preceded them. Unfortunately, all of these drugs work about the same and have similar side effects (read more about benzodiazepines in chapter 6).

In the 1960s Merck introduced the tricyclic antidepressant drug Amitriptyline (Elavil). Tricyclic drugs were promoted as safer and more effective than benzodiazepines. Initially all the rage, they quickly fell out of favor (read about their side effects in chapter 6) when the newer—supposedly safer, but largely overhyped—selective serotonin re-uptake inhibitors (SSRIs) became available.

The first SSRI to hit the American market was Prozac in 1987. It was quickly hailed as the wonder drug of the 20th century. But like so many of our "wonder drugs," Prozac and the rest of the SSRI drugs haven't live up to our dreams. The popularity of these medications is largely due to the false belief that SSRIs are safe and have relatively few risks. However, their side effects can be unbearable. Read more about them in chapter 6, too.

In December of 2006, the FDA warned that SSRI drugs cause increased chances of suicide in young adults. Suicide occurs more than twice as much on antidepressants than on sugar pills in individuals under age 25. Prozac alone has been associated with over 1,734 suicide deaths and over 28,000 adverse reactions. And to top it all off, studies show that up to 70% of those taking antidepressant medications do just as well by taking a placebo or sugar pill.

The newest class of "wonder drugs" for mood disorders are known as atypical antipsychotics. They include Zyprexa, Risperdal, Geodon, Ivega, Abilify, Clozril, and Seroquel. Originally used for schizophrenia and bipolar patients, atypicals have now become routine in the treatment of ADD, anxiety, depression, and Alzheimer's.

They're being marketed as safer and more effective than the older antipsychotic benzodiazepines. Of course, like their predecessors, they come with a steep cost: atypicals cost some 20 times more than do the older psychotic drugs. The FDA has gone on record warning that there's no proof that these drugs are safer or better and that any advertisement that promotes this is false. No problem. Even though they couldn't promote their drugs they way they wanted, the drug companies could and did hire academics and doctors to recommend them.

In an attempt to squelch the debate, the U.S. government funded a $60-million study in 2005 called CATIE (Clinical Antipsychotic Trials of Intervention Effectiveness). The study concluded that atypicals were generally no more effective than the older drug perphenazine (similar to Haldol) and that slightly fewer people on atypicals dropped out of the study due to tremors. But the atypicals had their own distinct side effects: weight gain and high blood sugar.

According to Harvard-trained psychiatrist Stefan Kruszewski, "the new generation of antipsychotics substantially increase the risk of obesity, diabetes type-2, hypertension, cardiovascular complications, heart attacks, and stroke." Persons on atypicals have been found to commit suicide 2–5 times more frequently than the schizophrenic population in general. Other potential side effects include tardive dyskinesia, low blood pressure (seen as dizziness and possibly fainting), increased heart beat, seizures, liver problems, difficulty swallowing, sleepiness, dry mouth, dizziness, restlessness, constipation, upset stomach, weight gain, increased appetite, and tremor.

I can't wait to see what the next "safer, more effective" antipsychotic drug is, can you? One in three doctor visits by women now involve a prescription for an antidepressant medication. And one in 10 American women take at least one antidepressant drug. Americans now spend more money on antidepressants than the gross national product of two-thirds of the world's countries.

The indirect and direct costs of mood-disorder illnesses total over 43 billion dollars a year. Depression and related mood disorders rank only behind high blood pressure as the most common reason people visit their doctors.

As much as 10% of the U.S. population has taken one of these medications. The largest increase in antidepressant use has been among preschoolers, aged 2–4. In 2003, over one million American children were taking an antidepressant medication.[1]

A NATURAL, NUTRITIONAL ALTERNATIVE

Fortunately for those looking for a safer, often more effective way to beat mood disorders, a group of progressive-minded physicians helped pioneer a new way of treating mental disorders known as **orthomolecular medicine.** (Read more about it in chapter 7).

In 1968, two times Nobel-Prize winner Linus Pauling originated the term "orthomolecular" to describe an approach to medicine that uses naturally occurring substances normally present in the body. "Ortho" means correct or normal, and orthomolecular physicians recognize that in many cases of physiological and psychological disorders, health can be reestablished by properly correcting (normalizing) the balance of vitamins, minerals, amino acids, and other similar substances within the body. **And unlike drug therapy, which attempts to cover up the symptoms associated with a mood disorder, orthomolecular medicine seeks to find and correct the cause of the illness.**

Amino-Acid and Nutritional Therapy: Neurotransmitters are produced from the amino acids in the foods we eat. Certain amino acids, along with B vitamins and minerals, make up these neurotransmitters. The neurotransmitters that cause excitatory reactions are known as catecholamines. The atecholamines epinephrine and norepinephrine (adrenaline) are derived from the amino acid phenylalanine and from tyrosine. The inhibitory (relaxing) neurotransmitter serotonin is produced from the amino acid tryptophan.

Essential Fatty Acids: Essential for our existence, these can not be manufactured by the body but must be obtained from the foods we eat. Essential fatty acids are made-up of polyunsaturated fatty acids (PUFAs). Research shows that the low blood levels of omega 3 essential fatty acids are associated with depression.[2]

Thyroid Hormones: Stress, depression, anxiety, and fatigue are all associated with low thyroid function. Thyroid hormones help regulate concentration, mental clarity, moods, and proper brain chemistry. Triiodothyronine (T3), one of the thyroid hormones, regulates the levels and actions of the brain chemicals serotonin, norepinephrine, and gamma-amino butyric acid (GABA). Serotonin is decreased when T3 levels become deficient, a more common occurrence than might be suspected.[3]

YOUR NEUROTRANSMITTERS

Neurotransmitters are brain chemicals that help relay electrical messages from one nerve cell to another. They are produced from **amino acids** (which we get from protein); vitamins B6, B3, and C; and the mineral magnesium. Amino acids, then, are the raw nutrients needed to manufacture the neurotransmitters.

Neurotransmitters help regulate pain, reduce anxiety, promote happiness, initiate deep sleep, and boost energy and mental clarity. **Excitatory** (stimulating) neurotransmitters include epinephrine and norepinephrine (adrenaline). **Inhibitory** (relaxing) neurotransmitters include serotonin and gamma-aminobutyric acid (GABA).

Serotonin, from the amino acid tryptophan (5-HTP), elevates mood, reduces food cravings, increases pain threshold, improves mental clarity, reduces IBS symptoms, promotes deep sleep, relieves tension, and calms the body.

Dopamine and norepinephrine are synthesized from the amino acid phenylalanine. They increase mental and physical alertness, reduce fatigue, and elevate mood.

Epinephrine, also synthesized from phenylalanine, helps increase energy and boost mental clarity. Low levels cause depression and fatigue. Prescription medications like Wellbutrin and Effexor attempt to boost the brain's levels. However, you can simply take L-phenylalanine or SAMe to increase your epinephrine levels.

GABA, formed from the amino acid glutamine, has a calming effect on the brain similar to Valium and other tranquilizers, without the side effects. You may have heard of prescription antidepressants called MAOIs, such as Nardil and Marplan. These work by increasing the effectiveness of GABA. Used in combination with niacinamide (a form of vitamin B3) and inositol (a vitamin-like member of the B complex), GABA can alleviate anxiety and panic attacks. Many of my patients are surprised by the effectiveness of GABA in treating their anxiety and panic attacks.

I've been using amino acid replacement therapy for several years and have treated thousands of patients with mood disorders. I've found this approach to be far superior to prescription medicines (in most cases) for mild to moderate mood disorders. Also over the years, I've used various questionnaires and tests to determine which amino acids need to be recommended for which patients.

BRAIN FUNCTION QUESTIONNAIRE

I've found the following Brain Function Questionnaire to be a quick and accurate assessment of a person's brain chemistry. And I've found very few problems with mixing the recommended supplements with prescription antidepressants. However, I advise you to seek out the guidance of a health professional familiar with orthomolecular medicine to direct your treatment if possible.

THE O GROUP: OPIOIDS

If three or more of these descriptions apply to your present feelings, you are probably part of the "O" group:

• Your life seems incomplete.
• You feel shy with all but your closest friends.
• You have feelings of insecurity.
• You often feel unequal to others.
• When things go right, you sometimes feel undeserving.
• You feel something is missing in your life.
• You occasionally feel a low self-worth or -esteem.
• You feel inadequate as a person.
• You frequently feel fearful when there is nothing to fear.

The "O" Group is named for the **opioid neurotransmitters** contained in the hypothalamus gland. These neurotransmitters have two primary functions:

First, opioids are released in small bursts when we feel a sense of urgency (stress). Some individuals seem to feed off of this adrenaline rush. A sense of urgency can also help us get out of bed in the morning or get the kids off to school. However, if you can never turn this sense of urgency off, you'll eventually deplete the opioids, along with other vital hormones including cortisol and DHEA.

As a way to turn off the constant mind chatter, those in the "O group" use stimulants and mind numbing chemicals (alcohol, marijuana, food, etc.) to escape the constant pressure they place on themselves to be more, do more, have more. These chemicals can temporarily relieve the anxious feelings associated with opioid overload by providing artificial opioids. Unfortunately, these artificial opioids also cause the opioid manufacturing cells in your brain to reduce their output. These cells then lose their ability to produce the needed opioid neurotransmitters. You then crave the artificial opioids, and an addiction has been born.

Second, when you exercise, your body releases extra opioids. This takes away the pain of sore muscles and may provide a feeling of euphoria. The opioids play an important role in pain modulation, so a deficiency of opioids can lower our pain threshold and make us more sensitive to painful stimuli.

DL-phenylalanine (a special form of the amino acid phenylalanine) can be extremely helpful in restoring proper opioid levels. Start with 1,000 mg. of DL-phenylalanine one–two times daily on an empty stomach. If you don't seem to notice any benefits, keep increasing the dose, up to 4,000 mg. twice a day. If you experience a rapid heart beat, agitation, or hyperactivity, reduce or discontinue the DL-phenylalanine. Phenylalanine in any form can increase blood pressure. So if you already have high blood pressure, consult your doctor before taking any form of it. It can be stimulating and should not be taken past 3:00 in the afternoon.

L-glutamine increases the effectiveness of DL-phenylalanine, so when taking DL-phenylalanine, take 500 mg. of L-glutamine one–two times daily on an empty stomach.

Continue to the next page to complete the questionnaire.

THE G GROUP: GABA

If three or more of these descriptions apply to your present feelings, you are probably part of the "G" group:

• You often feel anxious for no reason.
• You sometimes feel "free-floating" anxiety.
• You frequently feel "edgy," and it's difficult to relax.
• You often feel a "knot" in your stomach.
• Falling asleep is sometimes difficult.
• It's hard to turn your mind off when you want to relax.
• You occasionally experience feelings of panic for no reason.
• You often use alcohol or other sedatives to calm down.

The "G" group symptoms are from the absence of the neurotransmitter **gamma-aminobutyric acid (GABA).** GABA is an important neurotransmitter involved in regulating moods and mental clarity. Tranquilizers (Xanax, Ativan, Klonopin, etc.) used to treat anxiety and panic disorders work by increasing GABA.

GABA is made from the amino acid glutamine. Glutamine passes across the blood-brain barrier and helps provide the fuel needed for proper brain function.

L-glutamine supplementation has been shown to increase IQ levels in some mentally deficient children. That's because L-glutamine is brain fuel! It feeds the brain cells, allowing them to fire on all cylinders. That's why a deficiency in L-glutamine can result in foggy thinking and fatigue. Individuals with fibro-fog may benefit tremendously from supplementing this essential amino acid. Even a small shortage of L-glutamine will produce unwarranted feelings of insecurity and anxiousness. Other symptoms include continual fatigue, depression, and occasionally, impotence. A normal dose is 500–1,000 mg. once or twice daily on an empty stomach.

But you can also just supplement directly with GABA. Usually only a small dose is needed, 500–1,000 mg. twice daily. Some individuals may need to take it three–four times a day. Like most amino acids, GABA needs to be taken on an empty stomach.

However, some individuals may not notice much improvement from taking GABA or have unwanted side effects (burning in the stomach or a flushing sensation). For these individuals I recommend the amino acid **L-theanine.** Found also in green tea, it has a calming effect on the brain. It easily crosses the blood-brain barrier and increases the production of GABA. L-theanine also helps boost dopamine. Like GABA supplements, L-theanine doesn't cause drowsiness.

L-theanine has been shown to increase Alpha waves, which are associated meditative states of mind. Individuals taking L-theanine report feeling calm and relaxed. Research with human volunteers has demonstrated that L-theanine creates its relaxing effect in approximately 30 to 40 minutes after ingestion. Recommended dose of L-theanine is 100–200 mg. taken as needed, or 2–3 times a day on an empty stomach.

Continue to the next page to complete the questionnaire.

THE D GROUP: DOPAMINE

If three or more of these descriptions apply to your present feelings, you are probably part of the "D" group:

• You lack pleasure in life.
• You feel there are no real rewards in life.
• You have unexplained lack of concern for others, even loved ones.
• You experience decreased parental feelings.
• Life seems less "colorful" or "flavorful."
• Things that used to be fun aren't any longer enjoyable.
• You have become a less spiritual or socially concerned person.

Dopamine is a neurotransmitter associated with the enjoyment of life: food, arts, nature, your family, friends, hobbies, and other pleasures. Cocaine's (and chocolate's) popularity stems from the fact that it causes very high levels of dopamine to be released in a sudden rush.

A dopamine deficiency can lead to a condition known as anhedonia. Anhedonia is the lack of ability to feel any pleasure or remorse in life. It also reduces the person's attention span. The attention span of a person who has taken cocaine for some time is often reduced to two–three minutes, instead of the usual 50–60 minutes. Learning, for such a person, is nearly impossible.

Brain fatigue, confusion, and lethargy are all by-products of low dopamine.

The brain cells that manufacture dopamine use the amino acid **L-phenylalanine** as raw material. Like most cells in the hypothalamus, they have the ability to produce four–five times their usual output if larger quantities of the raw materials are made available through nutritional supplementation.

Start with 1,000 mg. of L-phenylalanine one–two times daily on an empty stomach. If you don't seem to notice any benefits, keep increasing the dose, up to 4,000 mg. twice a day. If you experience a rapid heart beat, agitation, or hyperactivity, reduce or stop taking L-phenylalanine. L-glutamine increases the effectiveness of L-phenylalanine, so take 500 mg. of L-glutamine one–two times daily on an empty stomach.

Phenylalanine can increase blood pressure. If you already have high blood pressure, consult your doctor before taking any form of it. Phenylalanine can be stimulating and shouldn't be taken past 3:00 in the afternoon.

An alternative to L-phenylalanine is S-adenosyl-methionine (SAMe). It works rather quickly and seems to provide the needed pep that many of my patients are looking for. SAMe has been shown to be as or more effective than tricyclic antidepressant drugs in treating depression. See chapter 15 for a description of using SAMe for pain relief.

Continue to the next page to complete the questionnaire.

THE N GROUP: NOREPINEPHRINE

If three or more of these descriptions apply to your present feelings, you are probably part of the "N" group:

• You suffer from a lack of energy.
• You often find it difficult to "get going."
• You suffer from decreased drive.
• You often start projects and then don't finish them.
• You frequently feel a need to sleep or "hibernate."
• You feel depressed a good deal of the time.
• You occasionally feel paranoid.
• Your survival seems threatened.
• You are bored a great deal of the time.

The neurotransmitter **norepinephrine,** when released in the brain, causes feelings of arousal, energy, and drive. On the other hand, a short supply of it will cause feelings of a lack of ambition, drive, and/or energy. Deficiency can even cause depression, paranoia, and feelings of apathy. Norepinephrine is also used to initiate the flow of adrenaline when you are under psychological stress.

The production of norepinephrine in the hypothalamus is a two-step process. The amino acid L-phenylalanine is first converted into tyrosine. Tyrosine is then converted into nor- epinephrine. Tyrosine, then, can be supplemented to increase norepinephrine (and dopamine). But too much tyrosine can cause headaches, so I usually recommend L-phenylalanine replacement first.

Start with 1,000 mg. of L-phenylalanine one–two times daily on an empty stomach. If you don't seem to notice any benefits, keep increasing the dose, up to 4,000 mg. twice a day. If you experience a rapid heart beat, agitation, or hyperactivity, reduce or stop taking L-phenylalanine. L-glutamine increases the effectiveness of L-phenylalanine, so take 500 mg. of L-glutamine one–two times daily on an empty stomach.

L-phenylalanine can increase blood pressure. If you already have high blood pressure, consult your doctor before taking any form of it. Phenylalanine can be stimulating and shouldn't be taken past 3:00 in the afternoon.

An alternative to L-phenylalanine is S-adenosyl-methionine (SAMe). It works rather quickly and seems to provide the needed pep that many of my patients are looking for.

You learned in chapter 15 about using SAMe for pain relief, but did you know that several well-designed studies have shown SAMe to be one of the best natural antidepressants available? More than 100 peer-reviewed studies reveal SAMe as an effective natural medication for depression. And it's faster acting with fewer side effects than prescription antidepressants. Unlike them, SAMe works quickly, within 30 minutes once you've taken the right dose. An analysis of the studies to date concluded that SAMe is *as effective as* any of the available prescription antidepressants on the market today.

SAMe increases the action of several neurotransmitters (dopamine, serotonin, and norepinephrine, for example) by facilitating the binding of these hormones to their cell receptors. It also increases the production of the body's own glutathione, a strong antioxidant involved in many brain processes. SAMe helps maintain mitochondrial function at peak levels, thus increasing energy production in the brain, and its antioxidant properties protect the brain and liver against free-radical damage. Normally the brain manufactures all the SAMe it needs from the amino acid methionine. However, low protein diets, malabsorption, and deficiencies, due to excess methionine use in certain detoxification pathways, can create a need for SAMe replacement.

I'm recommending SAMe more and more these days. SAMe seems to work faster and perhaps even better than L-phenylalanine to boost norepinephrine levels. I've had several patients comment that after they started taking SAMe, something kind of "shifted" and they felt better overall—better than they had felt in a long time.

But remember that not all SAMe is created equal. See p. 232 if you're tempted to buy your SAMe at a discount store! Like most amino acids, SAMe should be taken on an empty stomach. I recommend starting with 200–1200 mg. of SAMe in the morning and, if needed, 200–400 mg. in the early afternoon. Some individuals may need to take up to 1200 mg. in divided doses. For most individuals, lower doses will be all they need to notice a change in their depression. SAMe can cause dry mouth and may increase blood pressure. It shouldn't be taken past 4:00 in the afternoon, since its stimulating effects may interfere with your sleep.

Continue to the next page to complete the questionnaire.

THE S GROUP: SEROTONIN

If three or more of these descriptions apply to your present feelings, you are probably part of the "S" group:

- It's hard for you to go to sleep.
- You can't stay asleep.
- You often find yourself irritable.
- Your emotions often lack rationality.
- You occasionally experience unexplained tears.
- Noise bothers you more than it used to; it seems louder than normal.
- You flare up at others more easily than you used to; you experience unprovoked anger.
- You feel depressed much of the time.
- You find you are more susceptible to pain.
- You prefer to be left alone.

Serotonin is a hypothalamus neurotransmitter necessary for sleep. A lack of serotonin causes difficulty in getting to sleep as well as staying asleep. It is often this lack of sleep that causes the symptoms mentioned above.

Serotonin levels can easily be raised by supplementing with the essential amino acid L-tryptophan, but dietary supplements of L-tryptophan are banned in the United States. However, **5-hydroxytryptophan (5-HTP)**, a form of tryptophan, is available over-the-counter and works extremely well for most patients. When taken correctly, 5-HTP turns right into serotonin. Therapeutic administration of 5-HTP has been shown to be effective in treating a wide range of health problems including anxiety, depression, fibromyalgia, insomnia, binge eating, pain, and chronic headaches.

Studies (including double-blind) comparing SSRI and tricyclic antidepressants to 5-HTP have consistently shown that 5-HTP is as good as—if not better than—prescription medications. Furthermore, 5-HTP doesn't have some of the more troubling side-effects associated with prescription medications. One study evaluating the effects of 5-HTP in individuals with uni- and bipolar depression showed that patients had a 50% reduction in their mood-disorder symptoms. 5-HTP has also been shown to be as effective as SSRI drugs in relieving both anxiety and depression. A study comparing 5-HTP to the SSRI Luvox (fluvoxamine) revealed the following results: Anxiety improved in 48.3% of those on Luvox and in 58.2% of those on 5-HTP. Depression improved in 61.8% of those on Luvox and 67.5% of those on 5-HTP.

SSRI antidepressant drugs are 25%–60% effective for depression disorders. This means that on average, four out of ten patients will not respond to their SSRI medications. Of these 40% who then switch to older tricyclic drugs, 70% will respond. This still leaves a subgroup of patients who just don't respond to any of the prescription medications. Fortunately, the administration of 5-HTP to these nonresponders helps 50% of them become depression free.

This is a pretty dramatic finding, since these nonresponders had been suffering from depression for an average of nine years. Many of my patients with depression have tried dozens of drugs over the years, and nothing helped. But 5-HTP does!

One European study showed that the combination of MAOIs, such as Nardil or Parnate, with 5-HTP significantly improved FMS symptoms, whereas other antidepressant treatments were not effective. The doctors conducting this study stated that a natural analgesic (pain-blocking) effect occurred when serotonin and norepinephrine levels were enhanced in the brain. And more norepinephrine means more energy and improved mood. The pain relief certainly helps with the depression, too. (That's an understatement!)

I've explained in chapter 10 how to take 5-HTP if you're having trouble sleeping. **Individuals who aren't having problems with sleep but want to use 5-HTP to boost serotonin should take 100–200 mg. at dinner and then again at bedtime.**

Most people will notice an improvement in mood symptoms within a couple of weeks of starting 5-HTP. However, a minority find that after being on 5-HTP for several weeks or months, their improvement starts to taper off. This is most likely due to an increased awareness of deficiency in their other neurotransmitters—such as norepinephrine, GABA, or dopamine. If this happens to you, add 200–1200 mg. of SAMe once or twice daily on an empty stomach.

I have a small percentage of patients who don't notice much improvement on 5-HTP. If this happens, I recommend that they add St. John's Wort (if under the age of 50) or Ginkgo biloba (if age 50 or older) to their 5-HTP therapy. For any other problems experienced by using 5-HTP, refer to chapter 10.

This ends the Brain Function Questionnaire.

OTHER FACTORS AS CAUSES FOR DEPRESSION

Sure, the brain needs the amino acids discussed above, but it also relies on certain hormones, vitamins, minerals, and essential fatty acids. A deficiency in any of these can be cause for a mood disorder.

Poor sleep depletes mood-controlling neurotransmitters, including serotonin. Decreased serotonin leads to depression, mental fatigue, lowered pain threshold, and sugar cravings.

Q: I checked five items in the O group, three in the N group, and three in the S group. What do I do first?

A: The S group trumps all, if three or more S-group items are checked. Start or increase 5-HTP therapy. Hold off on treating the other categories; see if the 5-HTP will take care of them.

So in your case, I'd recommend taking 5-HTP for two weeks. Then add DL-phenylalanine or SAMe if needed. If you are already on 300 mg. of 5-HTP per day (from the jump-start plan), then don't increase your dose. Go ahead and start with the DL-phenylalanine or SAMe.

Another example: if you check five G-group items and three S-group items, start or increase 5-HTP first—for two weeks—rather than jumping to GABA. Then add GABA L-theanine if needed. One more example: you checked five N-group items and two S-group items. Since you didn't check three S-group items, go with the N group. Start taking L-phenylalanine or SAMe. Here's a good rule of thumb: always treat deficiencies in the calming amino acids (5-HTP, GABA, or L-theanine) first before supplementing the energizing ones (L-phenylalanine, DL-phenylalanine, or SAMe).

Q: *I checked nearly all the statements in all of the catagories! Do I need to take all of these amino acids?*

A: This is a sign that your brain chemistry is in need of a major overhaul. You may actually be deficient in more than one amino acid or neurotransmitter. But before you start trying to figure out how you're going to take three different amino-acid supplements—all on an empty stomach—let's look at your options. First, make sure that you are well into your jump-start plan, (including a vitamin-and-mineral supplement with a free-form amino acid complex, and 5-HTP).

Make sure that you are sleeping through the night. If not, stop right now and turn to chapter 10! Also, find ways to reduce your stress. Clean up your diet; avoid processed foods. If you are still checking items in multiple categories, then call my office (1-888-884-9577).

Low-protein diets, poor digestion, and malabsorption syndromes contribute to amino acid deficiencies. Remember, amino acids—along with certain vitamin and mineral cofactors—create the neurotransmitters (brain chemicals).

Magnesium deficiency affects 50% of the population. Magnesium and vitamin B6 are cofactors in the production of several neurotransmitters.

Chromium deficiency, especially common among those taking cholesterol-lowering drugs, can cause hypoglycemia and mood disorders.

Birth control pills and Premarin can deplete vitamin B6, which is needed to transform amino acids (tryptophan and phenylalanine) into neurotransmitters (serotonin and epinephrine.)

Vitamin C deficiency hurts the production of dopamine, norepinephrine, and serotonin. Vitamin C plays a major role in the production of the adrenal "fight-or-flight" hormone, adrenaline. A deficiency in adrenal function can contribute to fatigue, depression, and confusion.

A deficiency of essential fatty acids (or any essential nutrients) can create a chain reaction leading to all sorts of mood disorders, anxiety, depression, and panic disorders. Nutritional deficiencies are quite common in America. In one study, up to 50% of patients admitted for hospital care had nutritional deficiencies. You'll learn in chapter 29 that essential fatty acids can not be manufactured by the body but must be obtained from the foods we eat. Research shows that low blood levels of omega-3 essential fatty acids are associated with depression. So take your fish oil (in your CFS/Fibro-Formula)!

Emotionally stressful situations cause the body to release adrenaline, cortisol, and insulin. These stress hormones stimulate the brain to secrete serotonin. The more stress, the more serotonin needed to deal with the stress. Long-term stress, along with poor dietary habits, can deplete the body's serotonin stores. Stress can also deplete the body of magnesium (a common occurrence in FMS and CFS patients), B6, dopamine, norepinephrine, and GABA.

> *Q: Can I take 5-HTP or some of the other amino acids if I'm taking anti-depressants or sleep medications?*
>
> A: Yes. And you'd be in good company. Ninety percent of my patients are taking prescription antidepressant drugs. Of course you should know by now what I think about that. Yes, please take amino acids along with your medications. The amino acids can't do anything but *help* these drugs do their jobs by giving them some neurotransmitters to actually work with!

Stimulants like caffeine, diet pills, sugar, and nicotine cause a rapid rise in blood-insulin levels. This is followed by the brain's release of serotonin. Serotonin helps a person feel better and think clearer, but only temporarily. A stimulant high is always followed by a low. This then leads to further use of stimulants to keep serotonin levels high, and an addiction is created. People become dependent on stimulates to help raise serotonin levels, and this addictive process causes further depletion of serotonin.

Low thyroid function is associated with stress, depression, anxiety, and fatigue, because thyroid hormones help regulate concentration, mental clarity, moods, and proper brain chemistry. The thyroid hormone triiodothyronine (T3) regulates the levels and actions of serotonin, norepinephrine, and gamma-aminobutyric acid (GABA). Serotonin is decreased when T3 levels are deficient, which is more common than might be suspected. So if you suffer from depression, be sure to investigate your thyroid as a possible cause. See chapter 16 for more information.

DHEA deficiency has been linked to depression, as DHEA helps counter elevated levels of cortisol. In one study, women with the least DHEA were more likely to be depressed. Interestingly, their levels of DHEA correlated with their moods, even within the normal range. Research shows that the lower the DHEA, the more depressed a person becomes.

Enough DHEA, however, helps promote feelings of calmness. People who practice transcendental meditation have higher levels of DHEA than those who don't. People who took part in a stress-reduction program were able to increase their DHEA by 100%. At the same time, they reduced their stress hormones by 23%.

Low levels of DMAE (dimethylaminoethanol), a naturally occur-ring nutrient found in sardines and other foods, can cause depres-sion and/or fatigue. DMAE supplementation has been shown to elevate mood, improve memory and learning, and increase intelli-gence. It can actually raise your IQ and is even more effective when taken along with vitamin B5. DMAE has also been used with great success in the treatment of attention deficit disorder (ADD) in children and adults.

Depression often manifests itself as fatigue. By directly increasing energy levels and also alleviating depression, DMAE attacks fa-tigue on two levels. It decreases daytime fatigue, allowing for more natural sleep at night, and even increases longevity, as measured in lab animals.

Q: Should I stop taking my prescription antidepressants?

A: Definitely not until after you start feeling a lot better on my program, which might take a few months. When you're ready, and with the help of your doctor, slowly wean off the medications, all the time keeping up the amino-acid therapy. Most antidepressant medications can then be weaned off and never missed. But some will have to be restarted until you become stronger or find other less-toxic options.

Low levels of vitamin D are associated with low moods and depression as well as pain. That's why I recommend that anyone with FMS or CFS have their vitamin D levels checked. For more information, see chapter 26.

B-VITAMIN DEFICIENCIES

Neurotransmitters, the very same one that we are trying to augment here, owe their existence to adequate amounts of B vitamins—especially B1, B2, B3, and B5—which join with amino acids to make serotonin, GABA, dopamine, and norepinephrine. A deficiency of vitamin B12 can lead to inadequate amounts of acetylcholine, an important neurotransmitter involved in learning and memory. In fact, B vitamins are so important for producing and maintaining optimal neurotransmitters, that a deficiency in any of the B vitamins can lead to host of symptoms associated with anxiety and depression disorders.

Low levels of vitamin B9—folic acid—have been linked to depression and bipolar disorder in a number of studies. Insufficient folic acid is one of the most common nutritional deficiencies, and one-third of depressed adults are low in it. Also known as folate, it is needed to create dopamine, norepinephrine, and epinephrine. Low levels are associated with an increase in homocysteine, an amino acid by-product linked to cardiovascular disease and depression. An increase in homocysteine levels also indicates a potential deficiency in SAMe.

Q: I think that I also have fibro-fog...I'm sorry, what was I saying?

A: Decreased mental clarity, forgetfulness, and mental fatigue usually start to disappear when an individual starts sleeping through the night. If after a few weeks of sleeping well and treating whatever else showed up on your Brain Function Questionnaire, you're still experiencing mental fatigue, depression, low moods, or lethargy, make sure that you are taking 1000 mg. of adrenal cortex each day.

Then consider beginning on my Fibro Fog Formula. It contains 16 mental boosters, including ginkgo biloba, Siberian ginseng, and an assortment of amino acids. To order, visit www.TreatingAndBeating.com or call 1-888-884-9577.

Several studies have demonstrated the effectiveness of folic acid in helping to reverse depression. One of these studies evaluated the use of folic acid in a group of patients suffering from either depression or schizophrenia. Results showed that 92% of those on both folic acid and a standard prescription drug therapy made a full recovery, compared with only 70% of the control group, who took only the drug. Those who received the folic acid spent only 23 days in the hospital, while those on prescription therapy alone averaged 33 hospital days.

One British study shows that depressed individuals with low folic acid were often poor responders to prescription antidepressant drug therapy. The addition of folic acid increased the recovery time of these depressed individuals.

Another study showed that women who received folic acid plus Prozac had a greater reduction in depression symptoms than did women who took Prozac alone. This study didn't find any change in men who took folic acid along with Prozac compared to Prozac alone, but research shows that men often need to double the amount of folic acid used in this study anyway. The women in the study who took folic acid were able to see a drop in there homocysteine levels, and the men didn't. But these men took only 500 mcg. of folic acid, and I usually recommended that men with elevated homocysteine levels take 800–1,000 mcg. There is 800 mcg. of folic acid in our CFS/Fibro Formula. You can read more about folic acid in chapter 26.

Vitamin B3—niacin—helps convert the amino acid tryptophan into serotonin. This, as you can imagine, plays an important role in mental illness. Vitamin B3 has been used by orthomolecular physicians to treat schizophrenia, anxiety, and depression. It acts as a wonderful sedative to calm nerves and help with sleep.

Vitamin B3 is a by-product from the metabolism of tryptophan, and some psychiatric disorders—characterized by aggression, restlessness, and insomnia—are caused by a genetic inability to breakdown or absorb tryptophan. For the rest of us, a deficiency of vitamin B3 can cause weakness, dry skin, lethargy, headaches, irritability, loss of memory, depression, delirium, insomnia, and disorientation. For psychiatric disorders, including anxiety, depression, and insomnia, it is best to use a special version of vitamin B3 known as niacinamide, which doesn't cause flushing.

The drug company Hoffman LaRoche, which make Valium, reports that their research shows that niacinamide acts like a benzodiazepine (tranquilizer). Fortunately niacinamide doesn't have the side effects associated with benzodiazepine drugs. Still, some individuals with a sluggish liver may experience nausea on high doses of niacinamide. If this happens, I have them switch to the herb milk thistle, which helps optimize liver function. After a couple of weeks of taking milk thistle, they can usually add a low dose of niacinamide and slowly increase it over a period of weeks. If the nausea returns, then they should simply stop taking niacinamide.

The 200 mg. of niacin (150 mg. as niacinamide) in our CFS/Fibro Formula shouldn't cause any nausea or flushing. Read more about niacin in chapter 26.

Vitamin B6 is needed to convert amino acids into their respective neurotransmitters. Also known as pyridoxine, it is involved in more bodily functions than any other vitamin and is crucial for making serotonin, epinephrine, dopamine, norepinephrine, etc. So of course we include it in our CFS/Fibro Formula: 50 mg. More information on B6 is in chapter 26.

Vitamin B12 acts just like an MAOI drug in that inhibits mono-amine oxidase (MAO), an enzyme that metabolizes some of the neurotransmitters that help to elevate mood. Unlike MAOI drugs, however, vitamin B12 doesn't include the negative side effects. Although B12 deficiency is not as common as folic acid deficiency, it is more common than people— including most doctors—suspect. Even low normal levels can contribute to depression, particularly in the elderly. Read more about B12 in chapter 26.

Taking my CFS/Fibro Formula gives you 100 mcg. of vitamin B12 each day. But those with anxiety and/or depression may benefit from additional sublingual (melts under the tongue) vitamin B12.

The vitamin-like nutrient choline is essential for brain development. With the help of vitamin B5, it converts into the neurotransmitter acetylcholine, which plays an important role in learning and memory. A deficiency in choline may cause poor memory and mental fatigue. Read more about choline in chapter 26.

HYPOGLYCEMIA

Hypoglycemia (low blood sugar) can contribute to depression. Numerous studies have demonstrated that depressed individuals have faulty glucose-insulin regulatory mechanisms. Other studies have clearly shown the relationship between low blood sugar and decreased mental acuity.

Hypoglycemia is a complex set of symptoms caused by faulty carbohydrate metabolism. Normally, the body maintains blood-sugar levels within a narrow range through the coordinated effort of several glands and their hormones. If these hormones, especially glucagon (from glucose) and insulin (produced in the pancreas), are thrown out of balance, hypoglycemia can result.

This imbalance of glucose and insulin (in people not taking insulin by injection) is usually the result of consuming too many simple carbohydrates (sugars). Excessive insulin secretion then leads to glucose intolerance, and this condition is followed by decreased insulin sensitivity, elevated cholesterol levels, obesity, high-blood pressure, and type-2 diabetes or its precursor, syndrome X.

AVOIDING HYPOGLYCEMIA

Eat breakfast. No excuses. Cortisol levels are at their highest around 8:00 a.m., and in an attempt to keep otherwise low cortisol levels elevated in the morning, you may find that you prefer not to eat breakfast. That's because low adrenal function may cause you to feel nauseated, mentally and physically drained, jittery, and headachy, so eating is the last thing you want to do. Eat anyway! A small healthy snack is all you need until hunger comes, usually a couple of hours later. At that time, another balanced snack should tie you over until lunch. Then, don't skip lunch!

It's best to eat little meals throughout the day. Don't let your blood sugar drop too low, and avoid simple sugars. As any "sugarholic" can attest, a soda, doughnut, or pastry can provide a quick energy fix. But this rapid rise in blood sugar is followed by an equally rapid nosedive. And low blood sugar produces all the unwanted symptoms associated with mood disorders: fatigue, irritability, anxiety, mental fog, depression, and more. To avoid the ups and downs of blood-sugar swings, eat a balanced diet of whole, unprocessed foods. Aim to combine protein, fat, and carbohydrate in each snack or meal. One simple snack that combines these beautifully is a handful of nuts along with an apple, pear, or whole-wheat crackers.

If you're diabetic, check your blood sugar regularly. Watch for drops below the normal range, and treat them as your endocrinologist recommends.

Use the glycemic index to treat hypoglycemia. The glycemic index is a measurement of how quickly a carbohydrate elevates a person's circulating blood sugar. *The lower the glycemic index, the slower the rate of absorption and the less likely the food is to contribute to hypoglycemia.* If a food contains no carbohydrates (such as meat), then its glycemic index is zero.

The glycemic index is a great tool for any type-2 diabetic to learn to use, especially if you hope to control your disease by diet alone. Type-1 diabetics, through, who must always depend on injected insulin, will benefit less from the glycemic index.

See the next page for a short summary of some of the most common foods and their range of glycemic index. Think of the low-index foods as safe and the high-index foods are risky, as far as your blood sugar levels are concerned.

Check the labels on your foods! And don't be fooled by clever nomenclature. Look especially for what kind of sugar is in sweetened foods. Fructose has a low glycemic index, but sucrose and lactose have a high one! "Sugar," "turbinado," or "cane juice" listed on a label means basically the same as sucrose. Artificial sweeteners have a very low or zero index. "Wheat flour," "bleached flour," "white

High-index Foods (Risky)	Moderate-index Foods (Better)	Low-index Foods (Best)
• sucrose, glucose, maltose, lactose • cakes, sweets • pancakes, waffles • muffins, croissants, scones • nearly all breads • white potatoes • white rice, rice cakes, rice pasta • most breakfast cereals • corn, corn flakes, corn meal, corn chips, corn tortillas (taco shells) • most pizza • wheat flour • oats and oat flour • rolled oats, oat bran • gnocchi pasta • macaroni and cheese • couscous • low-fat ice cream • carrots • dried fruits, such as raisins and apricots • sweeter fruits, such as banana, pineapple, mango, watermelon	• milk • most pastas, including spaghetti • some breads: sourdough, rye, whole-grain pumpernickel, pita • wild rice, brown rice • noninstant oatmeal • Special K breakfast cereal • no-sugar-added Muesli • fruit juices • some beans: pinto beans, garbanzo beans (chickpeas), baked beans, navy beans, peas • canned lentils	• fructose (fruit sugar) • slow-cooking oatmeal • barley flour • rye flour • less-sweet fruits (eat all of the fruit, including the peel if normally edible, to keep the index low) • beans not listed in the moderate group • uncanned lentils • tomatoes, tomato soup • regular ice cream • yogurt • cream • nuts and seeds • nearly all vegetables

flour," "white wheat flour" and "enriched flour" all means the same thing: high index! "Whole-wheat flour" or "whole-grain flour" is somewhat lower on the index, though still moderate to high.

If you just must eat a high-index food like a bagel, muffin, or pizza, make it from whole-wheat flour and use fructose to sweeten it. And don't eat the high-index food by itself! Add some high-fiber vegetables or unpeeled fruit to the mix to lower the index of your total meal. You can sometimes find lower-index versions of baked goods at stores: look for "whole-grain" or "whole-wheat" on the label, and shoot for no more than one or two grams of sugar per serving.

To look up a particular food on the glycemic index, visit www.glycemicindex.com.

SUPPLEMENTS TO COMBAT HYPOGLYCEMIA

If you're following my adrenal restoration protocol (see chapter 11), you'll probably not need any of the following supplements. However, some individuals with severe hypoglycemia may benefit from them.

- **Chromium** is a trace mineral that works with insulin to facilitate the uptake of glucose into the cells. Glucose levels remain elevated in the absence of chromium.
- **Vitamin B3 (niacin)** helps regulate blood sugar levels and may help alleviate the symptoms of hypoglycemia. It is included in the CFS/Fibro Formula.
- **Magnesium** levels must be sufficient in order to avoid hypoglycemic reactions. So it's in the CFS/Fibro Formula.
- **Zinc** levels must be sufficient in order to avoid hypoglycemic reactions. It's also in the CFS/Fibro Formula.
- **L-glutamine,** an amino acid, helps regulate blood sugar levels. I've found it to be very effective in eliminating sugar cravings and hypoglycemic episodes. See p. 255 for dosage.
- **Gymnema Sylvester** is a climbing plant found in Asia and Africa. It's used in ayruvedic medicine, an indigenous healing practice from India, for the treatment of type-2 diabetes. Scientific studies have shown this herb to be a valuable addition in preventing the symptoms of hypoglycemia. It's also routinely used to reduce sugar cravings.

ST. JOHN'S WORT FOR DEPRESSION

The following supplements aren't amino acids, but they are definitely worth a try, no matter what group(s) you fit into.

St. John's wort has been incredibly successful in treating depression. In Germany, it is covered by health insurance as a prescription drug, and some 20 million people take it for depression. Seventy percent of German physicians prefer St. John's wort over other options for treating depression and anxiety. A review of 23 randomized double-blind, placebo- controlled studies involving 1757 people with mild or moderately severe depressive disorders showed that St. John's wort was *nearly three times superior to* a placebo in relieving depressive symptoms. A perennial plant native to Great Britain and northern Europe, St. John's wort has antibacterial, antidepressant, antiviral, and anti-inflammatory abilities but has received the most attention for its use in treating depression. (It's been described as "natural Prozac.") Hypericin, along with other chemicals contained in St. John's wort, acts as both a weak MAOI and an SSRI.

The ideal dose of St. John's wort is 300 mg. of standardized .3 hypericin. I usually don't start my patients on St. John's wort initially, though. They begin the jump start program and the appropriate amino-acid replacement therapy based on their Brain Function Questionnaire. If they aren't responding as quickly as I'd like, I'll add St. John's wort.

St. John's wort should not be taken along with prescription antidepressant medications, unless you are working with a knowledgeable physician. It may also increase the potential for sunburn, especially if taken with Propulsid, Prevacid, Feldane, or sulfa drugs. Consult your physician about taking St. John's wort along with Ultram. St. John's wort may decrease the effectiveness of certain medications, including digoxin, Coumadin, theophylline, birth control pills, and cyclosporine.

For an even more in-depth look at anxiety and depression, see my book *Treating and Beating Anxiety and Depression With Orthomolecular Medicine* available from Harrison and Hampton Publishing (2005) or from my office (1-888-884-9577).

NOTES
1. Rob Waters, "Drug report barred by FDA Scientist links antidepressants to suicide in kids," *Special to The Chronicle* (Sunday, February 1, 2004).

2. M.Maes et al., "Fatty acid composition in major depression: decreased omega-3 fraction in cholesteryl esters and increased C20:4 omega 6/C20:5 omega 3 ratio in cholesteryl esters and phospholipids," *Jour Affect Disord* 38 (1996): 35–46.

3. C. Kirkegaard and J. Faber, "The Role of Thyroid Hormone in Depression," *European Journal of Endocrinology* 138 (1998): 1–9.

FOR FURTHER READING AND RESEARCH

• J.E. Alpert and M. Fava, "Nutrition and depression: the role of folate," *Nutr Rev* 55(5) (1997): 145–9.

• J. Angst et al., "The treatment of depression with L-5-hydroxytrptophan versus imipramine: results of two open and one double-blind study," *Archiv fur Psychiatrie und Nervenkrankheiten* 224 (1997): 175–86.

• E. Barrett-Connor E et al., "Endogenous levels of dehydroepiandrosterone sulfate, but not other sex hormones, are associated with depressed mood in older women: the Rancho Bernardo study," *J Am Geriatr Soc* 47(6) (1999): 685–91.

• C. Berlanga et al., "Efficacy of S-adenosyl-L-methioninc in speeding the onset of action of imipramine," *Psychiatry Res* 44(3) (1992): 257–62.

• T. Birdsall, "5-hydroxytryptophhan: a clically effective serotonin precursor," *Altern Med Rev* 3(4) (1998): 271–80.

• M. Bloch ct al., "Dehydroepiandrosterone treatment of midlife dysthymia," *Biol Psychiatry* 45 (1999): 1533–41.

• G.M. Bressa, "S-Adenosyl-l-methionine (SAMe) as antidepressant: meta-analysis of clinical studies," *Acta Neurol Scand Suppl* 154 (1994): 7–14.

• V.I. Bukreev, "Effect of pyridoxine on the psychopathology and pathochemistry of involutional depressions," *Zh Nevropatol Psikhiatr Im. S. S. Korsakova* 78(3) (1978): 402–8 (in Russian).

• M.W. Carney, "Neuropsychiatric disorders associated with nutritional deficiencies. Incidence and therapeutic implications," *CNS Drugs* 3(4) (1995): 279–90.

• B.M. Cohen et al., "Effects of the novel antidepressant SAMe on alpha-I and beta adrenoceptors in rat brain," *Eur J Pharmacol* 170(3) (1989): 210.

• A. Coppen and J. Bailey, "Enhancement of the antidepressant action of fluoxetine by folic acid: a randomized, placebo-controlled trial," *J Affect Disorders* 60 (2000): 121–30.

• Costa and Greengard, "Frontiers in biochemical pharmacological research in depression," *Advances in Biochemical Psychopharmacology* 39 (1984): 301–13.

• J.P. de la Cruz et al., "Effects of chronic administration of SAMe on brain oxidative stress in rats," *NaunynSchmiedebergs Arch Pharmacol* 361(l) (2000): 47–52.

• J.L. Glaser et al., "Elevated serum dehydroepiandrosterone sulfate levels in practitioners of the (TM) and TM-Sidhi programs," *J Behav Med* 15(4) (1992): 327–41.

• K. Ito et al., "Effects of L-theonine on the release of alpha brain waves in human volunteers." *Nippon Nogeikagaku Kaishi* 72 (1998): 153–7.

- L.R. Juneja et al., "L-theonine-a unique amino acid of green tea and its relaxation effect in humans," *Trends Food Sci Tech* 10 (1999): 199–204.
- G.S. Kelly, "Folates: supplemental forms and therapeutic applications," *Altern Med Rev* 3(3) (1998): 208–20.
- C. Kirkegaard and J. Faber, "The role of thyroid hormone in depression," *European Journal of Endocrinology* 138 (1998): 1–9.
- J. Laporte and A. Figueras, "Placebo effects in psychiatry," *Lancet* 334 (1993): 1206–8.
- K. Linde et al., "St. John's wort for depression: an overview and meta-analysis of randomised clinical trials," *Br Med J* 313(7052) (1996): 253–8.
- M. Maes et al., "Fatty acid composition in major depression: decreased omega-3 fraction in cholesteryl esters and increased C20:4 omega 6/C20:5 omega 3 ratio in cholesteryl esters and phospholipids." *Jour Affect Disord* 38 (1996): 35–46.
- D. Mischoulon and M. Fava, "Role of 5-adenosyl-L-methionine in treatment of depression: a review of the evidence," *Am J Clin Nutr* 76(5) (2002): 11585–615.
- P. Pancheri et al., "A double-blind, randomized parallel-group, efficacy and safety study of intramuscular S-adenosyl-L-methionine 1, 4-butanedisulpho-nate (SAMe) versus imipramine in patients with major depressive disorder," III Clinica Psichiatrica, Universita La Sapienza Viale dell'Universita 30:00185, Rome, Italy, *Int J Neuropsychopharmacol* 5(4) (2002): 287–94.
- W. Poldinger et al., "A functional-dimensional approach to depression: Serotonin deficiency as a target syndrome in comparison of 5-HTP and fluvoxamine," *Psychopathology* 24 (1991): 53–81.
- J.J. van Hiele, "L-5-hydroxytryptophan in depression: the first substitution therapy in psychiatry?" *Neuropsychobilogy* 6 (1980): 230–40.
- H. Woelk, "Comparison of St. John's wort and imipramine for treating depression: randomized controlled trial," *Br Med J* 321 (2000): 536–9.
- Wolkowitz OM et al. "Double-blind treatment of major depression with dehydroepiandrosterone," *Am J Psychiatry* 156(4) (1999): 646–9.
- Yokogoshi H, Kobayashi M, Mochizuki M, et al. "Effect of theonine, r-glutamylethylamide, on brain monoamines and striatal dopamine release in conscious rats." *Neurochem Res* 23(5) (1998): 667–73.

· 17 ·
BOOSTING YOUR IMMUNE SYSTEM

Research reveals that CFS is strongly associated with lowered immune function. Boosting immunity helps contain and eliminate the viruses associated with CFS, including Epstein-Barr, cytomegalovirus, and the herpes viruses.

The human immune system is nothing short of amazing. It's so complex and sophisticated that we only now know a very small fraction, say 1%–2%, of how it all works. What we do know is that the strength of our immune system determines the state of our health. When our immune system is strong and functioning properly, we tend to be healthy. When it becomes compromised, we are susceptible to all sorts of illnesses.

Special cells known as **white blood cells** patrol the body, seeking invading organisms. Proteins in the form of **antibodies** help us identify and resist repeated infections. In addition to the circulatory system that regulates our blood flow, we also have a separate circulatory system for the immune cells, known as the **lymph system**. This system houses lymph—water, dissolved proteins, and other waste fluids that leak through the capillaries into the spaces between the body tissues. Lymph is collected and rerouted through the body's **lymph nodes**, small pea-like structures that contain a large number of immune cells. These nodes are distributed throughout the body and can be found in the armpits, in the groin, behind the ears, and in the thorax and abdomen. Lymph nodes may become enlarged when our bodies are fighting off an infection. Those with CFS may have chronically inflamed and enlarged nodes that can be felt in the armpits or along the throat just below the chin.

IT'S NOT THE SEED; IT'S THE SOIL

Pathogens (disease-producing microorganisms) are ever present in our environment. They are in the air we breathe, in the food we eat, and on the surfaces to which we are exposed. In fact, if our skin, throat, or other mucous membranes were cultured, most all of us would be found to contain one type of pathogen (disease-causing bug) or another. At any given time, 5%–40% of us have pneumococcus bacteria in our nose and throat, yet we rarely develop pneumonia, because our immune system keeps these pathogens under control.

So why does one person come down with the flu but her co-worker or family member doesn't? There are many factors, but the strength of our immune system ultimately determines our fate. To put it figuratively, it's not the planted seed that determines who gets sick, but the state of the soil it's in.

When a foreign invader enters the body or a cell becomes cancerous, the immune system handles it with two types of defenses.

NONSPECIFIC IMMUNITY: CELL-MEDIATED

Nonspecific defenses are called **cell-mediated immunity**. This type of immunity attempts to either prevent the invader from entering the body or quickly destroy it once it does enter. It involves special white blood cells—typically T-cell lymphocytes and neutrophils—which immediately organize an attack against the pathogen. Cell-mediated immunity is best suited to resisting infection by yeast, fungi, parasites, and viruses, including those associated with CFS, herpes simplex, Epstein-Barr and cytomegalovirus. Cell-mediated immunity is also critical in protecting against the development of cancer and is commonly involved in allergic reactions.

THE THYMUS GLAND

The thymus gland is the master gland of the immune system. Immune cells originate in the bone marrow, but then about half of them are transported to the thymus gland. The thymus gland it is especially susceptible to free radicals, stress, infection, chronic illness, and radiation. Located just underneath the breast bone, it's the size of a walnut. But when it's overly stressed, it becomes smaller. **It is in charge of cell-mediated immunity and is the source of powerful hormones that transform newly formed immune cells into mature T-cells.**

T-CELLS

T-cells, which make up the majority of the cell-mediated immune system, patrol the body for foreign invaders. These specialized cells help prevent cancer by destroying abnormal cells before they can proliferate. There are many different kinds of T-cells. The most important ones are:

- **Killer T-cells** destroy invaders, including viral and cancerous cells.
- **Helper T-cells** enhance the action of the other T-cells. They "sound the alarm."
- **Suppressor T-cells** dampen or turn down the immune system. They "signal the all-clear."

SPECIFIC IMMUNITY: HUMORAL

Specific defenses are known as **humoral immunity.** It relies on special molecules—including white blood cells—to form antibodies to match the surface cells of foreign invaders. It may take several days before these antibodies can be produced and delivered to the offending microorganisms.

B-CELLS

Agents of the humoral immune system, B-cells help manufacture antibodies and release them into the blood steam, where they are carried to the specific site of infection.

NATURAL KILLER CELLS

Natural killer cells (NK cells) seek out and destroy virally infected cells. They are especially important for those with CFS, as research has shown that CFS is associated with lowered NK-cell levels. Boosting NK-cell function helps contain and eliminate the viruses associated with CFS, including Epstein-Barr, cytomegalovirus, and the herpes viruses.

ANTIBODIES

Antibodies can perform in various ways. Some neutralize the poisons produced from bacteria. Others coat the bacteria and allow scavenger cells (phagocytes) to engulf and digest them.

MACROPHAGES

Macrophages are large scavengers that help clean up any leftover debris from the destruction of pathogens.

HOW THE IMMUNE SYSTEM WORKS

The body's first lines of defense are simply the surfaces of the body, which work to prevent pathogens from entering. Obviously, your skin helps quite a bit to protect you and hold you together! And mucus—you know, the sticky stuff—traps pathogens and moves them off the membranes and away from the body (or into the intestines where they are destroyed by the stomach acid. Chemicals bound to the pathogens keep them from penetrating the mucus. These chemicals are released by **secretory IgA.**

Once a pathogen gets past the surface defenses, it invades the tissues, spreads, and damages the cells. When this happens, the cells secrete a wide range of special chemicals including histamine, bradykinins, and serotonin. These chemicals alert the immune system that the body is under attack and trigger an increased blood supply to the area (this causes inflammation and fevers). Now the cell-mediated defense team is activated to attack the invaders. As a pathogen sustains damage, parts of it leak out of the cell. These "antigens" activate the humoral defense team. B cells produce specific antibodies antagonistic to the antigens. Then along come the macrophages which, like gobbling Pac-men, finish off the enemy. You didn't know there'd be so much violence in this book, did you?

IMMUNE SYSTEM ZAPPERS

I am indebted to Dr. Joseph Pizzorno, author of *Total Wellness,* for the following handy list of immune zappers, to which I've added my own explanations:

Sugar and other simple carbohydrates reduce white-blood-cell activity. One tablespoon of sugar in any form—white sugar, honey, or even fruit juice—results in a 50% reduction for up to five hours. There are four classes of simple sugars: sucrose (table sugar), fructose (fruit sugar), honey, and malts.

Drinking fruit juice is like mainlining sugar; it's too much sugar at one time. Think about it this way: you'd have a hard time eating ten apples, but you could easily drink a glass of apple juice, which may contain the sugar of up to 10 juiced apples. If fruit juice were marketed honestly, they would say, "All the sugar, none of the fiber!" Help yourself, however, to all the whole fruits you want.

Too much sugar—whether it's juice, honey, maple syrup, evaporated cane juice, brown sugar, fructose, or white table sugar—is never a healthy choice. Sugar depletes the body of B vitamins, calcium, and magnesium. One tablespoon of sugar, in any form, results in a 50% reduction in white-blood-cell activity for up to five hours. Hope a nasty virus doesn't travel your way during that time! **Sugar lowers our immune function!** Unfortunately, the average American consumes over 150 oz. of sugar a day. A can of Coke has 9–10 teaspoons, which is at least *three* tablespoons!

Occasional, moderate use is fine. But **too much sugar** has a number of other extremely damaging effects on the human body:

- it can suppress the immune system,
- contribute to mood disorders, including hyperactivity, anxiety, depression, and concentration difficulties—especially in children,
- produce a significant rise in triglycerides,
- cause drowsiness and decreased activity in children,
- cause symptoms associated with ADHD, especially in children,
- cause hypoglycemia (low blood sugar),
- increase the risk of coronary heart disease,
- lead to chromium deficiency,
- cause copper deficiency,
- upset the body's mineral balance,
- promote tooth decay,

- raise adrenaline levels in children,
- lead to periodontal disease,
- speed the aging process, causing wrinkles and grey hair,
- increase total cholesterol, increase systolic blood pressure, reduce helpful high density cholesterol (HDLs), promote an elevation of harmful cholesterol (LDLs),
- contribute to weight gain and obesity,
- contribute to existing diabetes, osteoporosis, or kidney damage,
- cause free-radical formation in the bloodstream,
- cause atherosclerosis,
- cause depression,
- increase the body's fluid retention,
- cause hormonal imbalance,
- interfere with absorption of calcium and magnesium,
- and increase the risk of Crohn's disease and ulcerative colitis.

OK, I think I made my point. An occasional sweet treat is acceptable and even encouraged. Moderation is the key. There's no reason to totally abstain from sugar unless you're fighting off an infection, have yeast overgrowth, or are battling diabetes. Just go easy. Considering artificial sweeteners? Read the boxes on the next few pages.

Alcohol can reduce the amount and activity of white blood cells.

Brown or Raw Sugar

It is often said that brown sugar is a healthier option than white sugar. But you can chalk that claim up to clever marketing. In reality, brown sugar is most often just ordinary table sugar that is turned brown by the reintroduction of molasses. (Normally, molasses is separated and removed when sugar is created from sugarcane plants.) In some cases, brown sugar—particularly when it is referred to as "raw sugar"—is merely sugar that has not been fully refined. But more often than not, manufacturers prefer to reintroduce molasses to fine white sugar, creating a mixture with 5%–10% molasses. This process allows them to better control the color and size of the crystals in the final product.

Because of its molasses content, brown sugar or raw sugar does contain certain minerals not present in white sugar: calcium, potassium, iron, and magnesium. But since these minerals are present in only minuscule amounts, there is no real health benefit to using brown sugar.

Food allergies cause the immune system to "ramp-up" and become overstimulated, and chronic immune challenges from food allergies may overwhelm secretory IgA reserves. Research has shown that allergic foods can cause a 50% drop in a person's white-blood-cell count. Daily intake of allergic foods can inflame intestinal cells, causing white blood cells to die and then release digestive enzymes into the surrounding tissue. When these enzymes damage the normally impermeable intestinal lining, the result is intestinal permeability. You learned from chapter 12 about how intestinal permeability can trigger autoimmune reactions. These reactions can

An Unexpected Immune Zapper: Splenda

A new study done at Duke University and published recently in the *Journal of Toxicology and Environmental Health* has some interesting news about the sugar substitute known as Splenda (sucralose). Splenda is an artificial sweetener derived from raffinose, a starch derived from sugar beets. The chemical sucralose, which contains chlorine, is marketed this way: "It comes from sugar, so it tastes like sugar." But it isn't natural at all. According to the study, the use of Splenda has several effects on the body:

• It reduces the amount of good bacteria in the intestines by 50%. The bacteria in your bowels, some 100 trillion of them—about three pounds worth—outnumber the cells in your body by a factor of 10 to one. These bacteria, also called gut flora, line your intestinal tract and serve as your first line of defense against potential pathogens (viruses, bad bacteria, and yeast). They play a crucial role in estab

lishing an overall healthy immune system. When bad bacteria and or yeast become overgrown in your intestinal tract, you have a condition called dysbiosis. Dysbiosis has been linked with disorders like yeast infections, irritable bowel syndrome, and autoimmune disorders—including rheumatoid arthritis.

• It increases the pH level in the intestines. The stomach needs an acidic environment in order to digest food and destroy potentially harmful pathogens, including unwanted bacteria and yeast. Low stomach acid triggers a chain reaction of digestive disorders, including malabsorption. Foods may be incompletely digested and subsequently absorbed into the bloodstream, where they can lead to food allergies, triggering pain and inflammation throughout the body.

• It contributes to increases in body weight.

The study researched male rats over a period of 12 weeks.[1]

start a cascade of unwanted consequences including inflammation, infection, and pain.

Hypothyroid can reduce the speed and effectiveness of enzymes associated with supporting immune functions.

Adrenal dysfunction causes lowered resistance to all forms of stress and leads to lowered immune resistance.

Chronic stress eventually leads to adrenal exhaustion.

Being overweight causes a reduction in bacteria-killing white blood cells.

Heavy metals, including cadmium, lead, and mercury, inhibit the formation of antibodies and reduce the bacteria-killing ability of white blood cells.

Pesticides and other environmental toxins can overwhelm the immune system and its supporting cast (liver, kidneys, etc.). Pesticides depress T- and B-cells and place a drain on the lymph system, especially the thymus gland.

Drugs, including acetaminophen, aspirin, ibuprofen, and corticosteroids, decrease antibody production.

NutraSweet (Aspartame)

Aspartame has been associated with a multitude of health risks and has largely lost favor around the world. Consider that the FDA had its concerns and denied approval of aspartame for 16 years before it finally gave in to political/economic pressure. This controversial artificial sweetener was approved through an interesting chain of events. When then-president Ronald Reagan brought Don Rumsfeld, former CEO of the aspartame manufacturer, Monsanto, to Washington, a new FDA commissioner was also hastily appointed. The new commissioner approved the artificial sweetener and then went on to become a consultant for NutraSweet's public-relations firm, receiving $1,000 a day for the next 10 years!

Aspartame, commonly known as NutraSweet or Equal, is an artificial sweetener. The body breaks it down into methanol and formaldehyde to metabolize it. Methanol toxicity causes depression, brain fog, mood changes, insomnia, seizures, and similar symptoms associated with multiple sclerosis. Formaldehyde is grouped into the same class of drugs as cyanide and arsenic. When the temperature of aspartame exceeds 86 degrees F, the wood alcohol in it is turned into formaldehyde and then into formic acid. Formic acid is the poison contained in the sting of a fire ant.

There are over 92 symptoms documented from using aspartame.

Inadequate rest suppresses natural-killer cell activity.

Candida **overgrowth** may allow toxins to be released directly into the body. These toxins cause the immune system to become overwhelmed and can initiate a host of immune-disrupting symptoms.

Severe trauma, including accidents, surgeries and burns, are extremely stressful to the body as a whole. Traumas can cause vitamin, mineral, and other essential nutrients to become deficient. Any inflammatory responses from the trauma can also overload the immune system.

Chronic antibiotic use can increase overgrowth of *Candida,* making bacteria more resistant to immune-system attacks.

TREATING CFS WITH ANTIVIRAL DRUGS

Recent tests of antiviral agents such as Zovirax (acyclovir), Valtrex (valcyclovir HCl), and Gamimune (immune globulin human) have been inconclusive, working no better than placebo in some tests. While these studies aren't very promising, I've had numerous patients experience substantial improvements in their CFS when taking antiviral medications. And at one time, I had nearly all of my CFS patients taking antiviral medications.

Of course, there are potential side effects to these medications, including upset stomach, vomiting, diarrhea, dizziness, tiredness, agitation, pain—especially in the joints, hair loss, and changes in vision. Although rare, other side effects can be serious. Talk with your prescribing doctor about these.

A Natural Alternative: Stevia

For an alternative to sugar, I recommend the natural sweetener Stevia. It is a South American herb that has been used as a sweetener by the Guarani Indians of Paraguay for hundreds of years. The leaves of the small, green *Stevia rebaudiana* plant have a delicious and refreshing taste that can be 30 times sweeter than sugar, so a little goes a long way. For more info, visit www.stevia.com. You can find Stevia at any health-food store. While it may take time to get used to its taste, it won't deplete your good bacteria (like Splenda), increase your risk of cancer (like Sweet'N Low), or cause neurotoxicity (like NutraSweet).

One medication showing potential is Ampligen. This experimental antiviral medication stimulates the production of interferon, a protein that induces healthy cells to counter infection. In two studies, CFS patients treated with Ampligen demonstrated improvements in cognition and performance. The drug has not yet been approved by the FDA and is in various stages of approval around the world for a wide range of conditions.

HYPOTHYROID AND REDUCED IMMUNITY

A low-activity thyroid can lower metabolism and reduce enzyme activities associated with initiating proper immune functions. Chronic infections—especially sinus infections—usually improve drastically once low thyroid is corrected.

I cannot emphasize enough how important it is to your immune system to correct low thyroid function. My patients with low thyroid—especially those with CFS, who typically battle constant yeast and viral infections—notice that most of their infections disappear once their thyroid (measured by temperature; see chapter 14) normalizes. By raising their metabolism and immune function, patients create an environment inhospitable to viruses, bacteria, yeast, and mycoplasma.

Many hypothyroid patients experience a nasty sinus infection once they start thyroid replacement therapy. It's the pathogen's final fight, and it's usually the last sinus infection they get.

IMMUNE-SYSTEM BOOSTERS

Since our CFS/Fibro Formula contains several effective immune boosters, including thymus extract, it may be all a patient needs to significantly improve her immune function. And a healthy diet and plenty of rest can go a long way toward fixing a sluggish immune system. Avoid simple sugars and trans-fatty acids, and eat balanced meals. Beyond that, consider these other immune boosters.

COENZYME Q10

This potent antioxidant aids in metabolic reactions, including the formation of ATP, the molecule the body uses for energy. CoQ10 can't be manufactured by the body; we must obtain from the foods we eat or from supplements. Meat, dairy spinach, and broccoli, for instance, contain high concentrations of CoQ10. Modern agricultural and livestock practices, however, make obtaining adequate CoQ10 through diet a challenge for most adults. And we tend to absorb and utilize less CoQ10 as we age, right when we need more it of. Researchers have estimated that as little as a 25% reduction in bodily CoQ10 can trigger immune-system dysfunction. I've found CoQ10 to be very helpful for my CFS patients.

In one study of 20 female patients with CFS (who required bed rest following mild exercise), 80% were deficient in CoQ10. After three months of CoQ10 supplementation (100 mg. per day), the exercise tolerance of the CFS patients more than doubled: 90% had reduction or disappearance of clinical symptoms, and 85% had decreased post-exercise fatigue.

DHEA

DHEA has been shown in preliminary studies to improve symptoms in some patients with CFS, and the DHEA levels of many CFS patients are low compared to optimal ranges. You may remember from the chapter on adrenal fatigue (11) that DHEA is responsible for several important immune- boosting functions. While I typically start fibromyalgia and CFS patients on adrenal cortex glandular supplements, I may also add additional DHEA 25–50 mg. to my CFS patients' routine.

NADH

Also called reduced B-nicotanamide dinucleotide, it is essential—along with CoQ10—for the production of cellular energy. A randomized, double-blind, placebo-controlled crossover study examined the use of NADH in treating CFS: 26 eligible patients diagnosed with CFS received either 10 mg. of NADH or a placebo for four weeks. Eight of the 26 (31%) responded favorably to NADH, in contrast to two of the 26 (8%) to placebo. I've had patients report some benefit from taking NADH, but it can be pricey, and I prefer the consistently positive results of taking CoQ10.

EFAs

Essential fatty acids have direct antiviral effects and are lethal at surprising low concentrations to many viruses. The antiviral activity of human mother's milk seems to be largely attributable to its EFA content. Further, interferon is dependent on EFAs and in their absence will be compromised.

Viral infections lower the blood levels of EFAs. This has been confirmed in the case of the Epstein-Barr Virus. Of particular interest is the observation that at eight and twelve months, those who have recovered from EBV show normal or near-normal EFA blood levels. In contrast, those who are still clinically ill persistently show low EFA levels. This study and others like it are one of the reasons that my CFS/Fibro Formula contains 2,000 mg. of EFAs.

THYMUS EXTRACTS

These have proven to be one of the best immune-boosting agents for treating CFS. A recent study published in the *Journal of Nutritional and Environmental Medicine* showed that patients taking "ProBoost" a patented thymus extract, obtained dramatic improvements in their CFS symptoms. The increase in their immune function, as demonstrated by blood tests, resulted in a broad range of improvements, including a 47% improvement in sleep quality, a 43% reduction in food sensitivities, a 53% reduction in chemical sensitivities, a 47% improvement in short-term memory, a 79% improvement in depression, and a 100% improvement in panic disorders.

A substantial amount of other clinical data also supports the effectiveness of using thymus extracts. They may provide the answer to chronic viral infections and low immune function. Double-blind studies reveal not only that orally administrated thymus extracts were able to effectively eliminate infection, but also that year-long treatment significantly reduced the number of respiratory infections and improved numerous immune parameters.

Thymus glandular extracts (like other glandular extracts) are able to raise T-cells when needed but will lower T-cells when an autoimmune disease is present. This balancing act is the big advantage that glandular extracts and many natural herbs have over prescription (synthetic) drugs.

I've added an **oral thymus spray called Xtra-Cell** to my CFS immune-boosting protocol. This spray is available from Douglas Labs by referral from your physician, or you can order it from my office.

For my most challenging CFS immune-compromised patients, I've begun using a CFS Frozen Glandular Formula, also from Douglas Labs. This high-tech glandular is extremely potent and yields positive results when other methods fail. It's rather expensive ($150 or more for a month's supply) but typically increases immune function, boosts energy, and provides relief from many of the symptoms of CFS. It is also available from your physician or from my office (visit www.TreatingAndBeating.com or call 1-888-884-9577).

OTHER IMMUNE BOOSTERS

Zinc is an important cofactor in the manufacture, secretion, and function of thymus hormones. When zinc levels are low, T-cell numbers go down. This may help explain why zinc lozenges, when used at the first sign of a cold, can reduce the number of sick days.

Antioxidants help protect the thymus gland from free-radical damage. Vitamins A, C, and E, along with the minerals zinc and selenium, play a vital role in reducing the damage associated with free-radical toxicity.

Astragalus membranaceus is a Chinese herb used to treat a wide variety of viral infections. Clinical studies have shown it be effective when used on an ongoing basis against the common cold. Research in animals has shown that *Astragalus* apparently works by stimulating several factors of the immune system, including enhancing activity of macrophages, increasing interferon production in natural-killer cell activity, enhancing T-cell activity, and potentiating other antiviral mechanisms. *Astragalus* appears particularly useful in cases where the immune system has been damaged by chemicals or radiation.

Selenium supplementation to individuals with normal selenium levels resulted, in one study, in a 118% increase in ability of white blood cells to kill tumor cells and an 82.3% increase in the activity of natural-killer cells.

Echinacea is one of the most popular herbal medicines in the United States and Europe. In 1994, German physicians prescribed *Echinacea* more than 2.5 million times. And there are over 200 journal articles written about this herb from the sunflower family that can be found in many perennial gardens across the United States. *Echinacea* is thought to stimulate the immune system by increasing the production of and activity of white blood cells, especially natural-killer cells. The German Commission E monograph suggests that persons with autoimmune illnesses (such multiple sclerosis, Lupus, or tuberculosis) should avoid *Echinacea*. A typical dose is up to 900 mg. three times a day. Some physicians suggest discontinuing *Echinacea* after two–three weeks and then restarting as needed after a week's rest.

Goldenseal *(Hydrastis canadensis)* is a perennial herb native to eastern North America. It has been shown to be a potent immune stimulator. It increases the blood flow to the spleen and the number and activity of macrophages. A typical dose is 250–500 mg. one–three times a day.

MGN-3, an arabinoxylan compound, is a polysaccharide composed of the hemi-cellulose-B extract of rice bran, modified by enzymes from Shiitake mushrooms. What? MGN-3 is a nutritional supplement with special patented chemicals, especially those derived from the immune-boosting Chinese Shiitake mushroom. Research has shown that MGN-3 supplementation triples the amount of natural killer cells. And I've had good results when recommending it to CFS patients. The main deterrent for taking this product is its cost: $60–$70 for 50 capsules. Usual dose is two–four capsules a day. It's costly, but I have no doubt it does in fact help raise NK cells, which are notoriously low in CFS patients.

Nature's Way *SystemWell* **Formula** is an extremely comprehensive product. I've been impressed with our patients' response to this supplement. It contains over 33 nutrients designed to boost the circulatory, systemic, cellular, digestive, respiratory, lymphatic, and epidermal (skin) systems. *SystemWell* contains vitamins A, C, and D and the minerals selenium and zinc. The herbal extracts include garlic, *Echinacea, Astragalus,* olive leaf, shiitake mushroom, and goldenseal. For the price, this is an incredible product.

PROTOCOL FOR CHRONIC SINUSITIS

Chronic sinus infections may be the result of bacterial or fungal infections. Sinus infections are usually treated with antibiotics and steroids. However, antibiotics will only make fungal sinus infections worse. I've found instead that many of my patients find relief from chronic nasal congestion and infections with the following protocol.

1. **Rinse nasal passages daily.** You can use a nasal rinse kit from Neil Med Pharmaceuticals (available from my office—call 1-888-884-9577—or by calling Neil Med directly at 1-877-477-8633.) Patients simply add warm water and one of the (50 to a box) buffered-sodium packets into the plastic six-ounce bottle. For stubborn infections, I encourage patients to add several drops of liquid Betadine. A topical antiseptic, Betadine kills viruses, bacteria, and yeast. You can also create your own nasal rinse kit by mixing together 1 t. of Betadine, 1 t. of baking soda, 1 t. of liquid glycerin, and 15–20 oz. of warm water. Draw the solution up into a bulb syringe (found in the baby-diaper aisle), and flush each nostril several times. Don't inhale through your nose; just let the mixture rest in your nose for a few seconds, and then gently blow your nostrils clean. (Betadine will stain your clothes, so be careful.) Use this rinse once a day for two weeks and then as needed at the first sign of a cold, the flu, or sinusitis.

2. **Avoid all dairy products until you become congestion free.** Dairy products increase mucous production.

Unfortunately, some of you won't truly feel well until after you uncover and correct some of the other "layers of the onion" that may be holding you back. In the following chapters, we'll look at how toxins, food allergies, yeast overgrowth, and parasitic infections can sabotage you from a complete recovery from your illness.

NOTES

1. B. Mohamed et al, *Journal of Toxicology and Environmental Health* A-71(21) (2008): 1415–29.

RESOURCES

• Xtra-Cell thymus spray and CFS Frozen Glandular Formula are available from Douglas Labs through a referral from your physician or by contacting my office (1-888-884-9577).

FOR FURTHER READING AND RESEARCH

• P. Cazzola et all, "In vitro modulating effects of a calf thymus acid lysate on human T lymphocyte subsets and CD4+\CD8+ ratio in the course of different diseases," *Curr Ther Res* 42 (1987): 1011–17.

• H.M. Chang and P.P.H. But (eds), *Pharmacology and Applications of Chinese Materia Medica* (Singapore: World Scientific, 1987): 1041–6.

• P. de Becker et al., "Dehydroepiandrosterone (DHEA) response to i.v. ACTH in patients with chronic fatigue syndrome," *Horm Metab Res* 31(1) (1999): 18–21.

• A. Fiocchi et al., "A double-blind clinical trial for the evaluation of the therapeutic effectiveness of calf thymus derivatives (thymomodulin) in children with recurrent respiratory infection," *Thymus* 8 (1986): 831–9.

• L.M. Forsyth et al., "Therapeutic effects of oral NADH on the symptoms of patients with chronic fatigue syndrome," *Ann Allergy Asthma Immunol* 82(2) (1999): 185–91.

• W.M. Jefferies, "Mild adrenocortical deficiency, chronic allergies, autoimmune disorders and the chronic fatigue syndrome: a continuation of the cortisone story," *Med Hypotheses* 42(3) (1994): 183–9.

• W. Judy. Presentation to the 37th Annual Meeting of the American College of Nutrition, Southeastern Institute of Biomedical Research, October 13, 1996.

• L. Kiremidjia-Schumacer et al., "Supplementation with selenium in human immune cell functions: effect on cyotoxic lymphocytes and natural killer cells." *Biol Trace Elem Res* 41 (1994): 115–127.

• M. Kouttab et al., "Thymomodulin: biological properties in clinical applications," *Med Oncol Tumor in Pharmacother* 6 (1989): 5–9.

• H. Kuratsune, "Dehydroepiandrosterone sulfate deficiency in chronic fatigue syndrome," *Int J Mol Med* 1(1) (1998): 143–6.

• W. Ringsdorf et al., "Sucrose neutrophil phagocytosis in resistance to disease," *Dent Surv* 52 (1976): 46–8.

• A. Sanchez et. al., "Level of sugars in human neutrophilic phagocytosis," *Am J of Clin Nutrit* 26 (1973):1180–4.

• L.V. Scott, "Differences in adrenal steroid profile in chronic fatigue syndrome, in depression and in health," *J Affect Disord* 54(1–2) (1999): 129–37.

• K.S. Zhao et al., "Enhancement of the immune response in mice by Astragalus membranaceus," *Immunopharmacology* 20 (1990): 225–33.

· 18 ·
FOOD ALLERGIES

"I was very reluctant to start the elimination diet. What was I going to eat? I was especially dreading the idea of not having tomatoes for a month. I'm southern, for heaven's sake! Depriving me of garden fresh tomatoes just didn't seem fair! But everything else Dr. murphree had suggested had helped, so….sure enough, tomatoes had been making my hands and feet swell and ache! I had no idea!"—an actual account from patient Bobbi Anne

I find that many of my fibromyalgia and CFS patients suffer from unknown food allergies. Uncovering and avoiding these foods often yields substantial improvement in their lingering symptoms. Still, I don't start exploring food allergies until after my patient has been on the jump start program, consistently sleeping through the night, and building their stress-coping savings account. Avoiding potentially symptom-triggering foods can be extremely helpful in the long run. However, in the short run, those with paltry stress coping accounts are ill equipped to take on the added stress of elimination or rotation diets.

Food allergies are considered rare, or aren't even acknowledged, by many traditional doctors. However, research and better diagnostic tests are validating what many health-care experts have known for quite some time; food allergies play a major role in our health. Says James Braly, MD and author: "The thinking of the majority of health professionals, including allergists and dieticians, is some fifteen to twenty years out of date when it comes to food and allergy." Conservative estimates show that 20% of young children in industrialized countries have food allergies.

Compounding the problem are outdated tests and theories. Most doctors adhere to the Reagin theory of allergic reactions: around 1925, scientists in Europe discovered a substance they called reagin that was involved with allergic reactions involving the skin. Thus the beginning of allergic skin-prick testing. Myopic thinking has prevented modern allergists from acknowledging that there might be *another* response that validates the presence of allergies, besides skin sensitivity. Reagin later turned out to be a specific antibody known as IgE. IgE is the antibody that's measured with the skin prick test and the radioallergosorbent test (RAST). Both are able to detect acute or immediate allergic responses (mediated by IgE), but they're best for airborne allergens. They don't, however, measure delayed sensitivity responses to food, which account for 95% of all food allergies. These delayed responses occur one hour to three days after eating allergic foods and are measured using a different antibody, IgG1-4. For this reason, immediate IgE, RAST, and skin-prick testing are inferior testing methods in comparison to tests that measure both immediate IgE and delayed IgG1-4 sensitivities.

> **Allergy:** a hypersensitive state acquired through exposure to a particular allergen and subsequent re-exposure to the same allergen, which then triggers an inappropriate immune response. For example, sneezing when you breathe in hickory pollen.
>
> **Allergen:** any substance capable of inducing an allergic response, but allergens are usually protein molecules.

Food allergies can be the cause of:

- headaches
- eczema
- psoriasis
- diarrhea
- colitis
- asthma
- hyperactivity
- rheumatoid arthritis
- gout
- chronic pain
- edema
- ear infections
- anxiety
- depression

Intestinal permeability and food allergies go hand in hand. Undigested proteins can be deposited into any available bodily tissue. This can create an allergic inflammatory response at any site within the body: muscles, heart, brain, joints, etc. Read more about intestinal permeability in chapter 12.

Food allergies are not rare and are responsible for a wide variety of health problems! Many of my patients have been tested and told they had allergies, but unfortunately, they were only tested for IgE antibodies. So although their airborne allergies were detected, many of their food allergies were not.

Two tests that measure immediate IgE and delayed IgG1-4 reactions are the enzyme-linked immuno-absorbent assay (ELISA) test and the food immune complex assay (FICA) Test. Both of these tests offer the convenience and accuracy of measuring both types of antibodies, while costing hundreds of dollars less than RAST and skin-prick tests. To find out more about these tests, contact my office (1-888-884-9577).

THE ELIMINATION DIET FOR TESTING FOOD ALLERGIES

All allergy tests are associated with some degree of error. Even ELISA and FICA tests are no better than 85% accurate. False positives and missed allergic foods are a common occurrence on most tests, so the gold standard for uncovering allergen sensitivities is still the two-week elimination diet. I recommend that everyone try this diet. What have you got to lose but your pain? But wait until you've successfully followed the jump-start plan for one month before trying this diet.

Following the elimination diet is a challenge, so always have plenty of snacks available at home, in the car, in your briefcase or purse, and at work. Don't get discouraged in the short-term! If correcting your problem was an easy thing to do, it would have already happened, right? For the next two weeks, eliminate:

- **all dairy products** (except butter) including milk, cheese, yogurt, and ice cream.
- **all corn and related products:** corn syrup, popcorn etc.
- **all gluten products,** including wheat, oats, barley, kamut, spelt, and all flours.
- **all soy products** (check food labels for hidden soy).
- **all nightshade foods,** including white potatoes, peppers, tomatoes, tobacco, and eggplant. Nightshades contain a poison similar to belladonna that may cause muscle or joint pain.

THE FRUIT AND VEGETABLE DIET

Another way to approach this diet is "The Fruit and Vegetable Diet." In this approach, you can eat all the fruit and vegetables you want for five days, while avoiding all other foods. If *Candida* yeast overgrowth is an issue, reduce the fruit and add more vegetables. After five days, you can begin to challenge one food group at a time. Remember to wait three days before challenging a new food group.

PINPOINTING THE ALLERGIC FOOD

After two weeks of totally avoiding the foods listed above, begin to challenge one food group at a time, beginning with dairy. For one day only, eat three or more servings of dairy while still avoiding the other food groups. Then immediately return to the elimination diet for three days. Remember, most food allergies are delayed reactions and can take up to three days before any symptoms are experienced. Keep a diet journal on hand to record the foods you eat and any symptoms you experience while reintroducing the eliminated foods.

After challenging dairy (and waiting three days), challenge another food group: gluten, for instance. Have oatmeal for breakfast, a sandwich for lunch, and buttered toast for a snack. Don't eat any other eliminated foods; you're only challenging gluten. Wait three more days before challenging another forbidden food group.

If you have a severe reaction, totally eliminate the offending food group for six months. Then slowly reintroduce it back into your diet: eat one small serving and wait a minimum of four days before eating another. Reactions may be avoided by slowly rotating these foods back into your diet.

In the case of a mild or moderate reaction, avoid the food group for one–three months (depending on the severity of your reaction) and then begin to reintroduce it.

DR. COCA'S PULSE TEST

The foods listed above are by far the most common allergic foods. However, practically any food can trigger an allergic reaction. For this reason you might want to dig a little deeper to pinpoint sensitivities to specific foods. Foods can actually be tested by merely tasting them. If a food elicits a rise in resting pulse rate, this indicates an allergic reaction. This is because the pulse is controlled by the autonomic nervous system, and stress causes this system to increase blood flow and pulse rate.

To use Dr. Coca's pulse test, you must first determine your resting pulse rate: count your pulse for a full minute while sitting still. (Sites commonly used to check the pulse are the underside of the wrist and the neck near the Adam's apple). It's best to check your pulse several times throughout the day and to notice if it changes at different times. Is it lower or higher in the morning? At night? To get the most accurate base line, take your pulse in bed before rising, before breakfast, after breakfast, in the middle of the morning, before lunch, after lunch, in the middle of the afternoon, before dinner, after dinner, in the middle of the evening, and before bed.

Keep a food diary and record your pulse rates and any symptoms. Does a pattern emerge? If there is no consistent pattern, there may be too many interfering substances undermining the process. If so, try the elimination diet for four–five days. Along with the obvious elimination foods, foods or chemicals in question should also be avoided during this time.

Your resting pulse is the pulse consistently found before eating, or an average of the lowest pulses most commonly recorded.

TESTING FOODS USING THE PULSE TEST

While sitting quietly, take your pulse. Then challenge this pulse by chewing a small amount of food or food supplement (don't swallow) for a full minute. Liquids can be held and swished around in the mouth. After one minute, take your pulse for a full minute. At the end of this time, expel the substance, and rinse out your mouth with pure water, which should also be expelled. Take your pulse again. If it returns to the resting value, you can repeat the process with another substance.

A positive-reaction food or supplement will elevate the pulse above six points. Avoid all such substances for two–three months. For someone who's been on a strict elimination diet for weeks, a rise of only one point may be significant. If other symptoms occur after testing, such as headache, sore throat, or fuzzy thinking, this is also a positive test, and the food should be avoided for three–six months. Severe-reaction foods should be avoided for at least three months.

THE ROTATION DIET

Once someone becomes sensitive to foods, damage to the intestinal tract has most likely occurred. Repetitive exposure to the same foods may initiate allergic reactions. Left untreated, intestinal permeability and overstimulation of the immune system can create an allergy to almost any food. A rotation diet helps reduce the chances of developing further allergies.

On this diet, you eat nonallergic foods every day for four–seven days. Allergic foods (as determined by testing or elimination dieting) are slowly reintroduced into the diet over a period of months. Consult a nutritionist for help in devising a suitable rotation diet.

FOOD GROUPS

- **Grains:** wheat, barley, oats, rice, rye, buckwheat, millet, and corn
- **Seeds:** sesame, sunflower, and pumpkin seeds
- **Nuts:** almonds, walnuts, pecans, pistachios, cashews, filberts, Brazil nuts, chestnuts, and coconut
- **Oils:** safflower, sunflower, soy, cottonseed, olive, sesame, corn, and peanut oils
- **Sweeteners:** maple sugar, beet sugar, cane sugar, corn syrup, and honey
- **Vegetables:** olives, eggplant, tomato, potatoes, peppers, paprika, sweet potatoes, yams, broccoli, cauliflower, kale, artichokes, cabbage, Brussels sprouts, radishes, turnips, parsnips, carrots, celery, zucchini, Swiss chard, spinach, winter squash, summer squash, cucumbers, lettuces, onions, garlic, chives, and asparagus
- **Legumes:** black-eyed peas, navy beans, pinto beans, wax beans, string beans, green beans, chick-peas, soybeans, lima beans, mung beans, peanuts, lentils, and carob

- **Fruit:** lemons, limes, oranges, pineapples, peaches, plums, pears, apples, tangerines, grapefruit, nectarines, bananas, grapes, prunes, papayas, figs, mangoes, kiwi, cherries, apricots, cranberries, strawberries, blackberries, and raspberries
- **Melons:** watermelons, cantaloupe, and honeydew melon
- **Dairy:** milk, cheese, yogurt, goat's milk, cream, butter, and ice cream
- **Poultry:** chicken, eggs, turkey, duck, pheasant, quail, and goose
- **Meat:** beef, lamb, and pork
- **Seafood:** fish, shrimp, oysters, clams, mussels, lobster, scallops, crayfish, and crab
- **Flavorings:** dill, comfrey, tarragon, coriander, pepper, cinnamon, mustard, caraway, ginger, vanilla, cocoa, thyme, basil, oregano, alfalfa, rosemary, sage, peppermint, clove, and nutmeg
- **Fungus:** mushrooms, hops, and bakers and brewers yeast

YOUR ROTATION DIET

The allergy testing labs we recommend in the appendix will supply you with a specific rotation diet based on your allergic foods. But if you elect not to be tested by a lab, use the elimination diet and/or the pulse test method to uncover any food allergies. Then using the food groups listed above, create your own rotation diet; write out four different breakfasts, lunches, snacks, and dinners. But make sure you're waiting three days before repeating a food. There's a sample menu on the next page.

Eating out can present a challenge, but I've found that most restaurants are able to accommodate your special needs once you mention your food allergies.

Visit your local health food store. Take this book, and explain your rotation diet. Ask them to help you shop for foods to make your diet more compliant. These stores are especially helpful in supplying hard-to-find grains, seeds, snacks, and nuts.

Most delayed food allergies resolve themselves after three months of avoidance. Don't fall off the wagon and begin repetitively eating the same foods day in and day out. Continue to rotate your foods.

Sample Rotation-Diet Menu for One Week

Monday
- Breakfast: eggs, wheat toast, orange
- Snack: apple and cashews
- Lunch: romaine lettuce with olive oil and vinegar; turkey breast with wheat bread, mustard, tomato, and mayo
- Dinner: egg omelet with cheddar cheese, broccoli, and onions
- Snack: cashews and strawberries

Tuesday
- Breakfast: pork bacon or sausage with oatmeal and raisins
- Snack: almonds and a pear
- Lunch: chicken salad (no bread or mayo), pear, and grapes
- Dinner: baked chicken, asparagus, and corn on the cob
- Snack: popcorn

Wednesday
- Breakfast: cream of rice topped with banana and blueberries; rice milk
- Snack: tangerine and Brazil nuts
- Lunch: corned beef on plain rye with sauerkraut and Swiss cheese (no mayo or mustard) and baked potato fries
- Dinner: steak with okra, wild rice, and pinto beans
- Snack: walnuts, blueberries, and dates

Thursday
- Breakfast: honeydew melon or cantaloupe, peanut butter on millet bread
- Snack: Pumpkin seeds and sunflower seeds
- Lunch: Baked fish with cauliflower, squash, and zucchini
- Dinner: Lobster, crab cakes, or shrimp salad and olive, artichoke, tomato, and yellow peppers
- Snack: cherries and pistachios

Friday
(Repeat Monday's menu.)

PROTOCOL FOR TREATING FOOD ALLERGIES

1. **Uncover any hidden food sensitivities** through the elimination diet, Coca pulse testing, or blood testing. Once uncovered, these foods should be avoided for one–six months, depending on the severity your reactions.

2. **Begin a rotation diet** as described above to reduce the chances of developing further food allergies.

3. **Treat any intestinal permeability.** See chapter 12 for how.

4. **Be sure you're using adrenal cortex glandular supplements as part of your jump-start plan.** They reduce allergic reactions.

5. **Make sure to take your digestive enzymes included in your jump-start plan.** Undigested food can lead to allergic reactions.

7. **Use my natural Inflammation Support Formula** to reduce or eliminate allergy symptoms.

OVER-THE-COUNTER AND PRESCRIPTION ALLERGY MEDICATIONS

Antihistamine medications like Benadryl or Zyrtec can offer welcomed relief from allergic reactions, and so can the leukotriene-blocking drug Singular. While these medications are relatively safe, they due have potential side effects, which are generally mild. Steroid nasal inhalers like Flonase may also be helpful. However, I encourage my patients to use the nasal rinse kit and formula described on page 293.

NATURAL REMEDIES

Several natural remedies can help relieve the symptoms of food and seasonal allergies. Below are some of the ones I find most helpful.

ESSENTIAL THERAPEUTIC'S INFLAMMATION SUPPORT

Available through my office, this contains the following:

• **Turmeric root extract** inhibits enzymes associated with PG-2 inflammatory hormones, major triggers for allergic reactions.

- **Rosemary leaf extract** helps block synthesis of leukotrienes (a cause of allergic inflammation) and PG-2 hormones. Singular also works by blocking leukotrienes.
- **Holy basil leaf extract** helps boost natural anti-inflammatory chemicals (PG-1 and PG-3).
- **Green tea leaf extract** is a potent antioxidant and increases the body's own anti-inflammatory activity.
- Ginger root extract reduces inflammation.
- **Chinese goldenthread root** helps regulate prostaglandins; it reduces the inflammatory PG-2 hormones and boosts the anti-inflammatory PG-1 and PG-3 hormones.
- **Barberry root extract** helps reduce the inflammatory PG-2 hormones and increases the anti-inflammatory PG-1 and PG-3 hormones.
- **Baikal skullcap root extract** reduces inflammatory chemicals.
- **Protykin** extract is a potent antioxidant and reduces inflammatory chemicals, including PG-2.

EXTRA VITAMIN C
This natural antihistamine may reduce the symptoms associated with allergic reactions. Take an additional 2,000 mg. above your CFS/Fibro Formula. Keep increasing by 1,000 mg. a day, until you experience a loose bowel movement. Then reduce your dose by 1,000 mg. or until you have a normal bowel movement once again.

STINGING NETTLE ROOT
This herb helps reduce allergic rhinitis (runny nose) and hay fever symptoms. It also helps prevent the bronchial spasms associated with asthma. Dosage is 500–1,000 mg. three times daily.

QUERCETIN
This bioflavonoid (plant pigment) is found in black tea, blue-green algae, broccoli, onions, red apples, and red wine. It inhibits the synthesis of certain enzymes responsible for triggering allergic reactions and is chemically similar to the allergy prevention medication Cromolyn. Dosage is 500–1,000 twice daily. It may take months

before quercetin reaches its peak of effectiveness. It can also interfere with the absorption of certain antibiotics, so don't take quercetin and antibiotics together.

METHYLSULFONYLMETHANE

This natural organic sulfur compound found in plant and animal tissues has proven beneficial in the treatment of allergic and inflammation disorders. It provides sulfur, an essential component in detoxification.

Due to its strong anti-inflammatory properties, it's included in my Essential Therapeutics Arthritis Formula. Normal dosage is 500 mg. three–four times daily. It's also called "MSM."

EXTRA FISH OIL

Studies have shown that supplementing with fish oils results in a dramatic reduction in a person's leukotrienes (one of the chemicals implicated in asthma and other allergic reactions) by 65%. This correlates with a 75% decrease in their clinical symptoms. Your CFS/Fibro Formula already contains 2,000 mg. of fish oil daily. But you can add this an additional 7,000 mg. per day.

DIETARY CHANGES

Reduce grains (wheat, breads, pasta, corn, etc.) and other high-omega-6 foods, including red meat. Omega-6 foods produce arachidonic acid, which leads to more inflammatory chemicals.

Consider reducing all caffeine consumption, including caffeinated teas (green tea is allowed), coffees, chocolate, and cocoa. The less caffeine, the better. To prevent withdrawal symptoms (headaches, mood disturbances, fatigue), slowly wean off. See pages 205–206 for suggestions on how.

RESOURCES
• Information on allergy testing labs, supplements, food allergy resources, and rotation diets can be found in the appendices.

FOR FURTHER READING AND RESEARCH

• A.P. Black, "A new diagnostic method in allergic disease," *Pediatrics* (May 1956): 171–6.
• J.H. Boyles, "The validity of using the cytotoxic food test in clinical allergy," *Ear, Nose and Throat Journal* (April 1977).
• W.F. Stevenson et al., "Dietary supplementation with fish oil in ulcerative colitis," *Ann Int Med* 11 (1992): 609–14.

· 19 ·
LIVER TOXICITY

We are constantly being exposed to potentially dangerous toxins through the food we eat, the air we breathe, and the water we drink.

Thankfully, our liver works to neutralize harmful chemicals, viruses, and bacteria. It's also first to process the nutrients delivered by the bloodstream. As the largest organ in the body, it filters two quarts of blood every minute and secretes a quart of bile each day. Bile is necessary for absorbing fat-soluble substances, including certain vitamins. It also helps eliminate toxic chemicals. Bile is then mixed with dietary fiber and voided through daily bowel movements.

An optimally functioning detoxification system is necessary for providing good health and preventing disease. Many diseases, including cancer, rheumatoid arthritis, Lupus, Alzheimer's, Parkinson's, and other chronic age-related conditions, are linked to a weakened detoxification system. A poor detox system also contributes to allergic disorders, asthma, hives, psoriasis, and eczema. It's associated with chronic fatigue syndrome, fibromyalgia, depression, and systemic candidiasis.

TWO PHASES OF DETOX

Unwanted chemicals, including prescription and nonprescription drugs, alcohol, pesticides, herbicides, and metabolic waste products are neutralized by the liver's enzymes. There are two enzymatic pathways, phase I and phase II.

Phase I detoxification enzymes are collectively known as cytochrome P450. The cytochrome P450 system is made up of 50–100 enzymes that attempt to neutralize toxic chemicals by transforming them into a less toxic form. Each enzyme is specially suited to certain types of toxins. Chemicals that can't be neutralized are changed into an intermediate form. As the phase I enzymes neutralize toxins, they spin off free radicals. If there aren't enough antioxidants to counter these free radicals, the liver may be compromised.

Phase I detoxification is inhibited by antihistamines, NSAIDs, azole drugs (antifungals), tranquilizers such as Valium and Klonopin, and antidepressants such as Prozac and Celexa. (Is it any wonder that FMS and CFS patients are told that their condition is "all in their head" when drugs make them sicker?)

Phase I is responsible for neutralizing most over-the-counter and prescription drugs, caffeine, hormones, yellow dyes, insecticides, alcohol, and histamine.

Phase II detoxification enzymes go to work on the toxins that the phase I enzymes turned into intermediate form. They do this by attaching minute chemicals to the structures. This process is called conjugation, and it neutralizes the toxins, making them more likely to be excreted through urination or defecation. Unfortunately, many of these intermediate forms are more toxic and potentially more damaging than in their original state. So an inadequate phase II detoxification system can cause all sorts of chronic illnesses.

A person suffering from poorly functioning phase II and overactive phase I detoxification is known as a pathological detoxifier. These individuals fill up doctors' offices on a regular basis, because they suffer from a variety of ailments that seem to never go away. One illness is replaced by another as the patient tries one prescription after another. Neither the doctor nor the patient realizes that a compromised detoxification system is being further aggravated by toxic prescription medications.

Phase II is responsible for neutralizing acetaminophen, nicotine, and insecticides. It is comprised of the following conjugation processes:

- **Glutathione conjugation** requires vitamin B6 and the tripeptide (made from three amino acids) glutathione.
- **Amino-acid conjugation** requires the amino acid glycine. Low-protein diets and deficient digestive enzymes inhibit this process.

Individuals with hypothyroidism, arthritis, hepatitis, and chemical sensitivities may suffer from poor amino-acid conjugation.

- **Methylation** requires S-adenosyl-methionine (SAMe). SAMe is synthesized from the amino acid methionine and dependent on folic acid, choline, and vitamin B12. Methylation detoxifies estrogen, testosterone, thyroid hormones, acetaminophen, and coumarin.

- **Sulfation** requires the amino acids cysteine and methionine and the mineral molybdenum. Sulfation is involved in processing steroids, thyroid hormones, food additives, certain drugs, and neurotransmitters. Individuals who can't take certain antidepressants or have reactions to certain sulfur-containing foods may benefit from taking extra molybdenum, taurine, cysteine, and methionine. (All these are included in our CFS/Fibromyalgia formula.)

- **Acetylation** requires acetyl-CoA and is inhibited by a deficiency in vitamin C, B2, or B5. This pathway is responsible for eliminating sulfa drugs, so individuals with sulfa allergies may benefit from extra vitamin C, B2, or B5.

- **Glucuronidation** requires glucoronic acid and detoxifies acetaminophen, morphine, benzoates, aspirin, and vanilla. Aspirin inhibits this process. Signs of deficiency include yellowish pigment in the eyes or skin not caused by hepatitis.

- **Sulfoxidation** requires molybdenum and detoxifies sulfites and garlic. You may be deficient in this enzyme if you have allergic reactions to sulfite foods or garlic, asthmatic reactions after eating, or a strong urine odor after eating asparagus. Individuals with a sluggish sulfoxidation pathway may benefit from taking additional molybdenum.

Fish oils, SAMe, broccoli, Brussels sprouts, and cabbage all stimulate phase I and phase II reactions. Choline, betaine, methionine, vitamin B6, folic acid, and vitamin B12 (altogether known as lipotrophic factors) stimulate bile production and its flow to and from the liver. Lipotrophic factors also increase SAMe and glutathione, which in turn spare the liver free-radical damage.

Free Radicals and Antioxidants

Free radicals are unstable atoms or molecules with an unpaired electron in the outer ring. They fill the void by taking an electron from another molecule, which then becomes unstable, needing another electron of its own. This sets up a destructive cycle that can cause damage to our bodies inside and out.

Internal metabolic activities, including immune and detoxification processes, generate free-radical molecules, but sometimes they come from our environment. External sources include radiation, alcohol, tobacco, smog, medications, and pesticides. Free radicals have been implicated in such conditions as rheumatoid arthritis, Alzheimer's, Parkinson's, cancer, and heart disease.

Believe it or not, oxygen is responsible for the creation of most toxic free radicals. Just like it causes rust on a car, excessive oxygen can cause premature aging and dysfunction in the body. That's why antioxidants, including vitamins A, E, and C, and beta carotene, are so important. Along with the amino acids cysteine, methionine, glycine, and glutathione (tripeptide), they help deter the effects of free-radical damage.

Have you ever cut open an apple and then left it out awhile? If so, you've witnessed free-radical damage. The once white inner meat of the apple turns brown when exposed to the oxygen in the air. Sprinkling lemon juice on the apple will turn the brown back to its normal color. This is an example of an antioxidant at work.

TOXIC WATER

A study released in 1988 by Ralph Nader's Center for Study of Responsive Law in Washington, DC, shows that much of the nation's drinking water is unsafe: Tests conducted in 38 states found over 2,000 toxic chemicals in the drinking water. About 10% of these chemicals are associated with causing cancer, cell growths, neurological damage, and birth defects. Thousands of chemicals found in our water supplies have never even been tested for safety.

> "No longer can anyone assume the 500 chemicals in the average U.S. municipal water supply are without side effects on the body....We now know, for example, that when the brain is unable to detoxify some of these chemicals, it actually manufactures chloral hydrate in the brain...[producing] the symptoms of brain fog."
>
> —Sherry Rogers, MD[1]

A joint study by the EPA and the National Academy of Sciences has attributed 200–1,000 US deaths each year to the inhalation of chloroform from water while bathing.

So what's in the water Americans are drinking? Here is a partial list of the unwelcome additions that have been found in drinking water.

- **arsenic** is a known carcinogen and poison
- **asbestos** is a known carcinogen
- **cadmium** causes arteriosclerosis, kidney damage, and cancer
- **lead** causes learning disabilities in children
- **mercury** causes nervous system and kidney damage
- **nitrites** are a possible carcinogen that also interferes with body's oxygen metabolism
- **viruses and bacteria**
- **toxic chemicals**
- **1,1,1-trichloroethane** causes liver damage and depression
- **1,1-dichlorethylene** causes depressed central nervous system and cancer
- **benzene** causes chromosomal damage in humans, anemia, blood disorders, and leukemia
- **chloroform** causes cancer
- **dioxin** is an extremely toxic carcinogen
- **ethylene dibromide** causes male sterility and cancer
- **polychlorinated biphyls** [PCB] causes liver damage, skin disorders, and GI problems and is highly suspected of causing cancer

Do I really need to continue? I think you get the message. Our drinking water is not safe! A hot shower or bath can increase your exposure to toxic chemicals by 400 percent. One thousand deaths occur every year from chloral hydrate poisoning while taking a shower.

Here's what you can do:

- **Have your water tested.** Several companies will run a laboratory test to see if your water is safe. Look in your local phone book under "water quality" or "laboratories, testing" or write to Water Test Corporation at 33 S. Commercial Street, Manchester, NH 03108.

- **Invest in a reverse-osmosis system.** This is the most effective way to remove unwanted chemicals. It does have its drawbacks though; prices start at $350 dollars and can go above $1,000 dollars. Activated carbon filter systems, either above or below the sink, remove impurities. Block and granular filter systems are superior to powdered filters.

- **Buy bottled water, preferably in glass bottles.** Plastic bottles can emit harmful chemicals. The best water is distilled spring water. Buying bottled water can get expensive, and you should always question the bottling source.

TOXIC "FOODS"

We are a social experiment in the making. Never in the history of mankind have we been exposed to so many man-made chemicals. We have traded good, wholesome foods for grocery store convenience. I don't deny the convenience of walking into a store and purchasing next week's dinner, but to be oblivious to the damaging chemical preservatives in our foods is myopic. Try setting a fruit or vegetable on your back porch, and notice it will be consumed in a matter of days, if not hours. Do the same with a lump of margarine, and it's still there a week later—no sane animal would touch it!

Tons of toxic industrial wastes, including heavy metals, are being mixed with liquid agricultural fertilizers and dispersed across America's farmlands.

Artificial dyes and preservatives are used in most of our processed foods. They are even found in both prescription and nonprescription drugs. Asthmatics are often allergic to sulfites, for instance, but some asthma inhalant medications actually have sulfites in them as a preservative! Examples of dangerous additives are benzoates, yellow dye (tartrazine), nitrites, sorbic acid, and sulfites. Allergic symptoms associated with them include hives, angioedema, asthma, sinusitis, headache, anxiety, depression, and chronic fatigue. The most notorious culprits are aspartame, monosodium glutamate, hydroxytoluene, and butylated hydroxyanisole.

Aspartame can be found in most diet sodas and in other artificially sweetened food products. Commonly known as NutraSweet or Equal, it is broken down by the body into methanol and formaldehyde. Toxic levels of methanol are linked to systemic lupus and now Alzheimer's disease. Methanol toxicity also causes depression, brain fog, mood changes, insomnia, seizures, and similar symptoms associated with multiple sclerosis. As for formaldehyde, it is grouped into the same class of drugs as cyanide and arsenic.

When the temperature of aspartame exceeds 86 degrees F, the wood alcohol in the product is turned into formaldehyde and then into formic acid. Formic acid is the poison contained in the sting of a fire ant.

The amino acid aspartic acid makes up 40% of aspartame. Aspartic acid is an excitatory amino acid and often contributes in children to attention deficit disorder. I always encourage my ADD patients to get off and stay off diet colas. There are over 92 documented symptoms from the use of aspartame.

Monosodium glutamate is often added to soups, stews, and Chinese food. **Benzoates, toluenes,** and **butylated hydroxyanisole** can be found in pickles, jams, jellies, and some sodas and cakes. **Sulfites** are added to salad bars, beer, frozen french fries, dried fruit, shampoos, conditioners, and some cosmetics. **Nitrites** are used to preserve luncheon meats, hot dogs, and other ready-to-eat meats.

Here's what you can do:

• **Avoid foods containing artificial dyes and preservatives.** If the ingredients list is hard to pronounce, it's probably even harder on your body. Organic meats are becoming more available at grocery stores around the country.

• **Consume whole, live foods.** Fruits, vegetables, and whole, unprocessed grains (unless you are gluten sensitive) are the healthiest foods to eat. These foods are loaded with antioxidant, cancer-fighting, and immune-boosting phytonutrients. They are easy on the digestive system and allow the body to generate more energy to fight diseases and build immunity.

TOXIC PRODUCTS

Toxic chemicals don't have to enter through the mouth. Many of the products we use on a daily basis in the form of shampoos, conditioners, lotion soaps, deodorants, and cosmetics are contaminated with toxic chemicals, especially heavy metals. Many of these metals have been implicated in causing or contributing to such conditions as Alzheimer's, ADD, depression, headache, hypertension, kidney failure, hearing loss, FMS, CFS, and tingling in the extremities.

Aluminum toxicity has been linked to Alzheimer's disease and mental dementia. Aluminum is found in some antacids, baking flours, baking soda, processed cheeses, toothpastes, shampoos and conditioners, deodorants, prescription and nonprescription drugs, and aluminum cans, pots, and pans.

Arsenic can cause central depression, headache, high fevers, decreased red blood cells, fatigue, diarrhea, and even death. Municipal or well water may get contaminated with arsenic.

I once treated a woman who had been diagnosed with multiple sclerosis, only to find through hair analysis and other testing that she had actually been poisoned with arsenic.

Cadmium levels, when elevated, are associated with hypertension, kidney failure, loss of coordination, numbness or tingling in the hands or feet, and loss of hearing. Common environmental sources include tobacco smoke and oil-based paints. A zinc deficiency exacerbates the effects of cadmium toxicity. If you are a smoker, please, please quit this destructive habit immediately. Many of my patients have had success with subliminal tapes and/or hypnosis.

Lead toxicity effects are numerous and include neurological disorders in children, chronic anemia, learning disturbances, and fatigue. Common sources of lead in the environment are lead-based paints, drinking water, industrial contaminants, airborne emissions, and occupations involving metal work and printing. It is also found in some personal care products. Lead absorption is higher when calcium intake is deficient.

Mercury toxicity can cause a wide variety of health problems: CFS, FMS, stunted growth, confusion and dementia, numbness in the extremities, depression, muscle and joint pain, allergies, chronic infections, and possibly brain damage. Mercury can suppress selenium absorption. Selenium blocks mercury absorption by binding with competing sulfur enzyme centers. Mercury can turn normal bacteria pathogenic (disease causing) and block the function of the nerve cells in the brain and peripheral nervous system. Mercury can also trigger autoimmune responses. Detoxifying from mercury requires oral herbs, mineral supplements, and prescription oral or intravenous medications.

One source of chronic, low-level mercury exposure is the eating of predatory fish. Mercury enters the water as a natural process of off-gassing from the earth's crust and as a result of industrial pollution. It is then routinely found in large predatory fish, such as swordfish, shark, salmon, and tuna.

Most of the mercury in our patients comes from the fillings in their teeth. Dental amalgams (silver fillings) contain a highly absorbable form of mercury that vaporizes at room temperature. And while mercury is poorly absorbed if taken orally, its vapors are readily absorbed through the lungs and quickly pass the blood-brain barrier. Once inside a cell, mercury is usually there to stay, so it accumulates in the kidneys, neurological tissue (including the brain), and the liver. Evidence of high mercury exposure has also been found in the heart, thyroid, and pituitary tissues of dentists. Animal research has shown that within 24 hours of having a silver filling placed, an animal has detectable levels of mercury in the spinal fluid, and in the brain within 48 hours. Patients with symptoms of mercury toxicity should have all dental amalgams removed by a dentist with knowledge of mercury poisoning. Some patients have had a worsening of their symptoms when their fillings were removed without the proper measures to prevent increased mercury exposure.

Other sources of mercury include the use of fossil fuels, fungicides, and some paints, and the production of chlorine, paper, and pulp.

Nickel is not as toxic as many of the other metals. It's associated with headache, diarrhea, blue gums and lips, lethargy, insomnia, rapid heart rate, and shortness of breath. It is found in some personal care products.

Copper toxicity has been implicated in learning and mental disorders and may contribute to increased systolic blood pressure. It is found in some personal care products.

Here's what you can do:

- **Use stainless steel pots and pans.** Also avoid aluminum- and lead-lined cans.
- **Switch to natural toothpaste, hair products, and deodorants.** Visit your local health-food store or browse online; you should find a wide selection of natural body products. Read the labels.
- **Never take antacids that contain aluminum.** Not only do they contain toxic aluminum, they block hydrochloric acid, preventing the body from synthesizing essential nutrients like vitamin B12. A deficiency of vitamin B12 can cause dementia, Alzheimer's, depression, and fatigue. Antacids also don't allow you to absorb calcium. So if you are taking Tums as a source of calcium, you have been duped by their marketing team.
- **Conduct a hair analysis.** These inexpensive tests can be done at home and are an accurate first step in uncovering heavy metal overload. See Appendix C for resources.

TOXIC BODIES

The body does its best to dispose of toxins by neutralizing them or voiding them in the urine or feces. The lungs help through respiration, and the skin through sweat. But whether they come from heavy metal poisoning, pesticides, artificial food additives, or metabolic activities, these chemical toxins are neutralized at a price: the creation of more free radicals.

Here's what you can do:

- **Test your liver.** I recommend phase I and phase II detoxification testing to my patients who can't seem to get well. (Ask your doctor to order this test, or contact my office at 1-888-884-9577.) Individuals plagued with unrelenting poor health are usually saturated with poisonous chemicals.

- **Explore alternatives to long-term prescription drugs like nonsteroidal anti-inflammatories.** Work with your doctor.

- **Severely reduce or eliminate alcohol, nicotine, allergic foods, and preservative-rich foods.**

- **Supplement with antioxidants to combat free radicals.** Include vitamins A, E, and C; the mineral selenium; and pycnogenol.

- **Enjoy foods from the Brassica family:** broccoli, cabbage and Brussels sprouts. They contain phytochemicals that stimulate phase I and phase II detoxification pathways.

- **Supplement with a formula containing an amino-acid blend.** (Our Essential Therapeutics CFS/Fibromyalgia formula is a good choice for this.) Glutathione is the most abundant and important liver-protecting antioxidant. Although it is readily absorbed from fruits, vegetables, and meats, depletion may occur during high or sustained exposure to toxins. Glutathione supplements are not readily absorbable, so supplement with its building blocks instead: cysteine, methionine, and glycine.

- **Supplement with silybum marianum (milk thistle).** The silymarin complex, particularly the silibinin component of milk thistle, protects the liver from free-radical damage. It prevents certain toxins from entering liver cells and stimulates regeneration of damaged liver cells.

Medical use of milk thistle can be traced back more than 2000 years. Over 30 years ago, intensive research on the liver-protecting properties of milk thistle began in Germany. Extensive research also may have led to the approval of a standardized milk thistle extract in Germany for the treatment of alcohol-induced liver disease and other diseases of the liver.

Milk thistle extract protects liver cells, both directly and indirectly. It is able to regenerate liver cells that have been injured, prevent fibrosis or fatty liver, bind to the outside of cells and block entrance of certain toxins, and even neutralize toxins that have already penetrated the liver. Milk thistle treatment can be effective even several hours after initial poisoning occurs, such as in the case of poisoning by death cap mushrooms. And there are no side effects.

Silymarin may also prevent the damage caused by certain drugs such as acetaminophen, antidepressants, and antipsychotic, cholesterol-lowering, and anticonvulsive drugs. One study showed that increasing the antioxidants in patients receiving psychotropic drugs reduced the production of potentially damaging free radicals in the liver.

Silymarin has been shown in animal studies to raise the glutathione levels in liver cells by as much as 50%. It also increases the activity of another antioxidant known as supraoxide dismutase (SOD).

Milk thistle may someday be the main treatment for hepatitis, a chronic viral infection of the liver that can lead to liver damage and, in some cases, liver failure. During a six-month treatment period in patients with chronic alcohol hepatitis, liver function test results normalized and liver enzymes improved over controls using placebo.

The normal dose is 420 mg. in three divided doses (80% silymarin content) daily.

- **Supplement with alpha lipoic acid.** This powerful antioxidant compound helps recycle glutathione. It is both fat and water soluble, so it works in both mediums. Manufactured by the body in small amounts, it needs to be also obtained through the diet. It can help prevent and repair damage to liver cells and is being studied for its regenerative properties in neurological diseases including Alzheimer's, multiple sclerosis, Lou Gehrig's disease, and Parkinson's disease. To increase liver detoxification and boost cellular energy, take between 200–400 mg. of ALA daily. I recommend Essential Therapeutics Liver Detox Formula, which contains both ALA and milk thistle, as well as methionine, n-acetyl-l-cysteine, L-cysteine, and taurine. To order, you can visit www.TreatingAndBeating.com or call 1-888-884-9577.

- **Supplement with coenzyme Q10.** CoQ10 is also known as ubiquinone, because of its nature to exist in all living matter. It is most abundant in the organs requiring the most energy: the heart and liver. It is a vital catalyst for energy; without it, the process of cellular energy ceases (which spells d-e-a-t-h). CoQ10, along with ALA, gives the spark to the power plants of the cells, the mitochondria.

CoQ10 plays a direct or indirect role in most systems of the body. Experiments have shown that supplementing the diet with CoQ10 can extend the life span of mice by 50%. It acts as a powerful antioxidant, helps stimulate white blood cells, protects heart muscle from disease, reduces blood pressure, boosts the metabolism, helps prevent periodontal disease, and protects the liver. Studies have shown that CoQ10 can raise the brain energy level by over 29%. This is good news for those with fibro-fog.

SPECIAL PROTOCOL FOR CHEMICALLY SENSITIVE PATIENTS

Chemically sensitive patients display evidence of sluggish detoxification processes. They may have had elevated liver enzymes on past blood tests, hepatitis, or a fatty liver. They tend to have adverse—even opposite—reactions to prescription medications. Strong odors tend to give them problems; newsprint, gasoline, copy machine toner, tobacco, perfumes, etc. The longer they've had the illness the more sensitive they've become. You already know if this applies to you; you've tried in the past to take supplements or medications, but you just can't tolerate them. This doesn't include allergic or funny reactions to *specific* types of medicines. Those with chemical sensitivities will have adverse reactions to most all drugs and supplements. Most also can't tolerate caffeine or alcohol.

I don't routinely use detoxification supplements or procedures on my new patients. However, since the severely chemically sensitive ones (usually CFS patients) aren't able to take any of the usual supplements (CFS/Fibro, 5-HTP, adrenal cortex, etc.), I'll start them slowly on the following protocol.

- **First, get as "cleaned up" as you can.** Explore alternatives to long-term prescription drugs like nonsteroidal anti-inflammatories (Celebrex, Mobic, Aleve, etc.), benzodiazepines (Xanax, Klonopin, Ativan, etc.), anti-depressants, and statins (Crestor, Lipitor, Zocor, etc.). Severely reduce or eliminate alcohol, nicotine, known allergic foods, and preservative-rich foods. Try to eat live foods with no additives or preservatives. Especially enjoy foods from the Brassica family: broccoli, cabbage, and Brussels sprouts. They contain phytochemicals that stimulate phase I and phase II detoxification pathways.
- **Then, uncover and address any food allergies** (chapter 18) **and intestinal permeability** (chapter 12).
- **Take a digestive enzyme with each meal,** which takes some of the burden off the liver.
- **Before starting any other supplements, use milk thistle and alpha lipoic acid** (Essential Therapeutics Liver Detox Formula) for one week. As discussed earlier in the chapter, milk thistle protects the liver from free-radical damage, prevents certain toxins from entering liver cells, and stimulates regeneration of damaged liver cells. Milk thistle also helps prevent the damage caused by certain drugs such as acetaminophen, antidepressants, cholesterol-lowering drugs, and tranquilizing drugs. One study showed that increasing the antioxidants (including milk thistle) in patients receiving psychotropic drugs (Prozac, Celexa, Paxil, Klonopin, Ativan, Xanax, etc.) reduced the production of potentially damaging free radicals in the liver.
- **One week later, start a hypoallergenic multivitamin-and-mineral powder formula.** I use Douglas Labs' (pea protein) Protein Powder. I have the patient start with half the recommended daily dose and gradually increase up to the normal dose.
- **Two more weeks later,** begin 5-HTP if needed according to the Brain Function Questionnaire in chapter 16 or if needed for sleep. Rather than the protocol outlined in chapter 10, start with 50 mg. of 5-HTP at lunch. After a few days, try 100 mg. at lunch and 50 mg. with dinner. Keep increasing (as long as you don't have any problems) until you are taking 300 mg. in divided doses, with food, each day.

- **Add 100 mg. of CoQ10 to your daily supplementation routine.** It plays a direct or indirect role in most systems of the body. (Experiments have shown that supplementing the diet with CoQ10 can extend the life span of mice by 50%.) It acts as a powerful antioxidant, helps stimulate white blood cells, protects heart muscle from disease, reduces blood pressure, boosts the metabolism, can raise brain energy levels by over 29%, helps prevent periodontal disease, and **protects the liver.**

NOTES
1. *Tired or Toxic* (Syracuse: Prestige, 1990).

RESOURCES
- Liver detox functional testing, liver detox kits, and hair test for toxic chemicals—including heavy metals—are available from my office (1-888-884-9577) or by referral from your doctor.
- For analysis of drinking water, air filters, water filters, and other products, contact the American Environmental Health Foundation at 1-800-428-2343 or www.aehf.com.
- Protein Powder is available from Douglas Labs by referral from your doctor or from my office (1-888-884-9577).

FOR FURTHER READING AND RESEARCH

- Blot W, Li JY, and Taylor P. "Nutrition intervention trials in Linxian, China; supplementation with specific vitamin mineral combination." Cancer Incidence and Disease-Specific Mortality in the General Population. *Journal of the National Cancer Institute* 1993;85:1483–92.
- Cerutti PA. "Oxy-radicals and cancer." *Lancet* 1994;344:862–3.
- Chang LW. "Toxico-neurology and neuropathology induced by metals." In: Chang LW, ed. Toxicology of Metals. Boca Raton:CRC Press 1996;511–535.
- Cross CE, Halliwell B et al. "Oxygen radicals and human disease" *Annals of Internal Medicine* 1987;107:526–45.
- Dalenzuela A, Aspillaga M et al. "Selectivity of silymarin on the increase of glutathione content in different tissues of the rat." *Planta Med* 1989;55:420–422.
- Feher J, Lange I et al. "Free radicals and tissue damage in liver disease and therapeutic approach." *Tokai Je Exp Clin Med* 1986;11:121–134.
- Flora K et al. "Milk thistle (Silybum marianum) for the therapy of liver disease." *Am J Gastroenterol* 1998;93:139–43.
- Goldsmith J et al. "Evaluation of health implications of elevated arsenic in well water." *Water Res* 1972;6:1133–36.
- Knoll O et al. "Consequences from EEG findings and aluminum encephalopathy." *Trace Element Med* 1991;8-s:18-s:20.

- Lorscheider Fl, Vimy MJ, and Summers AO. "Mercury exposure from 'silver' tooth fillings: emerging evidence questions a traditional paradigm." *FASEB J* 1995;504–508.
- McKinnon R A and Nebert DW. "Possible role of cytochrome in lupus erythematosis and related disorders" *Lupus* 1994;3:473–78.
- Muzes G, Deak G et al. "Effected bile flavonoids silymarin on the in vitro activity and expression of supraoxide dismutase (SOD) enzyme." *Acta Physiol Hung* 1991;78:3–9.
- Nylander M, Frieberg L, and Lind B. "Mercury concentrations in the brain and kidneys in relation to exposure from dental amalgam fillings." *Swed Dent J* 1987;11:179–187.
- Palasciano G, Portincasa B, et. al. "Effective silymarin on plasma levels of malondialdhide in patients receiving an antioxidant treatment with psychotropic drugs." *Curr Ther Res* 1994;55:537–545.
- Quick AJ. "Clinical value of the test for hippuric acid in cases of diseases of the liver." *Arch Int Med* 1936;57:544–556.
- Rifat SL. "Aluminum hypothesis lives." *Lancet* 1994;343:3–4.
- Rigden S. "Entero-hepatic resusicitation program for cfids, Charlotte, NC." *Chronic Fatigue and Immune Deficiency Syndrome Chronicle* Spring 1995:46–49.
- Sargent JD, Meveres A, and Weitzman M. "Environmental exposure to lead and cognitive deficits in children." Letter. *New England Journal of Medicine* 1989;320(9):595.
- Suzuki T and Yamamoto R. "Organic mercury levels in human hair with and without storage for eleven years." *Bull Environ Contam Toxicol* 1928;28:186–188.

· 20 ·
PARASITES

Parasites are living organisms that survive off of a host. And parasitic infections are often discovered as the primary cause of many chronic illnesses, including autoimmune diseases, allergies, candidiasis, and other diseases that don't correspond nicely with a textbook remedy.

Unlike some naturally oriented doctors, I don't believe that every patient who walks through my door suffers from a yeast or parasitic infection. Although this simple, comprehensive philosophy is tempting to embrace, it's just not shown reliable. I've found that my much more complex jump-start program usually reduces or completely vanishes the symptoms of FMS and CFS. But if your symptoms persist beyond the jump-start, then parasites must be ruled out as a cause.

Parasitic infections, once mainly associated with third-world countries, have become a common occurrence in the United States. Though the primary mode of transmitting parasites is fecal to oral contamination, water contamination is often the culprit. In fact, Milwaukee's water supply was found to be contaminated with *Cryptosporidium,* a parasite that caused one hundred deaths and infected over 400,000 people. Shockingly, most municipal water supplies are contaminated with parasites like *Cryptosporidium.* Each year, 1 million Americans become ill due to contaminated drinking water, and 10,000 of them die.

Now, parasites don't have to be so deadly. In fact, 99% of those living in undeveloped countries are infected with parasites. Humans and parasites are able to coexist, as long as the human intestinal tract lining is intact, keeping the parasites where they can't do damage. But a permeable intestinal lining allows parasites to penetrate into the body and cause allergic and inflammatory reactions. Many people with FMS or CFS already have damaged intestinal linings and are susceptible to parasitic infection.

World travel and increased immigration have contributed to a rise in parasitic infections with in the US. One 1991 study of an immigrant population showed that 74% of them had parasites. In the US, the most common parasites include *Giardia lamblia, Blastocystis hominis,* and *Dientamoeba fragilis.*

G. lamblia is highly contagious and carried by most animals, including dogs and cats. Consequently, it has infested most of the ground water in North America. Children in day care programs are especially vulnerable to *Giardia* and *Dientamoeba.* It is estimated that between 21%–44% of children in day care are infected with one or both of these parasites. These parasites can then spread to the rest of the family.

Other parasites include intestinal worms, such as roundworms, tapeworms, hookworms, and pinworms. Roundworms are most prevalent in the Appalachian Mountains.

RECOGNIZING AND TESTING FOR PARASITES

Not all patients infected with intestinal parasites display gastrointestinal problems; they can have other symptoms that improve once their infection is treated. Everyone with a chronic illness, especially FMS/CFS, should be tested for intestinal parasites. Notice how many of the symptoms below—characteristic of parasitic infection—are found in individuals with FMS/CFS:

- abdominal pain
- anorexia
- autoimmune disease
- chronic fatigue
- constipation
- fever
- bloating
- gas
- indigestion

- headaches
- nausea
- vomiting
- diarrhea
- colitis
- IBS
- Crohn's disease
- arthritis
- weight loss
- bloody stools

- rash
- skin/rectal itching
- low back pain
- food allergies
- malabsorption syndrome
- intestinal permeability
- chemical intolerance

Parasite Symptom Checklist

Consider being tested for parasites if you check "yes" to more than half of the statements below.

_____ Have you ever traveled outside the United States?

_____ Do you have foul-smelling stools?

_____ Do you experience any stomach bloating, gas, or pain?

_____ Any rectal itching?

_____ What about unexpected weight loss?

_____ What about food allergies that continue to get worse despite treatment?

_____ Do you feel hungry all the time?

_____ Have you been diagnosed with irritable bowel syndrome?

_____ What about inflammatory bowel disease?

_____ Do you have sore mouth and gums?

_____ Do you experience chronic low-back pain that's unresponsive to treatment?

_____ Do you have digestive disturbances?

_____ Do you grind your teeth at night?

_____ Are you frequently around animals, including any pets?

Most local laboratories may miss parasitic infections. For this reason, I recommend using a lab like Genova, which specializes in stool-testing procedures. They provide a discreet take-home stool-test kit, and patients send their samples directly to Genova. There it is tested for parasites as well as bacterial and yeast overgrowth. To order such a test for yourself, see Appendix C.

TREATING PARASITES WITH PRESCRIPTIONS

Metronidazole (Flagyl) is usually used for *Amoeba, Blastocystis* and *Giardia* infections. Side effects may include nausea, headache, dry mouth, metallic taste, occasional vomiting, vertigo, diarrhea, parathesia, and rash. Rare side effects include seizures, encephalopathy, pseudomembranous colitis, peripheral neuropathy, and pancreatitis.

Iodoquinol (Yodoxin) is also used for *Amoeba* and *Dientamoeba* parasites. Side effects may include rash, acne, nausea, diarrhea, and cramps. Rare side effects include optic atrophy, loss of vision and peripheral neuropathy after prolonged use (months).

Paramomycin (Humantin) is used to treat *Amoeba* infections. Side effects may include GI disturbances and occasional auditory nerve damage or renal damage.

Quinacrine HCl (Atabrine) is mainly used for treating *Giardia*. Side effects include dizziness, headaches, vomiting, diarrhea, occasional toxic psychosis, psoriasis-like rash, and insomnia. Rare side effects include acute liver disease, convulsions, and severe exfoliative dermatitis.

TREATING WITH NATURAL REMEDIES

Citrus seed extract is used through the world to treat a variety of viral, bacterial, fungal, and parasitic infections. It is not absorbed by the body but works within the intestinal tract. It is quite safe and relatively nontoxic, even when used for months at a time.

Artemisia Annua (Wormwood) is a Chinese herb that I find extremely effective in treating most parasitic infections. Artemisia can be toxic if used in large doses or for long periods of time. It works best when combined with other natural parasite supplements.

Allium sativum (Garlic) is a perennial plant used as food seasoning. It is also used around the world in treating such health conditions as cardiovascular disease, immune deficiencies, and viral, bacterial, fungal, and parasite infections. Garlic is a potent remedy for most intestinal parasites, especially roundworms and hookworms.

Berberine is the active ingredient in Goldenseal *(Hydrastis canadensis),* Oregon grape root *(Mahonia aquifolium)* and barberry *(Berberis vulgaris).* It is effective against *E. coli* (sometimes called "traveler's diarrhea"), shigellosis (dysentery caused by *Shigella),* food poisoning (from *Salmonella paratyphi),* Klebsiella, giardiasis (from *Giardia lamblia),* and cholera (from *Vibrio cholerae).*

In one study cited in *The Textbook of Natural Medicine,* 40 children ages 1–10, who were infected with *Giardia,* received either the prescription drug metronidazole, berberine, or a placebo. After six days, those on berberine had reduced their symptoms by 48%. And their stool samples showed that 68% were clear from *Giardia.* Those taking metronidazole also had stool samples that showed them to be completely free of infection. However, they enjoyed a modest 33% reduction in their symptoms. This study demonstrates that berberine is more effective in eliminating the symptoms of *Giardia,* and perhaps a larger dose of berberine administered over a longer period of time would result in identical stool-sample results.

AVOIDING PARASITES

• Always wash your hands after using the bathroom, handling animals, or working in the yard.
• Drink bottled, filtered, or distilled water.
• Always wear shoes outside.
• Don't allow your pets to lick your face.
• Deworm your pets as recommended by your veterinarian.
• Wash fruits and vegetables before eating them.
• Don't eat raw fish or meat. Make sure all meats are thoroughly cooked.
• Don't drink from lakes, streams, or rivers without first treating the water.

PROTOCOL FOR PARASITIC INFECTION

• **Supplement with *Lactobacillus acidophilus.*** It has proven effective in treating IBS, *H. pylori,* diarrhea, and colitis. It's especially helpful in treating yeast overgrowth. For more information on *acidophilus,* see chapter 22.
• **Get plenty of fiber in your diet.** Consistent daily bowel movements help keep your digestive system clean. Constipation, on the other hand, increases your chances for hemorrhoids and contributes to an unhealthy colon environment (see more about

a poorly functioning colon in ch. 12). Dietary fiber can help this situation in a number of ways. **Cellulose** is a nondigestible carbohydrate that makes up the outer layer of fruits and vegetables. It is found in apples, carrots, pears, broccoli, green beans, grains, and Brazil nuts. **Hemicellulose** is a nondigestible complex carbohydrate that absorbs excess water. It is found in apples, beets, corn, bananas, and pears. **Lignin** is found in Brazil nuts, carrots, green beans, peas, tomatoes, peaches, strawberries, and potatoes. This form of fiber binds with bile acids, helping to lower cholesterol and prevent gallstone formation. **Glucomannan** is found in the tuber amorphophallis plant. It removes excess fat from the colon walls, and may help with weight loss. It is a bulk-forming laxative that helps curb the appetite. **Psyllium** is a good intestinal cleanser and stool softener. Another bulk-forming laxative, it can help with colitis and other intestinal conditions. There are many other sources of natural fiber. Used properly, fiber can help regulate bowel movements, lower cholesterol, detoxify the body of harmful chemicals, reduce varicose veins, lose excess water, regulate glucose-insulin levels, prevent gallstones and certain cancers, and help with weight loss. Some herbs can be used for intestinal cleansing as well, but I don't recommend using cascara sagrada or Senna for extended periods, since both may cause a dependency.

- **Get tested.** If you suspect you have intestinal permeability (as do most individuals with FMS/CFS), yeast overgrowth, or a parasitic infection, contact my office or Genova Diagnostics for a stool-test kit.

- **Take your digestive enzymes with each meal** (see more about these in chapter 12).

- **Consider supplementing magnesium for persistent constipation.** The amount in my Essential Therapeutics CFS/Fibro Formula will probably be enough to have you experiencing normal bowel movements in 2–3 weeks. If not, add an additional 140 mg. of magnesium citrate daily until you start to have loose bowel movements. Then simply reduce the magnesium until you are having a normal bowel movement once again.

RESOURCES

• Private stool parasitology tests (mailed to your home) are available by referral from your doctor to Genova Labs or from my office. See Appendix C.

FOR FURTHER READING AND RESEARCH

• J.F. Goncalves et al., *Rev Inst Med Trop Sao Paulo* 32(6) (1990): 428–35.
• D. Juranek, "Giardiasis," Centers for Disease Control: Division of Parasitic Infection, Atlanta, Georgia.
• R. Wajsman et al., "Prevalence of *B.hominis* and other parasites in an immigrant population," Presentation at American College of Gastroenterology, 56th Annual Meeting, October 13–15, 1991.

· 21 ·
THE BODY'S URINARY SYSTEM

Urinary tract disorders are another "layer of the onion" that might need to be peeled away to make you better. Of my FMS patients, 25% have chronic UTIs or interstitial cystitis.

The human urinary system produces, stores, and carries urine. The urinary system includes two kidneys, two ureters, the urinary bladder, two sphincter muscles, and the urethra. The kidneys are small, bean-shaped organs, that rest on either side of the spinal column, just below the rib cage. They consist of about 1 million filtering units known as nephrons. Each unit consists of a glomerulus, ball-shaped network of capillaries, and a network of tubules. Blood is filtered by the glomerulus, and the filtered matter then passes through the tubular system where water, electrolytes, and nutrients are reabsorbed.

The kidneys play a crucial role in regulating electrolytes (such as sodium, potassium, and calcium) in the human blood. In addition, they clear urea, a nitrogenous waste product from the metabolism of amino acids, as well as other unwanted by-products, from the blood.

The kidneys make urine when they filter the blood. The urine flows from the kidneys through a pair of thin tubes, called the ureters, to the bladder. There it is stored until a person urinates. During urination, muscles in the wall of the bladder contract, forcing urine out of the bladder and into a tube called the urethra. One end of the urethra is connected to the bladder; the other end is open to the outside of the body. In women, the opening is located just above the vagina. In men, it's at the tip of the penis. When the bladder muscles tighten and the sphincter muscles relax, urine leaves the body by passing through the opening of the urethra.

The bladder, which stores urine, swells into a round shape when it is full. A normal bladder can hold up to 16 fluid oz. (500 ml.) of urine comfortably for 2 to 5 hours. Humans produce an average of 1.5 liters (about 50 oz.) of urine each day. Increased fluid intake generally increases urine production, while increased perspiration and usage of diuretics or other medications may decrease urinary volume.

Individuals with fibromyalgia and CFS often have problems with their urinary system. They may experience chronic urinary tract infections (UTIs), interstitial cystitis, incontinence (involuntary loss of urine), and urinary retention (inability to pass urine).

URINARY TRACT INFECTION

UTIs are more common in women who are sexually active, people with diabetes, and people with sickle-cell disease or anatomical malformations of the urinary tract. Also, women are more prone to UTIs than males, since a women's urethra is much shorter and closer to the anus than a man's. This is why proper hygiene is so important in females. UTI can be especially dangerous for infants and can cause permanent renal damage.

Symptoms and signs include painful, hesitant, frequent urination and high temperature lasting for more than three days. Nausea and vomiting along with pain and temperature may indicate a more complicated UTI, in which a kidney is infected.

Some urinary tract infections are asymptomatic. Others may have quite dramatic symptoms including confusion and associated falls, which are common for elderly patients with UTI who show up at the emergency room.

DIAGNOSIS OF UTI

The diagnosis of UTI is confirmed by a urine culture. A negative urine culture suggests the presence of other illness, such as chlamydia or gonorrhea.

CAUSES OF UTI

Common organisms that cause UTIs include *E. coli* and *S. saprophyticus*. Less common organisms include *P. mirabilis, K. pneumoniae,* and *Enterococcus spp.*

Over 90% of UTIs are caused by *E. coli*. This bacteria is normally found in everyone's gut and, with the exception of a few rare dangerous forms, it is a healthy part of our normal bowel bacteria. The problems begins when *E. coli* escapes the bowel and enters the bladder. The bladder is able to remove most infections through the process of urination, but *E. coli* are quite resilient and able to use projections to help them stick to the bladder wall.

PREVENTION OF UTI

- Drink 70 ounces of water a day.
- Avoid excess alcohol and caffeinated beverages.
- Don't resist the urge to urinate; visit the bathroom as soon as you feel compelled.
- If you have frequent UTIs, avoid taking baths; take showers instead.
- Practice good hygiene by wiping from the front to the back to avoid contamination of the urinary tract.
- Sexually active women—and to a lesser extent, men—should urinate within 15 minutes after sexual intercourse to allow the flow of urine to expel the bacteria before specialized extensions anchor the bacteria to the walls of the urethra.
- Clean the urethral meatus (the opening of the urethra) after intercourse.
- Clean genital areas prior to and after sexual intercourse.

CONVENTIONAL TREATMENT OF UTI

Most uncomplicated UTIs can be easily treated with oral antibiotics such as trimethoprim, cephalosporins, Macrodantin, or a fluoroquinolone (such as ciprofloxacin or levofloxacin).

Symptoms consistent with pyelonephritis, a serious kidney infection, may call for intravenous antibiotics.

Patients with recurrent UTIs may need further investigation such as ultrasound scans of the kidneys and bladder or intravenous urography (X-rays of the urinary system following injection of contrast material).

Often, long courses of low-dose antibiotics are prescribed to help prevent otherwise unexplained cases of recurring UTI.

NATURAL TREATMENT OF UTI

Taking antibiotics will usually kill the bacteria that is causing a bladder infection, but will also kill the healthy "good bacteria" in your body. Always combat this side effect of antibiotics by taking probiotics along with them, 12 hours apart from each other.

Another option, which I prefer, is to try natural remedies before resorting to antibiotic therapy. If the symptoms don't clear up within a couple days, then you can always start antibiotic therapy then. Natural therapies can also be used while you're waiting for your tests results to confirm a UTI.

- **Cranberry juice** can end a UTI. In addition to acidifying urine, cranberries contain substances that inhibit bacteria from attaching to the bladder lining and, as such, promote the flushing out of bacteria with the urine stream. Dosage is one to two cups of pure cranberry juice (no sugar added) or 2–4 cranberry capsules (standardized to 11%–12% quinic acid) a day for 1–2 weeks. This may well be all you need to eliminate a UTI.

- **D-mannose** is a naturally occurring sugar similar in structure to glucose but metabolized differently. (Because the body metabolizes only small amounts of D-mannose and excretes the rest in the urine, it doesn't interfere with blood-sugar regulation, even in diabetics.) Though D-mannose doesn't kill bacteria, it prevents bacteria from attaching to the bladder wall. D-mannose is safe, even for long-term use, although most people will only need it for a few days. Those who have frequent recurrent bladder infections may choose to take it on a daily basis. I've found it to be the best option for stubborn, chronic UTIs.

INTERSTITIAL CYSTITIS

Recurrent UTI symptoms may point at a problem known as interstitial cystitis (IC).

Interstitial cystitis is a chronic inflammatory condition of the bladder that causes frequent, urgent, and painful urination and pelvic discomfort. The lining of the bladder breaks down, allowing toxins to irritate the bladder wall, and the bladder becomes inflamed and tender and does not store urine well. The condition does not respond to antibiotics, since it is not associated with a bacterial infection like is UTI. Like UTI, IC is much more common among women than among men. Although the disease previously was believed to be a condition of menopausal women, growing numbers of men and women are being diagnosed in their 20s and younger. Data released just this year suggests that up to 12% of women may have early symptoms of IC.

Symptoms: The symptoms of IC are basically the symptoms of UTI, only more stubborn. IC is often misdiagnosed as UTI, until it refuses to respond to antibiotics. IC symptoms may also initially be attributed to prostatitis or epididymitis (in men) and endometriosis or uterine fibroids (in women).

Causes: The cause of interstitial cystitis is unknown, though several theories are being investigated, including autoimmune, neurological, allergic, and genetic. Regardless of the disease's origin, IC patients clearly struggle with a damaged bladder lining. When this protective coating is compromised, urinary chemicals can leak into surrounding tissues, causing pain, inflammation, and urinary symptoms.

Diagnosis: IC diagnosis has been greatly simplified in recent years with the development of two new methodologies. The "Pelvic Pain Urgency/Frequency (PUF) Patient Survey," created by C. Lowell Parsons, is a short questionnaire that helps doctors identify if pelvic pain could be coming from the bladder. The KCL test, also called the potassium sensitivity test, uses a mild potassium solution to test the integrity of the bladder wall. Though the latter is not specific for IC, it has been determined helpful in predicting the use of compounds designed to help repair the bladder lining. Previously, IC was diagnosed by visual examination of the bladder wall after stretching it. This test, however, can contribute to the development

Foods that Contribute to IC Symptoms

Drinks
- coffee
- tea
- soda (particularly diet)
- carbonated water
- chocolate milk
- soy milk
- cranberry juice
- most fruit juices
- beer
- wine

Protein
- bologna
- ham
- hot dogs
- most sausages
- smoked fish
- hazelnuts
- macadamia nuts
- peanuts
- pecans
- pistachios
- English and black walnuts
- many common cheeses
- soy cheese
- tofu

Carbohydrates
- bread or cereal w/preservatives
- soy flour
- sorbet

Fruits and Veggies
- bananas
- apricots
- citrus fruit
- cantaloupe
- cherries
- dried fruit w/preservatives
- peaches
- most plums
- most dried figs
- golden raisins
- grapes
- guava
- kiwi fruit
- most berries
- passion fruit
- papaya
- persimmon
- starfruit
- chili peppers
- pickles
- raw onions
- sauerkraut
- soybeans
- tomato
- tomato sauce
- tomato juice
- fava beans
- lima beans

Other
- multivitamins
- MSG (monosodium glutamate)
- chocolate
- mayonnaise
- most salad dressings
- bouillion
- most packaged and canned soups
- ascorbic acid
- autolyzed yeast
- BHA and BHT
- benzoates
- caffeine
- cloves
- chili powder
- red pepper
- hot curry powder
- citric acid
- hydrolyzed protein
- meat tenderizers
- miso
- paprika
- soy sauce
- vinegar
- worcestershire sauce
- metabisulfites
- sulfites
- cesulfame K
- aspartame
- mustard
- mincemeat
- saccharine
- sour cream
- yogurt

of small hemorrhages, making IC worse. Thus, a diagnosis of IC is made by excluding other illnesses and reviewing a patient's clinical symptoms.

Treatment of the bladder lining: Traditional medications work to repair and hopefully rebuild the wounded bladder lining, allowing for a reduction in symptoms. But FDA-approved therapies for IC have had recent setbacks in various research studies. **Elmiron** (pentosan polysulfate) is supposed to provide a protective coating in the bladder. But data released in late 2005 by Alza Pharmaceuticals suggests that 84% of Elmiron is eliminated—intact—in the feces. Another 6% is excreted in the urine. **DMSO,** a wood-pulp extract, can be instilled directly into the bladder via a catheter, yet it is much less frequently used in urology clinics. Research studies presented at recent conferences of the American Urological Association have demonstrated that at the FDA-approved dosage of a 50% solution of DMSO, irreversible muscle contractions and damage may occur. DMSO therapy has yielded mixed results, and long-term benefits appear fleeting.

Recently, the use of a new therapeutic instillation—implemented like DMSO—has generated considerable excitement in the IC community. And rightly so. Published studies report a 90% effectiveness in reducing symptoms. This treatment is called a "rescue instillation" and can be conducted with any number of "cocktails" to treat specific symptoms.

Another bladder-coating treatment, Cystistat, is believed to replace the deficient layer on the bladder wall. The primary component of Cystistat is sodium hyaluronate, a derivative of hyaluronic acid, which occurs naturally in the fluids of the eye, in the joints, and in the bladder-lining layer that is deficient in many patients with interstitial cystitis. This layer is believed to provide the bladder wall with a protective coating. Cystistat, however, is still in the process of approval and not yet available to the public.

Treatment of the pelvic floor: Pelvic-floor dysfunction may also be a contributing factor to IC symptoms. Thus most major IC clinics now evaluate the pelvic floor and/or refer patients directly to a

physical therapist for a prompt treatment of pelvic floor muscle tension or weakness. The tension is often described as a burning sensation, particularly in the vagina.

Muscle tension is the primary cause of pain and discomfort in IC patients who experience pain during intercourse. Tender trigger points (small tight bundles of muscle) may also be found in the pelvic floor.

Exercises such as Kegels can be helpful as they strengthen the muscles, but they can provoke pain and additional muscle tension. A specially trained physical therapist can provide direct, specific evaluation of the muscles, both externally and internally.

OTHER TREATMENTS FOR IC

Bladder distention (a procedure done under general anesthesia that stretches the bladder capacity) has shown some success in reducing urinary frequency and giving pain relief to patients. Unfortunately, the relief achieved by bladder distentions is only temporary (weeks or months) and consequently is not really viable as a long-term treatment for IC. It is generally only used in extreme cases.

Pain control is important in the treatment of IC, as the pain of this condition has been rated equivalent to cancer pain. A variety of traditional pain medications, including opiates, can be used to treat the varying degrees of pain. Electronic pain-killing options include TENS (a machine that sends electrical impulses to the skin through sticky pads) and PTNS (similar to a TENS treatment, except a needle is used).

Alkalinizing the urine through diet seems to help reduce the burning pain and urinary urgency of IC in some patients. See the facing page for a list of common foods that seem to make IC worse. I know that the list can be intimidating, but I encourage my cystitis patients to conduct a modified elimination diet for 2–3 weeks, avoiding all the foods above. Then they challenge one of these foods at a time. If you do this, be sure to keep a food diary to keep up with what you learn about your body.

For more information about IC and your diet, visit www.ic-net-work.com/handbook and click under "Living with IC—Diet."

Prelief by AkPharma, Inc. is calcium glycerophosphate, a food-grade mineral classified as a dietary supplement. It's a natural treatment for IC and also a good source of calcium. In a retrospective study conducted by AkPharma, over 200 patients consumed acidic foods and beverages with and without Prelief. Seventy percent of the patients had a reduction in IC pain and discomfort with the use of Prelief when consuming acidic foods. Sixty-one percent of them reported a reduction in urinary urgency after using Prelief. For more information or to order Prelief, visit www.prelief.com or call 1-800-994-4711.

Bioflavonoids are naturally occurring substances that act as mast-cell inhibitors (similar to an antihistamine), anti-inflammatories, and antioxidants. Since IC is associated with an increased number and activation of mast cells and inflammation in some patients, it has been suggested that bioflavonoids—quercetin in particular—have potential in the treatment of IC.

Cysta-Q, distributed by Farr Labs, is a quercetin-based dietary supplement that was specifically developed to target the symptoms of IC. Cysta-Q also contains bromelain, papain, nonacidic cranberry powder, nonacidic black cohosh, skull cap, wood betony, passionflower, and valerian in order to enhance the effectiveness of the quercetin. The quercetin used in Cysta-Q is derived from grape skin, onion skin, grapefruit rind and green algae. Initial studies have shown promise, but additional research is needed to access the long-term benefits of this natural formula. To find out more about Cysta-Q, visit www.CystaQ.com or call 1-877-284-3976.

Polysaccharides are long chains of sugar molecules. These naturally occurring substances may work by replacing the defective lining in the bladder, and they are thought to have a protective effect on the bladder. Elmiron is a synthetic polysaccharide. Examples of natural polysaccharides include glucosamine, chondroitin, marshmallow root, spirulina, and aloe vera. Desert Harvest, Inc., manufacturers a special IC-specific formula of aloe vera available in capsule form. It contains freeze-dried, whole-leaf aloe vera with no additives or fillers. Desert Harvest designed a double-blind, placebo-controlled study in which patients ingested three capsules twice a day with eight oz. of liquid for three months. Of the eight patients who completed the study, seven received relief from at least some of their symptoms. Of those seven, four experienced significant relief from all or most of their symptoms. Only one patient had no response after completing all six months of the study. For more information about Desert Harvest Aloe Vera products, visit www.desertharvest.com or call 1-800-222-3901.

Algonot-Plus combines polysaccharides (glucosamine and chondroitin) with quercetin and also adds an organic, unrefined olive seed oil from the island of Crete which increases absorption and adds its own antioxidants.

No formal research on this combined type of treatment for IC has yet been published, but several studies indicate that these supplements may be helpful, on their own, in the treatment of IC. Glucosamine and chondroitin have previously been given to many IC patients in an open-label study with very good results when taken for a few months.

TC Theoharides, MD, and Grannum Sant, MD, have been involved in IC research and patient care for over 10 years. Their recent studies are encouraging for the benefits of combined therapies such as Algonot-Plus. For more information on Algonot-Plus, visit www. algonot.com, or call 1-800-254-6668.

FOR FURTHER READING AND RESEARCH
- Avorn J, Monane M, Gurwitz JH, Glynn RJ, Choodnovskiy I, and Lipsitz LA. "Reduction of bacteriuria and pyuria after ingestion of cranberry juice." *JAMA* 1994;271:751–754.
- Bar-Shavit Z, Goldman R, Ofek I, Sharon N, and Mirelman D. "Mannose-binding activity of Escherichia coli: a determinant of attachment and ingestion of the bacteria by macrophages." *Infect Immun* 1980;29:417–24.
- Bodel PT, Cotran R, and Kass EH. "Cranberry juice and the antimicrobial action of hippuric acid." *J Lab Clin Med* 1959;54:881–888.
- Chiang G, Patra P, Letourneau R, Jeudy S, Boucher W, Green M, Sant GR, and Theoharides TC. "Pentosanpolysulfate inhibits mast cell histamine secre-

tion and intracellular calcium ion levels: an alternative explanation of its beneficial effect in interstitial cystitis." *J Urol* Dec 2000;164(6):2119–25.

- Galli SJ. "New Concepts about the mast cell." *New Engl J Med* 1993;328:257–265.
- Herman RH. "Mannose metabolism." *Am J Clin Nutr* 1971;24:488–98.
- ICA UpdateAutumn 1998;13(3):9.
- *ICA Update* Spring 1997;12(1):3.
- Katske F, Shoskes DA, Sender M, Poliakin R, Gagliano K, and Rajfer J. "Treatment of interstitial cystitis with a quercetin supplement." *Tech Urol* Mar 2001;7(1):44–6.
- Koziol JA, Clark DC, Gittes RF, and Tan EM. "The natural history of interstitial cystitis:a survey of 374 patients." *J Urol* 1993;9:465–469.
- Kuzminski LN. "Cranberry juice and urinary tract infections: is there a beneficial relationship?" *Nutr Rev* 1996;54(11 pt 2):S87–S90.
- "Metabolism of [3H]pentosan polysulfate sodium (PPS) in healthy human volunteers." *Xenobiotica* Aug 2005;35(8):775–84.
- Meyhoff H, Nordling J, Gammelgaard P, and Vejlsgaard R. "Does antibacterial ointment applied to urethral meatus in women prevent recurrent cystitis?" *Scand J Urol Nephrol* 1981;15(2):81–3.
- Middleton E, Kandaswami C, and Theoharides TC. "The effects of flavonoids on mammalian cells: implications for inflammation, heart disease and cancer." *Pharmacol Rev* 52;673–751:2000.
- Ofek I, Goldhar J, Zafriri D, Lis H, Adar R, and Sharon N. "Anti-Escherichia coli adhesion activity of cranberry and blueberry juices" (letter) *N Engl J Med* 1991;324:1599.
- Ofek I and Beachey EH. "Mannose binding and epithelial cell adherence of Escherichia coli." *Infect Immun* 1978;22:247–54.
- Ofek I, Goldhar J, Eshdat Y, and Sharon N. "The importance of mannose specific adhesins (lectins) in infections caused by Escherichia coli." *Scand J Infect Dis Suppl* 1982;33:61–7.
- Ofek I, Crouch E, and Keisari Y. "The role of C-type lectins in the innate immunity against pulmonary pathogens." *Adv Exp Med Biol* 2000;479:27–36.
- Shoskes DA, Zeitlin SI, Shahed A, and Rajfer J. "Quercetin in men with category III chronic prostatitis: a preliminary prospective, double-blind, placebo-controlled trial." *Urology* 1999;Dec:54 (6):960–3.
- Theoharides TC, Patra P, Boucher W, Letourneau R, Kempuraj D, Chiang G, Jeudy S, Hesse L, and Athanasiou A. "Chondroitin sulphate inhibits connective tissue mast cells." *Brit J Pharmacol* 2000;131:1039–1049.
- Theoharides TC, Pang X, Letourneau R, and Sant DR. "Interstitial cystitis: a neuroimmunoendocrine disorder." *Annals NY Academy Sciences* 1998;840:619–634.
- Theoharides TC, Kempuraj D, and Sant GR. "Mast cell involvement in interstitial cystitis: a review of human and experimental evidence." *Urology* Jun 2001;57(6 s.1):47–55.

- Theoharides TC, Kempuraj D, and Sant GR. "Massive extracellular tryptase from activated mast cells in interstitial cystitis." *Urology* 2001.
- Theoharides TC. "The mast cell: a neuroimmunoendocrine master player." *Int J Tissue Reactions* 1996;18:1–21.
- Theoharides TC and Sant GR. "Preliminary findings on the beneficial use of a glucosamine-chondroitin preparation in interstitial cystitis patients." *Intern J Immunopathol and Pharmacology* 2001.
- Theoharides TC and Sant GR. "New agents for the medical treatment of interstitial cystitis." *Expert Opin Investig Drugs* 2001;Mar:10(3):521–46.
- Walker EB, Barney DP, Mickelsen JN, Walton RJ, and Mickelsen RA Jr. "Cranberry concentrate: UTI prophylaxis." *J Fam Pract* 1997;45:167–168.
- Whitmore K, Bologna R, et al. "Survey of the effect of prelief on food-related exacerbation of IC symptoms." 1998–99 (unpublished).

· 22 ·
YEAST OVERGROWTH SYNDROME

An overgrowth in the gastrointestinal tract of the usually benign candida albicans is becoming recognized as a complex medical syndrome called chronic candidiasis or yeast overgrowth syndrome.

An overgrowth of the usually benign *Candida albicans* in the gastrointestinal tract is now recognized as a complex medical syndrome called chronic candidiasis, or yeast overgrowth syndrome. Although it has been clinically defined for some time, it was not until recently that the public and many physicians realized the magnitude of the problem. As many as one-third of the Western world's population may be affected by Candidiasis. And unfortunately, there is no shortcut to getting yeast under control.

WHAT IS CANDIDIASIS?

Candida albicans is a yeast that can be found living in the intestinal tracts of most individuals. Yeasts cohabitate there in a symbiotic relationship with over 400 healthy bacteria. These bacteria help with digestion and absorption of certain nutrients, and they keep the yeasts in check. When these good bacteria die or are suppressed, the yeasts are allowed to grow to unhealthy levels, causing candidiasis.

SIGNS AND SYMPTOMS

Candidiasis commonly infects the ears, nose, and the urinary and intestinal tracts. Typical symptoms are constipation, diarrhea, irritable bowel, abdominal pain, bloating, gas, indigestion, rash, bladder spasms and infection, and ear and sinus infections.

Yeast overgrowth is similar to allergies in that there are a plethora of symptoms. This can lead to skepticism in many doctors; the symptoms are tough to define. It's not uncommon for yeast over-growth to cause or contribute to such complex conditions as de-pression, asthma, fatigue, mental confusion, weakened immunity, allergies, chemical sensitivities, hyperactivity, chronic ear and sinus infections, and adrenal fatigue.

Like most opportunistic infections, *Candida* and other yeasts may increase during times of stress. This overgrowth leaks toxins into the bloodstream or other tissues, allowing antigens (foreign invad-ers) to set up residence in various bodily tissues. Antigens then trigger complex allergic reactions. (This might explain why most individuals with chronic yeast overgrowth develop food, inhalant, and environmental allergies). Allergic reactions can manifest in a variety of symptoms: fatigue, brain fog, depression, joint and muscle pain, digestive disorders, headache, rash, and breathing problems. Inflammation of the nose, throat, ears, bladder, and intestinal tract, can lead to infections of the sinus, respiratory, ear, bladder and intestinal membranes. In an attempt to arrest these infections, your physician might prescribe a broad-spectrum anti-biotic. Such antibiotics promote yeast overgrowth and often times, additional symptoms.

CAUSES

The most common cause of candidiasis is medication overuse, especially of antibiotics but also of birth-control pills and corti-costeroids. These can suppress the immune system and the good intestinal bacteria. When used appropriately, antibiotics and corti-costeroids save lives, but if you are taking these medications, check with your doctor about possible alternatives.

A minor increase in intestinal yeast is usually not a problem, lead-ing possibly to infection of the mouth (thrush) or vaginal lining (vaginitis or "yeast infection"). The body's immune defenses are usually strong enough to keep the yeast from taking over the intes-tinal tract.

However, if yeast overgrowth is left unchallenged, more sinister symptoms appear. Yeasts can change into an invasive mycellial fungus with rhizoids (tentacle-like projections) that penetrate the lining of the intestinal tract. These projections can cause intestinal permeability and leak toxins across the cellular membranes. Penetration by these rhizoids and the resulting intestinal permeability cause a disruption in the absorption of nutrients and finally nutritional deficiencies. Deficient nutrients lead to reduced immunity and further weakening of the body's defense systems. This can lead to fatigue, allergies, decreased immunity, chemical sensitivities, depression, poor memory, and digestive complaints.

Your resistance to yeast overgrowth may be compromised by allergic reactions, more antibiotics, stress, fatigue, and poor nutrition. This sets the stage for environmental sensitivities. As the liver and adrenal glands become chronically overwhelmed, tolerance to the fumes of certain environmental chemicals is reduced: gasoline, diesel, other petrochemicals, formaldehyde, perfumes, cleaning fluids, insecticides, tobacco, pesticides, household cleaners, etc.

TREATMENT

The relationship of *Candida albicans* to many common health disorders was first described by a Birmingham, Alabama, physician, C. Orian Truss, MD. Dr. Truss is the author of *The Missing Diagnosis,* which reveals how a yeast-free, low-sugar diet, along with antifungal medications, helped many of his chronically ill patients get well. His book is definitely recommended reading.

Proper treatment of yeast overgrowth requires a comprehensive multidimensional approach. Used alone, prescription drugs or natural antiyeast supplements rarely produce significant long-term results.

PROTOCOL FOR YEAST OVERGROWTH

I don't treat yeast overgrowth until a patient has had time to implement the Jump-Start Program described in chapter 13. I want to make sure she is consistently going into deep sleep each night. And before I start killing off yeast and creating die-off reactions, I want her nutritional deficiencies shored up. She should be reporting more energy and enjoying more resilience to daily stress. For that reason, it is usually several weeks before I attempt to treat yeast overgrowth, and then only if she is displaying symptoms of the illness.

Treating yeast overgrowth requires a comprehensive, multidimensional approach. Used alone, prescription drugs like Nystatin, Nizoral, and Diflucan—or even natural antiyeast supplements—rarely produce significant long-term results.

If you do suspect yeast overgrowth, contact my office or Genova Diagnostics for a stool-test kit. The kit is simple, home-based, and discreet. Alternatively, you can take the yeast questionnaire in Appendix A to help you decide if you are suffering from candidiasis. If you suspect that you are, and especially if a stool test reveals a yeast overgrowth, follow the guidelines below: control yeast through diet, treat any intestinal permeability, improve digestion, replace good bacteria, consider prescription medications, supplement with natural remedies, and give your liver extra support.

CONTROL YEAST THROUGH DIET

Begin **the *Candida* diet,** which eliminates yeast-nourishing foods. A number of dietary factors appear to promote the overgrowth of *Candida.* Try eliminating all the foods below for three months:

• **Sugar** is the chief nutrient for *Candida albicans,* so restricted sugar intake is absolutely necessity to effectively treat chronic Candidiasis. Avoid refined sugar, honey, maple syrup, fruit juice, milk, white potatoes, corn, processed or bleached (white) flour, bakery goods, muffins, cereals, and anything containing sugar. Ice cream, cake, cookies, and other sweets should be avoided for at least three months.

• **Fruits** should also be avoided, along with fruit juice (except any fruit juice taken with 5-HTP). After the initial two weeks, try introducing apples and pears to see if you have any reactions. (Reactions might include fatigue, depression, aches and pain, rectal itching, itching of the ears or nose, and digestive disturbances.) If not, then try berries: strawberries, blueberries, blackberries, and raspberries. Avoid all other fruits.

• **Alcoholic beverages** should be avoided, as should malted-milk or other malted products.

• **Mold- and yeast-containing foods** are best avoided for two to three months. These include peanuts, dried fruits (including prunes, raisins, and dates), vinegar, pickled vegetables, sauerkraut, relishes, green olives, vinegar-containing salad dressings, catsup, mayonnaise and, pickles.

• **Milk** should be avoided for at least three months, since it is a simple carbohydrate.

• **Dairy products other than milk** present increased yeast problems for some people. Still every person is different, and some are able to be more liberal with their diet. Try these other dairy products, and seeing if you have any problems.

What Can I Eat on the *Candida* Diet?

• All vegetables are allowed, including fresh tomatoes and onions.

• Meats and proteins allowed include beef, chicken, clams, crab, eggs, ham, lobster, salmon, shrimp, tuna, turkey, veal, all game birds and animals. Limit nuts and seeds to limited amounts of walnuts, cashews, almonds, sunflower seeds, and pumpkin seeds.

• Cold-pressed nonhydrogenated oils are encouraged. Take one tablespoon of virgin olive oil each day on your salads or vegetables. Add a little lemon juice if you desire.

• Butter is fine; avoid margarine.

• Old-fashioned oatmeal is okay, but limit it to one serving daily.

• Alternate sweeteners will no doubt help you to cope with the lack of sugar in this diet. Try the artificial sweetener Splenda, or better yet, natural plant-based sweeteners like stevia or FOS.

After two weeks, reintroduce apples and pears to your diet and watch for any reactions such as fatigue; depression; aches and pain; itching of the ears, rectum, or nose; and digestive disturbances. If there are no symptoms from reintroducing apples and pears, try challenging berries: strawberries, blueberries, blackberries, and raspberries. If you don't have any reactions, then continue to enjoy berries, apples, and pears in moderate amounts. After at least three months, gradually reintroduce other forbidden foods. Go easy! Remember how hard it is to get rid of yeast overgrowth, and don't sabotage your efforts with yeast-feeding foods.

- **Most vitamin and mineral supplements purchased at a drug store** are contaminated with yeast. Look for yeast-free products, though even some of these vitamins contain yeast, because the B vitamins contained in them were derived from yeast-fermenting processes. All of the protects I recommend, including the Essential Therapeutics CFS/Fibro formula, 5-HTP, Liver Formula, etc. are yeast free.

TREAT ANY INTESTINAL PERMEABILITY

A leaky gut left uncorrected will sabotage your attempts to eliminate yeast overgrowth once and for all. You can even follow your *Candida* Diet at the same time as your Elimination Diet from chapter 12. *I've found that healing intestinal permeability is often the crucial step in ridding a person of persistent yeast infections.*

IMPROVE DIGESTION

This is an important step in treating candidiasis. Since yeast can't live in an acidic environment, a healthy level of stomach acid helps deter its growth. And patients on acid-blocking drugs increase their risk for developing yeast overgrowth. So follow the instructions in chapter 12 for building up healthy levels of gastric HCl and/or pancreatic enzymes.

REPLACE GOOD BACTERIA

Bacteria such as *Lactobacillus acidophilus, L. bulgaricus, L. catnaforme, L. fermentum,* and *Bifidobacterium bifidum* normally inhabit vaginal and gastrointestinal tracts; help digest, absorb, and produce certain nutrients; and keep potentially harmful bacteria and yeast in check. Use probiotics to replace these bacteria when taking antibiotics, but not at exactly the same time of day.

L. acidophilus has proven to be effective in treating irritable bowel syndrome, *H. pylori,* diarrhea, and colitis. And it's especially helpful in treating yeast overgrowth.

Yogurt contains certain strains of good bacteria, but it isn't standardized for a particular amount. Also, most yogurts are made from *L. bulgaricus* or *Streptococcus thermophilus.*

Both are friendly bacteria, but neither will help colonize the colon. So it's best to use live organisms that are shipped on ice and then kept refrigerated until purchase. Live *L. acidophilus* and *B. bifidum* powders or capsules are preferred.

Supplement with probiotics for three months: 5–10 billion organisms daily. Or take up to 20 billion if taking antibiotics. Some extremely resistant yeast infections may need continuous probiotic replacement therapy.

CONSIDER PRESCRIPTION MEDICATIONS

Take a prescription medication as indicated by the results of your stool test and prescribed by your physician. Typically used are Nizoral, Nystatin, and Diflucan. **Nystatin** is the safest of the three, as it doesn't penetrate the intestinal lining, but yeast overgrowth that's escaped the lining will need to be treated with something else. These medications are typically used from three–six weeks, though Nystatin can be used for longer periods. Since prescription antifungal medications are taxing to the liver's detoxification system, supplement them with milk thistle and/or alpha lipoic acid (ALA) in order to protect your liver. Side effects of these drugs are potentially serious, but so is chronic yeast overgrowth. Consider your benefits and risks; some individuals are so infected with yeast that treating with anything other than prescription medications is futile.

SUPPLEMENT WITH NATURAL REMEDIES

You can use natural remedies either by themselves or in combination with prescription medications. Most of our patients start with prescription medications for about three weeks and then switch to herbal antifungal supplements for one–two months. However, I've had lots of success just using herbals and diet to treat yeast overgrowth. Our patients who elect to take a natural remedy and no prescription medication take one tablet a day of my **Essential Therapeutics Yeast Formula** and slowly increase to three tablets a day with food for at least three months. (Difficult cases may require up to six months or more.) This concentrated, broad-spectrum formula combines specific natural agents useful in supporting a healthy balance of intestinal microflora, thus discouraging the overgrowth of yeast. Sustained-release and pH balanced, it is readily absorbed into both the small and large intestines. You should be able to find something similar at your local health-food store. My formula contains:

- **Calcium undecylenate:** 150 mg.
- **Undecylenic acid:** This is one of the most powerful antiyeast medications available. A fatty acid naturally found in sweat, it has been used as a topical (Desenex) and as an oral antifungal agent.
- **Sorbic acid:** 50 mg.
- **Beberine sulfate:** 200 mg.
- **Indian barberry:** 50 mg.; minimum 6% berberine
- **Chinese goldenthread:** 25 mg.; minimum 20% berberine
- **Green tea leaf:** 50 mg. The polyphenols in green tea kill harmful bacteria and promote the growth of the friendly form.

To order my Yeast Formula or other natural remedies (listed below), see page 461.

Caprylic acid is a naturally occurring fatty acid and a potent antifungal medicine. It should be taken as an enteric-coated timed-release capsule. Dosage is 500–1,000 mg. three times daily with food.

Berberine or Barberry *(Berberis vulgaris)* has a wide range of antimicrobial properties. It is a proven herbal medicine used successfully to treat fungal, bacterial, and parasitic infections. Dosage of standardized extract (4:1) is 250–500 mg. three times daily with food.

Garlic has been used for medicinal purposes for centuries. It is an effective treatment for the overgrowth of *Candida albicans* and other yeasts. It has shown to be more potent than Nystatin for *Candida albicans.* Dosage of standardized garlic (1.3% alliin) is 600–900 mg. two–three times daily with food.

Goldenseal *(Hydrastis canadensis)* is another berberine-containing plant. Dosage of standardized extract (4:1) is 250–500 mg. three times daily on an empty stomach.

Oleic Acid, the major component of virgin olive oil, hinders conversion of *Candida* to its more harmful, invasive form.

Citrus seed extract is a broad-spectrum antimicrobial used to successfully treat yeast and bacterial parasites. Dosage is 100–200 mg. twice daily after meals.

Tanalbit is used to treat intestinal parasites and yeast overgrowth. It should be taken in capsule form. Dosage is one capsule three times daily with food.

Fructo-oligosaccharide (FOS) is a short-chain polysaccharide used in Japan for dozens of years. It isn't digested by humans but does stimulate the growth of good bacteria within the intestinal tract. It also helps with liver detoxification, lowers cholesterol, and eliminates various toxins. Dosage for powder is 2,000–3,000 mg. daily.

If You Get Worse at First

Sometimes, when a lot of *Candida* organisms are killed off during initial treatment, a sudden release of toxic substances results in an immune response and intensified symptoms, called the Herxheimer reaction. The body becomes extremely acidic. Some doctors call this a die-off reaction; others call it a healing crisis. It normally lasts no longer than a week and is frequently confused as an allergic or adverse reaction to the antifungal treatment. Symptoms can be minimized by taking Alka-Seltzer Gold, or 2 tablespoons baking soda in 8 oz. of water, as a buffering agent two to three times daily as needed.

If the reaction is severe, you might need to reduce your antifungal medications—or take them every other day—for several days. I usually recommend that patients half the dosage for a week and then return to the original dose. Patients should then continue their antifungal medications for a minimum of three months. If treatment is discontinued too early, symptoms will gradually return.

GIVE YOUR LIVER EXTRA SUPPORT

Supplement with Essential Therapeutics Liver Detox Formula when taking antifungals, especially prescription medications. Or at the minimum, take milk thistle as directed by your nutritionally oriented physician.

AFTER YOU'VE HEALED

Once fungus overgrowth has subsided and the yeast have returned to a normal level (at least three–four months), medications and supplements can be gradually decreased over six–eight weeks, and the patient can gradually add previously forbidden foods to her diet. Be vigilant in monitoring your sugar and simple carbohydrate intake.

RESOURCES

• Essential Therapeutics Yeast Formula, Probiotics, and Liver Detox Formula are available by contacting my office (see p. 461). Similar products should be available from your local health food store or nutritionally oriented physician.

• A home-based stool test for yeast overgrowth is available through a referral by your doctor to Genova Diagnostics, or by contacting my office.

FOR FURTHER READING AND RESEARCH

• Abbasi KM, Amin AH, and Subbaiah TV. "Beberine sulfate: antimicrobial activity, bioassay, and mode of action." *Can J Microbiol* 1969:15:1067–76.
• Boreo M, Pera A, Andirilli A et al. "Candida overgrowth in gastric juice of peptic ulcer subjects on short- and long-term treatment with H-2 receptor antagonists." *Digestion* 1983:28:158–163.
• Diebel LN et al. "Synergistic effects of candida and Escherichia coli on gut barrier function." *J Trauma* 47(6):1045–50;discussion 1050-1, 1999.
• Keeney EL. "Sodium Caprylate: A new and effective treatment of moniliasis of the skin and mucous membrane." *Bull Johns Hopkins Hosp* 1946:78:333–9.
• Krause W, Matheis H, and Wulf K. "Fungaemia and funguna after oral administration of Candida albicans." *Lancet* 1969:1:598–99.
• Kudelo NM. "Allergy in chronic monilial vaginitis." *Ann Allergy* 1971:29:266–67.
• Masahan VM, Harma K, and Rattan A. "Antimyocotic activity of berberine sulphate: An alkaloid from an Indian medicinal herb." *Sabouraudia* 1982:20:79–81.
• Moore GS and Atkins RD. "The fungicidal and fungistatic effects of an aqeous garlic extract on medically important yeast-like fungi." *Myocologia* 1977:69:341–8.
• Neuhauser I. "Successful treatment of intestinal moniliasis with fatty acid-resin complex." *Arch Intern Med* 1954:93:53–60.
• Robinett RW. "Asthma due to candida albicans." *U Mi Med Ctr J* 1968:34:12–15.
• Romano TJ and Dobbins JW. "Evaluation of the patient with suspected malabsorption." *Gastroentero Clin N Am* 1989:18(3):467–83.

· 23 ·
WEIGHT LOSS THROUGH
A HEALTHY DIET

**Along with eliminating their chronic pain and fatigue,
many of my patients are eager to lose weight.
So I'm including this chapter to help you lose those pounds that
are holding you back from total wellness.**

Some of my overweight patients gained weight from the medications they were taking. Some gained weight from lack of sleep; studies show you need 6–8 hours of restorative sleep nightly in order to lose weight. Also, low serotonin states can create sugar cravings, so in an effort to self-medicate, you may have eaten an excess of starches and sweets.

Others, by bankrupting their stress-coping savings account, are now suffering from hypothyroid. All are suffering from a sluggish metabolism, and can't seem to lose weight no matter how many diets they try. I have patients tell me that they hardly eat anything and still gain weight. Many are unknowingly sabotaging their body's ability to lose weight by skipping meals or going on starvation, low-calorie diets, which slows their metabolism even more.

While I know you'll feel better after losing unwanted weight, prematurely starting a weight-loss program can be disastrous. You should first and foremost build up your stress-coping savings account through the jump-start plan. If this book has a theme, that's it! By increasing your stress-coping chemicals, including serotonin, you'll sleep better, reduce nervous eating, and stop the sugar cravings. Some form of weight loss will certainly result!

So until you start sleeping through the night, repairing your adrenal glands, and supplementing with a good optimal daily allowance vitamin-and-mineral formula, it's just too stressful for you to attempt any of the diets in this book. So, before starting the diet in this chapter, make sure you're well on your way to feeling better—mentally and physically.

It's no science that there are numerous weight loss programs to choose from. I've tried a number of them myself, with varying results. I've found that fad diets, where a person loses weight quickly, are always doomed to failure for FMS/CFS patients. They invariably gain the weight back, because the diet is too hard to maintain. Therefore I recommend for you a weight-loss program based on a healthy diet and increased exercise. Then it's only a matter of time before your weight will start to come off.

POPULAR DIETS

A low-fat or low-protein diet is a recipe for disaster! I strongly *dis*courage these diets. They don't allow for enough protein or fat, both of which the body needs to run optimally. A deficiency in fat and/or protein leads to a deficiency in essential hormones, amino acids, essential fatty acids, and enzymes. And in today's high-stress environment, adequate amounts of amino acids and the neurotransmitters they produce are crucial for optimal health. Likewise, fat is needed for proper metabolism, synthesizing hormones, and supplying the EFAs omega-3 and omega-6. So don't avoid eating fat. In fact, eating fat can *help* you to lose weight (read on).

We've already examined the importance of proteins and the amino acids that comprise them. Without these amino acids, our bodies just can't work properly. And low-fat diets usually results in protein deficiency. But proteins are the key building blocks of all life-forms. They makes up over one-half of the body's dry weight and are second only to water in abundance within the body. Muscles, skin, hair, brain, blood vessels, connective tissue, and nails are all made from protein. It's the main structural component of our cells and of the enzymes responsible for all bodily functions.

Antibodies, which fight off bacterial and viral infections, are made up of proteins. So are many of our hormones, including insulin. Protein and fat actually buffer the effects of insulin and allows the body to use glucose at a slower rate. So increasing protein and healthy fat consumption (within the allotted percentages) will actually *aid* in weight loss.

What's more, fat stimulates the hormone that signals your brain that you are full. This is why you can only eat so much fat at a time. Think about it: you can probably eat a whole bag of fat-free chips at one sitting. However, try eating a stick of butter (OK, imagine that it tastes good). You wouldn't get too far before you felt quite full.

Fats have become a nasty four-letter word, something to be avoided at all costs. Low-fat or no-fat foods are now common staples for many Americans. You know what I'm talking about. They dominate the grocery store shelves. But you can hardly call some of them foods—Fat-free potato chips are really nothing but a processed, simple carbohydrate. Many people think these fat-free products can be eaten with impunity, so it is not unusual for a child or adult to consume 1,000 fat-free calories in a single sitting. But a calorie is a calorie, and too many make you overweight.

That said, I don't believe in counting calories. And if you eat properly, you won't need to.

Low-calorie diets are insane! Starving the body on a low-calorie diet doesn't work; just ask Oprah. A low-calorie diet reduces the body's metabolism and its ability to burn fat. Some of these diets promise you'll lose ten pounds a week. But realistically you can only lose a pound or two of fat per week; anything else is just water or muscle loss.

And starvation diets are extremely hard on the body. Some of these dieters start to lose their hair and muscle tone, and their skin starts to sag. Starving the body is a sure way to cause unwanted health problems. So if you like being sick, be sure to not eat enough food.

Low-carb diets can be useful. Written by cardiologist Robert Atkins and published in 1972, *Dr. Atkins' New Diet Revolution* has had a profound affect on the way Americans eat. For over 30 years, Dr. Atkins and his legions of fans have been advocating a low-carbohydrate approach for improved health and weight loss. And this controversial diet has finally gained a foothold in mainstream medicine.

The National Institute of Health is about to begin a study based on Dr. Atkins's work, and recent studies have shown positive—sometimes dramatic—results. One study compared low-fat dieters with low-carb dieters. Over a six-month period, individuals on the two diets lost 20 pounds and 31 pounds respectively. Low-fat dieters had a 22% reduction in their triglycerides (blood fat levels), while those on the Atkins diet decreased their levels by a whopping 49%. The diet is based on consuming 10% of calories as carbohydrates, 60% as fat, and 30% as protein.

Many people had unsuccessfully tried countless other diets and finally lost weight on this one. For them, a low-carb diet has been a godsend. There are others who have tried this diet and either don't lose weight or—more commonly—can't stay on the diet for a long enough period of time. The diet is very limiting and usually only those with a strong will can stay on it long enough to lose weight and keep it off.

I like to use a form of this diet to help activate a person's metabolism; losing a quick 5–6 pounds can deliver a *big* psychological boost. But I don't recommend this diet long-term and don't agree with many of the toxic food choices Dr. Atkins endorses. People—especially those with FMS/CFS—shouldn't live off of fried pork skins, hunks of processed cheese, and excessive amounts of hormone-fed livestock! The diet is so limiting that most individuals have little choice but to subsist on a diet devoid of anything that comes from the ground (vegetables and fruits), at least at first. In Dr. Atkins's defense, he does allows most vegetables, but many people don't cook at home and find a very limited variety of vegetables to choose from when eating out. People need to eat live foods! We are only now learning of the far-reaching health benefits of plant-based flavonoids. And there is a big difference in the nutrition received from processed, preservative-rich, simple carbohydrates and that received from natural complex carbohydrates.

For these reasons, I advocate a diet that allows for up to 40% of calories from complex carbohydrates. Don't count calories or carbohydrate grams; instead, avoid the foods we now know sabotage any chance of losing weight: simple sugars!

ALL ABOUT CARBS

Carbohydrates are basically sugar molecules—sometimes arranged in long chains or pairs. They're found in fruits, vegetables, grains, and animal products, and they are divided into two groups: simple and complex.

Simple carbohydrates, sometimes called sugars, have either one or two connected sugar molecules. Examples include fructose (found in fruits), galactose (in dairy products), maltose (in grains), glucose (in corn syrup), sucrose (table sugar), and lactose (in milk). All of these act similarly in the body—they are digested quickly and dramatically effect blood-glucose levels.

The consumption of simple carbs, processed away from the whole foods in which they are naturally found, is extremely difficult on your pancreas. These processed foods are the number one source of "hidden" simple carbs; they are no different than mainlining pure sugar.

> Processed foods are also devoid of fiber, and low fiber intake is directly related to high cholesterol, digestive problems, and colon cancer.

For instance, fructose is found naturally in an apple, but it's accompanied there by fiber, which slows down the absorption of the fructose in your body. When an apple is processed into apple juice, the fiber is removed, and your body has no buffer between your pancreas and the straight sugar coming down the pipe! Similarly, a sweet potato is loaded with sucrose but also fiber and other fantastic nutrients. But when this sucrose is processed out of its source and pasted onto Fruit Loops, it becomes a poison to your body. It's not as if God gave us food that we couldn't eat...we're just supposed to mostly eat it like we find it.

Complex carbohydrates, sometimes called starches, are made up of long chains of three or more sugars. Complex carbohydrates can be found in most vegetables, unprocessed grains, and legumes.

Complex carbs are loaded with nutrients! They contain essential vitamins, minerals, and phytochemicals that help us combat and prevent disease. Cauliflower and broccoli contain powerful antioxidants. Eggplant contains substances used as a topical treatment for skin cancer. Figs contain antitumor chemicals, and cranberries are used to treat urinary tract infections (see more about that in chapter 21). Red grapes contain potent anti-oxidants and also have antibacterial and antiviral properties. Most nuts—including almonds, Brazil nuts, and walnuts—are high in nutrients and help lower high cholesterol. Onions and garlic have strong antibacterial, antiviral and anticancer chemicals and also help boost the immune system. Soybeans contain anticancer protease inhibitors and are loaded with natural estrogen, making them effective in the treatment of benign prostate hypertrophy, PMS, and menopause. These are just a few examples of the natural live foods essential for our good health.

In addition, complex carbohydrates take a considerable amount of time to be broken down and utilized by the body. This prevents the unwanted highs and lows associated with simple sugar consumption.

BRAIN FUEL

All carbohydrates provide glucose, the sugar that feeds the brain. If the brain doesn't get sufficient glucose, it will do whatever it can to keep from "starving" by pulling glucose out of muscle and then fat tissue. This explains why people on extended low-calorie or high-protein diets will actually lose muscle mass.

Hypoglycemia, by definition, is basically a glucose deficiency. It triggers fatigue, irritability, anxiety, depression, and mental lethargy.

Keeping the body fueled with adequate glucose is a challenge, since the liver, which stores broken-down glucose, can only accommodate the equivalent of two cups of pasta. New stores must be built up every five hours. However, eating excessive carbohydrate intake is unhealthy, too, since unused carbs—especially simple carbs—are stored as fat.

INSULIN AND WEIGHT GAIN

"If I don't eat fat, I won't gain weight" is one of the biggest misconceptions about dieting. Eating simple carbohydrates or too many carbohydrates will cause most people to gain weight!

That's because simple carbs or lots of carbs causes our **blood-sugar (glucose)** levels to rise, since all carbs are turned into glucose. The body must counter this rapid rise in blood glucose by having the pancreas release extra **insulin.**[1] This insulin then shunts the excess carbohydrate into the cells, where it is *stored as fat.*

The role of insulin traces its roots back to a time when man's very survival depended on bodily reserves of fat. Early man couldn't walk into the local grocery store and purchase that night's dinner. Often, man himself was being hunted. So fat was used as fuel when wild game was in short supply and man was not yet agriculturally inclined. These hunters and gatherers would go days—sometimes weeks—without eating. During these lean times, glucose stored in fat tissue served as bodily fuel.

But in today's fast-food, eat-until-you-flop world, insulin's efficiency leads to unwanted weight gain, and simple carbohydrates are the worst offenders. Not only do these sugars turn into fat, they also contribute to arteriosclerosis, depression, and malnutrition.

INSULIN RESISTANCE

Insulin's primary function is to regulate the blood-sugar levels. It stimulates the liver to release glycogen and make room for incoming sugar. It allows sugar to be transported into the cells where they provide energy, and it stores excess glucose as fat. The relationship between glucose, glucagon and insulin is a self-regulating system that serves us well until our metabolism starts to slow down.

Years of eating excess carbohydrates, especially simple ones, plus the effects of metabolic aging begin to take their toll in our mid-30s and

---

Can Sugar Cause Diabetes?

Not exactly. But increased insulin levels, decreased insulin receptors, and cells stuffed full of fat prevent sugar from reaching its intended destination, the cells. Instead, the sugar remains in the bloodstream where it can causes damage to the arterial walls and lead to high blood pressure, arteriosclerosis, high blood lipid levels, heart disease, and type-2 diabetes. Type-1 diabetes is a different illness where the pancreas actually makes no insulin at all. It's development is autoimmune and not related to weight, sugar, or diet.

40s. If we've used up our glucose storage space (we're overweight), our cells won't allow any more sugar in. The body attempts to remedy the sugar-storage problem by reducing the cells' insulin receptors. Unfortunately, this sends a message to the pancreas to release even more insulin, which results in **functional hyperinsulinemia.**

In functional hyperinsulinemia, there is more insulin produced than is required. Along with sugar-filled cells, a high-carbohydrate diet can contribute to its development. When a high concentration of sugar rapidly enters the bloodstream, the pancreas overreacts, protecting against the very dangerous hyperglycemia (high blood sugar).

> "After 26 years in medicine, if I had to choose the number one food that has caused the most depression, it would be sugar."
>
> —Sherry Rogers, MD

For example, you eat a candy bar. The sugar in the candy bar enters the small intestine and is rapidly broken down. Sugar is dumped into the bloodstream, and insulin is oversecreted in response to a large wave of sugar being released so fast. The excess insulin consequently lowers the blood sugar within a short period of time to a hypoglycemic (low) state. The individual then naturally desires more sugar, and the cycle is repeated. This is why a typical low-fat–high-carb diet causes yo-yo-ing blood sugar levels that go sky high and then plunge. This pattern can cause many of the same symptoms experienced by those with FMS/CFS: fatigue, depression, irritability, weight gain, decreased immunity, anxiety, poor concentration, and insomnia.

LOSING WEIGHT THE HEALTHY WAY

Americans are obsessed with losing weight. Unfortunately, 90% of all dieters fail in their quest to lose weight. Many dieters experience a yo-yo effect, losing weight and then gaining it all back, plus some.

The increase in weight as experienced in this country is due to several factors, including sedentary lifestyles, stress, poor eating habits, and the readiness of fast, preservative-enriched foods. Our great ancestors didn't eat 150 pounds of sugar a year as does today's average American. Nor did they eat processed breads and pastas that are designed to stay on store shelves for weeks at a time. A simple diet of lean meat (killed that day), fruits, vegetables, nuts, and berries (gathered), supported our ancient ancestors. Genetically, we haven't changed much in thousands of years; we are still pretty much as God designed. But while our internal bodily systems haven't changed, our external environment certainly has.

To lose weight, you're going to have to think counter-culture.

Eat a diet of approximately 40% complex carbohydrates, 30% fat (good fats!), and 30% protein. I know this doesn't sit well with many of you who have based your diets around the notion that all fat is bad, but remember, we need the good fats and their EFAs (If you still feel nagging doubts, read chapter 29)! Fat also delays the release of insulin, slowing down the rate at which carbohydrates are released into the bloodstream, and so helping you to not store sugar as fat.

Follow the Glycemic Index. This index is a measurement of how quickly a carbohydrate elevates circulating blood-sugar levels. The lower the glycemic index, the slower the rate of absorption. I've included a helpful sample from the glycemic index in chapter 16. You should choose your carbohydrates mostly from the "low" category and sometimes from the "moderate" category. Choose foods in the "high" category very infrequently. Or, if you tend to binge, consider avoiding them entirely.

The easiest way to follow these glycemic rules is to avoid the obvious culprits: white and red potatoes, white rice, white bread, corn chips, corn bread, corn pudding, corn on the cob, popcorn, cooked carrots, beets, cookies, pastries, and anything with refined sugar. Remember that honey is a simple sugar, and so is maple syrup, corn syrup, sucrose, and fructose. So read labels!

To satisfy your sweet tooth, use a plant-based sweetener like stevia or FOS. Both are available at health food stores. If you use an artificial sweetener, Splenda is the best choice.

ARE YOU CARB INTOLERANT?

Many people are carbohydrate intolerant. Their cells have become full of stored carbohydrates (turned into fat) and can no longer effectively metabolize large amounts of carbohydrates. This situation may cause fatigue, mental lethargy, confusion, depression, headaches, bloating, indigestion, and weight gain. A two-week trial on a low-carb diet is an easy way to see if you are carbohydrate intolerant. If you are, you'll feel significantly better after the two weeks. Be careful not to reduce your carbohydrate intake too quickly or severely, though. It could prove to be too much of a shock to your body.

THE TWO-WEEK, LOW-CARB CHALLENGE

Don't try this diet until you correct any sleeping disorders and normalize the adrenal gland.

For two weeks, choose only low-glycemic foods, and keep total carbohydrate intake at or below 20 grams a day. If after two weeks on this diet, you don't feel any better, then you are probably not carb intolerant. If you feel better after two weeks, then you most likely are, and you should stay on this regimen for another two–four weeks. Then you can slowly increase your carb intake, continuing to make as many low-glycemic choices as possible.

If you start to have sugar-withdrawal symptoms—such as feeling jittery, anxious, depressed, or foggy-headed—don't give up; they will subside. And when you're done, your sugar cravings will be weakened, and you'll have achieved better control of your food choices!

If you begin to feel absolutely miserable, then you are probably bottoming out your serotonin levels. Increase your (low-glycemic) carb intake, and wait until your serotonin levels are better shored up before trying again.

Long-term use of this diet, however, increases the risk of ketosis, which makes the blood more acidic than it should be. This increased acidity can cause headaches, bad breathe, dizziness, fatigue, and nausea. Long-term ketonic states are simply not healthy. So follow the two-week (or up to six-week) low-carb challenge test with the balanced diet described above. It might not be the fastest, but it truly is the *healthiest* way to lose weight. Here's some tips to help:

If you blow your diet every once in awhile, of course don't feel guilty. It's the long-term, day-in-and-day-out eating habits that matter. Try to do the best you can, but don't get discouraged if you can't avoid all the "bad foods" on a consistent basis—very few people can. It's OK to eat sweets every once in awhile. Just don't make it a habit! Also, keep your diet goals simple. Don't try to count calories! Simply avoiding high glycemic carbohydrates, going easy on moderate carbohydrates and eating balanced meals over time will allow you to lose weight.

Keep in mind the percentages. Look at your dinner plate. Is it about one-third protein with a little more carbs than protein? And are you getting a good hearty serving of healthy fat? If not, add some avocado, some oil-based salad dressing, or even a pat of butter.

Eat smaller meals. Eat healthy snacks throughout the day instead of three huge meals. Start with breakfast, and then have a piece of fruit or a handful of nuts a couple of hours later. Keep up the combination of carbs, fats, and protein even when snacking. After lunch, eat another healthy snack a few hours before dinner. This will help you avoid overeating at dinner. Smaller meals are also easier than larger ones to digest and allow the body more energy for other functions, like operating the immune system.

Don't skip meals. Many people have gotten into this bad habit. Then when they do eat, nothing is safe around them. Anything within reach that can be quickly consumed is fair game! That's because the brain, by that time, is screaming out for glucose. Your body might be trying to skip a meal, but your brain just won't let you! And the brain doesn't care whether it's a simple or complex carbohydrate; it just wants its glucose "fix."

Unfortunately this often means pre-packaged junk food, which are easy to grab and shovel in. The simple sugars in these foods, as you now know, have no nutritional value, rob the body of needed vitamins and minerals, contribute to obesity, high cholesterol, weakened immunity, and can lead eventually to type-2 diabetes. So don't skip meals!

Keep healthy snacks readily available in your purse, briefcase, or car. When you feel hungry, eat a small snack. Arriving home at night ravenous, and then eating a big dinner followed by snacking in front of the television while reclining in your La-Z-Boy just isn't going to cut it. If you're starving on the way home from work, you've already blown it. Instead, eat a small snack to tide you over until dinner.

Don't snack after dinner, since this requires the body to digest and use energy when it should be resting. You have a new stomach lining every five days, with the cells that contact food being replaced every few minutes. This new growth and repair takes place while you're asleep. So free your stomach up to heal by finishing your eating well before bedtime.

Treat any low thyroid function according to chapter 14. Hypothyroid can cause weight gain.

Consider the elimination diet outlined in chapter 12, because food allergies and intolerances can cause weight gain, too. (The elimination diet can be conducted at the same time as the low-carb challenge from p. 362).

If you feel better on the elimination diet, it will probably boost your weight loss, too. Some of patients feel (and look!) so great on the elimination diet that they make it their permanent eating plan.

Try a diet pill. No, not the latest "wonder drug" with who-knows-what side effects. Instead, try the following natural supplements and nutrients to help you lose weight. You might already be taking them as part of your healing plan.

NATURAL DIET PILLS

• **The amino acids DL-phenylalanine, L-phenylalanine, and L-tyrosine all act as natural appetite suppressants.** DL-phenylalanine also increases pain-relieving endorphins. L-tyrosine has the added benefit of stimulating thyroid and human growth hormones, both of which increase the body's metabolism. Even though L-tyrosine is used more rapidly than are the other two aminos, I usually start my weight-loss patients off with DL-phenylalanine. It has proven itself, time and time again, to be the most effective appetite suppressant. Remember that these amino acids can raise blood pressure or cause insomnia, headaches, and irritability when taken by sensitive individuals or in excessive doses. Just as important, these supplements should not be taken along with drugs known as MAOIs. Always take free-form amino acids on an empty stomach, and start with 1,000–2,000 mg. twice a day. Always start off slow and gradually increase the dosage, up to 8,000 mg. daily. Vitamin B6 is needed for these amino acids to work properly, so add 100–250 mg. of B6 per day. (You don't need to worry about this extra B6 if you are taking my CFS/Fibro Formula.) Don't take L-tyrosine in the evening, since it has a stimulating effect.

- **L-glutamine** can also be extremely helpful in eliminating sugar cravings. Animal studies have shown it quite effective in lowering both blood glucose and insulin levels. L-glutamine should be taken on an empty stomach, 500–1,000 mg. twice a day. It can be taken at the same time as DL and L-phenylalanine.

- **L-Carnitine** helps transport fatty acids to the fat-burning mitochondria. It helps the liver rid the body of unwanted waste products, increasing the body's cellular metabolism. I recommend 500–1,000 mg. of L-Carnitine twice a day. As with all amino acids, it should be taken on an empty stomach. There are no side effects to L-Carnitine.

- **5-HTP** is, as you should definitely know by now, the precursor to the neurotransmitter serotonin. Serotonin is—among many other things—an appetite regulator. (The drug combination Fen-Phen was prescribed to stimulate serotonin but had serious side effects—like heart damage—and has been recalled by the FDA.) 5-HTP also helps reduce or eliminate sugar cravings. It can help prevent binge eating when under stress or feeling depressed.

- **Chromium** is a mineral that helps control blood-sugar levels. It increases liver glycogen storage and allows for efficient uptake of glucose by muscle cells while inhibiting excessive storage of fat. Dosage is 200–400 mg. of chromium with glucose tolerance factor (a patented process) daily, 30 minutes before a meal. Nature's Way makes a supplement called **Blood Sugar** that combines chromium and an herbal extract, Gymnema Sylvestre. Gymnema Sylvestre is a plant from India that is used around the world to treat type-2 diabetes. It helps regulate blood sugar and reduce sugar cravings. Several studies have shown this herb to be quite effective for lowering blood sugar levels, even with diabetics taking insulin by injection.

• **CoQ10** is similar to L-carnitine in its effect on cellular metabolism. It aids in the production of ATP, the main energy compound generated within cells. I recommend 50–200 mg. daily.

NOTES

1. Just like insulin is released by the pancreas to keep blood sugar levels from rising too high, glucagon is secreted to prevent these sugar levels from becoming too low. Glucagon causes stored glucose (glycogen) to be released from the liver. During periods of fasting, exercise, or low-calorie/low-carb diets, the pancreas can also cause the protein in muscles to be converted to glucose.

· 24 ·
THE BENEFITS
OF EXERCISE

**You might not have felt up to exercising for years.
But soon you will, and you'll be on your way to
enjoying its fantastic "side effects."**

It might take a month or two of the jump-start program before
you feel like starting an exercise routine. And if you dive right in
and overdo it, you'll just have a "flare up," become discouraged,
and quit. Once you can get through a normal day with only mild
pain or fatigue, start by adding a simple five-minute walk around
the block during your best part of the day. Then after a few weeks,
begin increasing the time you walk each day.

A shopping mall is a great place for rainy-day walks, and you'll
probably see other folks there up to the same thing. OK, I'll admit
that step-aerobics, Stairmasters, and cross-country ski machines
may be more glamorous. But walking is the easiest form of exercise
to maintain on a consistent basis. Long after the stationary bike,
the treadmill, and the Soloflex have been abandoned, walking will
still be in vogue. And it requires only commitment and a good pair
of shoes! Walking six days a week will burn over two pounds of
fat a month, and a faster-paced walk will burn even more calories.
Running burns twice as much as moderate walking.

And here is even more good news: **your metabolism continues to
burn calories, even after you're through exercising.** Your metabolic rate increases 25% and remains elevated for several hours
after a workout.

**Exercise also decreases triglycerides (fats) in your blood and
LDL—the bad form of cholesterol—while increasing HDL
—the good form.** High blood pressure is lowered, and the heart
becomes stronger and more efficient, pumping more blood per

beat. Exercise increases the diameter of coronary arteries, greatly reducing the risk of heart attack. Exercise can even reduce the risk of a second heart attack. Among heart-attack survivors, those who choose not to exercise are over 20 times more likely to have another heart attack then are those who exercise.

In addition, **exercise is a wonderful stress reducer and mood elevator.** It helps relieve mild depression by generating endorphins, the body's natural pain killers that are associated with the "runner's high." Some researchers have said that exercise can raise levels of norepinephrine—a neurotransmitter associated with drive, ambition, energy, and happiness—by 200%. **Exercise also stimulates important neurotransmitters that help us combat insomnia; irritability; fatigue; and food, alcohol, and tobacco cravings.** Blood glucose and insulin levels are decreased, which is extremely beneficial for carbohydrate-intolerant individuals and type-2 diabetics. (Type-1 diabetics will need to adjust their insulin regimen to account for increased exercise.)

Exercise stimulates brown fat, found at the posterior base of the neck and shoulders, to burn more calories. It also increases human growth hormone, which burns fat and builds muscle while stimulating the thymus gland, the master gland of the immune system.

Allergy sufferers can benefit from regular exercise as well, since it raises levels of norepinephrine and cortisol, which help reduce inflammation and allergic reactions. Many of my asthmatic patients notice a drastic reduction in the frequency and severity of their attacks after being on a consistent exercise program that's medically right for them.

Exercise helps detoxify the body by ridding it of waste products (including carbon monoxide) and enhancing delivery of oxygen and nutrients to the cells. Exercise helps reduce insulin production, too, and too much insulin can cause excess carbohydrates to be stored as fat.

So once you start to feel better, go ahead and start your first 5-minute walk. The benefits of exercise are numerous.

· 25 ·
FEEDING THE SPIRIT

**We can't separate our minds from our body's health
any more than we can separate our eyes from seeing.
The connection is profound.**

Psychoneuroimmunology is the study of the interrelationships
between the mind, brain, and immune system. Four decades of
ongoing research in this area is just now making its way into the
medical and public arena. The research reveals how the brain uses
the nervous system to communicate with every system in the body,
including the immune system. But more importantly, it leads to
an understanding of how thoughts, emotions, and the experiences
they create can influence our overall health.

Just how does the mind control our health? Well, let's look at how
the body, brain, and mind interact. Think of the brain as a musi-
cal instrument and the mind as the musician. Nothing happens
until the musician picks up the instrument and begins to play. In
the same way, the brain is an instrument (in this case, an "organ")
under the influence of the mind.

A person's inner spirit is the conductor of the symphony. Like the
conductor, your spirit has the ability to control every note played
by the body. Although every one of us has an inner spirit, most
don't fully tap into its incredible positive energy. When you do
tap into this energy through prayer, meditation, and times of pure
mental clarity, you know that, without a doubt, you've experienced
a taste of bliss. Some people call this spirit our innate intelligence;
some call it Holy.

Since our minds undoubtedly influence our bodily functions, it is
only logical to ask, "How can we control our minds?" The self-help
movement has already educated us on positive thinking, affirma-
tions, resolutions, goal setting, and mission statements. These are

all valid tools to help you write your life script, which is a combination of genes, environment, thoughts, beliefs, and experiences. These make up your reality, your own little world. For instance, if you lived alone with a group of pygmies, you'd feel like a giant. You might think you're more attractive, stronger, or more powerful than everyone else. Or just the opposite, you might feel inferior, because you look so different. It is all about our beliefs, which turn into our reality.

WRITE A NEW LIFE SCRIPT

Rewriting your script from one of poor health, despair, and helplessness is crucial in overcoming your illness. This time is an opportunity to evaluate what was not (and probably still is not) working in your life.

We rarely question what is truly important in our lives. *Why are we here? For what purpose?* Normally, we live each day as the day before, sometimes "sleepwaking" through entire portions of our lives. But major life challenges are often catalysts for re-evaluating life. We may seek solace by tapping into our inner spirit. We may turn to God and ask for his guidance. (If we fail to recognize this opportunity, God will usually give us additional chances!)

> *For as a man thinketh in his heart, so is he.*
> —Proverbs 23:7

Your script might have read like this: "Hard working, perfectionist responsible for everybody around her. Long work hours, poor diet, too much real or imagined responsibility, negative thoughts, and unmanaged stress."

A 20-year study by George Engel, professor of medicine at University of Rochester, showed that 70–80% of all chronically ill patients had experienced extended periods of feeling helpless before the onset of their disease.

TRUE HEALTH IS A TRIANGLE

True health is made up of three pillars: physical, chemical, and spiritual. Picture a triangle in which each of these pillars interacts and supports one another. Our inner spirit makes up the bottom pillar (or line of the triangle). The other two pillars, physical and chemical health, join together at the pinnacle.

Physical health involves the mechanical aptitude of various moveable body parts, how well the muscles and joints move. How strong are the various bones that support our posture? Our dexterity, flexibility, and stamina are all associated with physical health.

Chemical health involves the nutrients, enzymes, hormones, white blood cells, neurotransmitters, and other biochemicals that perform the countless functions needed to run the body.

Spiritual health is determined by our inner self (conscious and unconscious mind) and our higher self (spirit, God within us, Universal intelligence, Holy Ghost, etc.). These act as the rudder that steers every facet of our lives, including the state of our bodies. This is the spiritual pillar.

If any one side of the triangle is removed or ignored, the entire structure weakens and begins to collapse onto itself.

THE HEALER WITHIN

We are born with an innate ability to heal ourselves. If this were not true, we would quickly succumb to the millions of deadly microbes that inhabit our lungs and digestive tracts. These bugs are monitored and kept in check by the inner healer, the autonomic nervous system. It also controls how fast your heart beats, the rate of your breathing, how you walk, how you stand, and how fast blood pumps through your veins. It coordinates all functions of the body, including the immune system. Do you have to think about healing a broken bone? No. Your inner self maintains a constant vigil, overseeing every bodily process. We are truly amazing organisms.

> *All that we are arises with our thoughts; with our thoughts we make our world.*
>
> —Gantama Buddha

You have a new liver every six weeks, and 98% of the atoms in our bodies are renewed every year. The power that made the body is ultimately the power that heals it.

Understanding this concept can be intimidating. Medicine has been blinded by science and has largely neglected the profound influence of our higher self. Health professions are known as the "healing arts," yet the art of medicine has been too often replaced with brain scans and drug therapies. But true health is more than the absence of disease. It is optimal physical, chemical, and spiritual well-being.

I suggest a new paradigm, one that considers the role of our inner self in determining our state of health.

MIND CHATTER AND RESPONSIVE THOUGHTS

Our minds never stop chattering. We—consciously or subconsciously—take in, sort, analyze, and respond to billions of thoughts each day. This constant chatter, if not checked, begins to take its toll on our mental and physical well-being. Negative thoughts can create a blueprint for the subconscious mind to rely on. A few negative thoughts a day aren't so bad, but 30 years of incessant worry shapes who we become as people, our personality. Your script is being written and rewritten every day by every thought you have.

I could write a lengthy chapter about all the mind-body studies and how they relate to emotional, mental, spiritual, physical, and chemical health, but I think it's really this simple. Do you feel better or worse when you are laughing? How about scowling? It doesn't take a scientific study of brain scans and heart monitors to know the answers.

Have you ever tried to stay sad or angry when smiling at yourself in the mirror? You can't do it. This is because the muscles in the face, when contracted into a smile, trigger the brain to release happy hormones. I've found I feel and look my best when I'm physically and mentally rested. When I make the time to tone down the mind chatter and begin to listen to my inner voice, health, vitality, and joy are the rewards.

I'm not implying that you can think, meditate, or even pray yourself free of ailments. I know how debilitating FMS and CFS can be. These are not illnesses to be taken lightly! However, finding and tapping into your inner self only increases your chances of getting and being well in its truest sense.

Sometimes we have to dig deep to find the courage to overcome life's tragedies. Consider Stephen Hawking, the famous physicist who has no use of his arms or legs. Some would have given up and been content to slowly die.

> *The greatest discovery of my generation is that human beings can alter their lives by altering their attitudes of mind.*
>
> —William James

We can't always control life's obstacles, but we can control how we respond to them. Neglecting your inner self—your life essence—while attempting to overcome something as potentially life squelching as FMS/CFS is like trying to use a magnifying glass to watch a big-screen movie. Remove the magnifying glass and take in the big picture. Don't just focusing on covering up symptoms with chemicals or physical therapies. That ignores the third pillar. Can you have optimal health without personally experiencing love and inner peace on a daily basis?

In order to heal yourself, you must begin to realize that true health comes from within. Your state of health is largely determined by how well you recognize this concept and your willingness to listen and trust your inner self.

THE HEALING POWER OF PRAYER

Although 95% of Americans believe in God, most doctors are uncomfortable discussing spiritual matters. This is sad, since 60% of the population would like to discuss spiritual issues with their doctors and 40% would like for their doctors to pray with them.

The effects of prayer are numerous: less anxiety, stress, and anger; lowered resting pulse rate and blood pressure; increased production of happy hormones; and increased pain threshold. In addition, prayer and other spiritual practices tap into the mind-body connection. They have a calming effect that involves every system in the body, including the nervous system, immune system, endocrine (hormonal) system, digestive system, and cardiovascular system.

One study involving individuals with HIV showed that participation in religious or spiritual activities substantially improved immune function.

One of the most talked-about studies evaluating the positive benefits of prayer was published in *The Southern Medical Journal* in 1988. It involved 393 hospitalized patients who were equally divided into two groups: one group served as the control and was treated with traditional medical care alone. The second group received prayer along with traditional medical care. Neither group, nor their doctors, knew who was receiving prayer from third parties. The group receiving prayer had these remarkable results: they had fewer congestive heart failures (8 versus 20), fewer of them needed diuretics (5 versus 15), they experienced fewer cardiac arrests (3 versus 14), they had fewer episodes of pneumonia (3 versus 13), fewer of them were prescribed antibiotics (3 versus 17), and they generally required less medication than the control group, who received no prayer from the volunteer third parties.

> *Everything can be taken from a man but one thing: The last of the human freedoms—to choose one's attitude in any given set of circumstances, to choose one's own way.*
>
> —Victor E. Frankl

TAPPING INTO YOUR INNER SELF

One of the healthiest things you can do in this lifetime is to learn to rise above the constant mind chatter by quieting your mind and allowing your inner self to flourish. You'll start to realize how negative and self-destructive thoughts sabotage your innate desire to be healthy. Life's true game is less about controlling your surroundings and more about letting go of unwanted negative thoughts—much like shedding layers of clothes when entering a warm room. The ability to control our minds by understanding, acknowledging, and choosing which thoughts, emotions, and feelings serve us best is perhaps the key that unlocks optimal health. Below are just a few ways to quiet the mind and tap into your inner self.

CONSCIOUS BREATHING

Conscious breathing is one way to integrate your mind and body. Focusing on breathing, using mantras (repetitive sounds), and/or visualizing a word or a soothing scene are central to most meditative practices. In basic breathing exercises, all you need is a quite place and a willingness to quiet the mind. Conscious breathing reduces stress and allows you to filter out the constant mind chatter. Quieting the mind offers the opportunity to get in touch with your inner self. A conscious breathing exercise can be done any time of day and as often as you wish. Use it as a powerful stress-busting tool when you are feeling overwhelmed:

> Those who are at peace with themselves and their immediate surroundings have far fewer serious illnesses than those who are not. The simple truth is happy people don't get sick.
>
> —Bernie Siegel, MD

Bring your attention to your breathing. Notice the flow of breath in and out of your lungs. Take a deep breath in through your nose, allowing the air to fill your lungs. Slowly exhale through your mouth. Observe the rhythm that naturally occurs. Acknowledge any distracting thoughts, and simply let them go when they appear. Return your attention to the rhythm of your breathing. Continue to take deep breathes in and out. When it feels natural, try allowing more time between each breath. Pause when appropriate, and feel the inner peace. Enjoy the freedom from mind chatter.

REFOCUSING TECHNIQUE

This technique is designed to allow you to take control of your mind. Too often we find ourselves at the mercy of our emotions and have knee-jerk reactions that don't serve our higher self. When facing a stressful situation that threatens to overwhelm your best intentions, stop and take time to consider the wisdom of your inner self. This allows you to avoid being at the mercy of old negative habits and to write a new positive script that serves you better.

1. **Stop.** Call time out. Take several deep breaths. Remember that with the help of your inner self, you can take control of a situation.

2. **Look.** Rise above the situation and just be an observer. Notice how you feel, your thoughts, your surroundings, any other people involved. Be objective. Take it all in.

3. **Listen.** Take a few minutes to focus on your breathing. Listen to what your inner self is saying. Pay attention to your chest area. Notice how you feel. Is this how you want to feel? Listen deeply. What is your inner self, your inner voice, telling you about this situation?

4. **Choose.** Make an affirmative statement about what you wish to choose in light of this situation "I choose to feel calm, balanced, and open to positive experiences."

5. **Let it go.** Choose happiness, peace, and serenity over having to be right. Choose acceptance of not knowing over having to understand. Choose love over hate. Choose thoughts of improving health over nagging reminders of disease.

MEDITATION

Meditation can generally be divided into two categories: concentration methods, which emphasize focusing on your breathing or a specific object, and mindfulness meditation, which usually uses chants, focused breathing, or repetitive thoughts. The goal in either case is to allow thoughts, feelings, and emotions to appear moment by moment without placing any attention on them. Simply let the thoughts enter. Acknowledge them and let them go, allowing yourself to tap into your inner self.

> *I've always liked the time before dawn, because there's no one around to remind me who I'm supposed to be, so it's easier to remember who I am.*
>
> —Brian Andreas[1]

Meditation may be especially helpful for chronic pain. Others studies have shown the effectiveness of meditation for anxiety, substance abuse, skin ailments, and depression.

YOGA

Yoga has been practiced in India for over 6,000 years. Hatha yoga, based on a system of physical postures, is the best-known form in America. Yoga means "yoke," or union of the personal self with the Divine source. Others describe yoga as a way to join mind, body, and spirit to enrich one's life. Yoga has made its way into several large hospitals around the country and continues to gain in popularity. Used on a regular basis, yoga offers a unique way to exercise and tone the physical body while at the same time quieting the mind.

THE HOUR OF POWER

Taking time on a daily basis to quiet the mind is a crucial component of living the lives we want to live. I try to find an hour of power every day. My hour of power involves prayer, meditation, and exercise. I also use some of this time to listen to positive subliminal tapes on such topics as abundant energy, laughter and happiness, and stress management.

NOTES
1. Brian Andreas is one of my favorite artists. You can view his imaginative and insightful works at www.storypeople.com.

FOR FURTHER READING AND RESEARCH
• G. Engel, "A Life Setting Conductive to Illness: The Giving Up–Given Up Complex," *Bulletin of Menninger Clinic* (1968).

PART FOUR

RESOURCES

· 26 ·
THE A-B-Cs OF VITAMINS

Vitamin A is a potent antioxidant with great immune-enhancing abilities. A deficiency in zinc ceases vitamin A metabolism, even when the vitamin is abundant. Too much vitamin A can lead to dry lips and skin, headache, thinning hair, and bone pain, but symptoms are quickly reversed when levels are reduced. **White spots on the fingernails indicate a zinc and vitamin A deficiency and suggest reduced immunity.** Especially important in FMS/CFS, vitamin A helps correct intestinal permeability (leaky gut), which is associated with migraines, asthma, rheumatoid arthritis, IBS, cystitis, sinusitis, rhinitis, ear infection, dermatitis, hives, and eczema. Vitamin A's other benefits include:

- **maintaining a healthy thymus gland, which controls the entire immune system.**
- developing and maintaining the surfaces of the mucous membranes, lungs, skin, stomach, and urinary, digestive, and reproductive tracts.
- helping to form bones and soft tissue, including tooth enamel.
- protecting against some cancers.
- treating acne (both orally and topically).
- enabling night vision.
- usefulness in calcium metabolism.
- protecting against asthma.
- reducing allergic reactions.
- helping prevent birth defects when taken by expectant mothers (a minimum of 2,000 IUs and no more than 8,000 IUs per day).

The body *stores* fat-soluble vitamins, which include vitamins A, D, E, K, and beta-carotene. Because of this, an overdose is possible when taking these vitamins. However, the side effects of vitamin toxicity are quickly eliminated once they are discontinued.

Vitamin B1 (thiamin) is needed to metabolize carbohydrates, fats, and proteins. It is important for proper cell function, especially nerve cell function. It is involved in the production of acetylcholine, a nerve chemical directly related to **memory and physical and mental energy.** A deficiency of Vitamin B1 can lead to fatigue, mental confusion, emaciation, depression, irritability, upset stomach, nausea, and tingling in the extremities.

Vitamin B1 has been reported to be deficient in nearly 50% of the elderly. This could possibly explain the dramatic increase in presenile dementia and Alzheimer's disease the past few decades. Diets high in simple sugars, including alcohol, will increase the chances of a vitamin B1 deficiency. The tannins in tea inhibit vitamin B1 absorption.

Vitamin B2 (riboflavin) is responsible for the metabolism of carbohydrates, fats, and proteins. Vitamin B2 is involved in producing neurotransmitters (brain chemicals) responsible for sleeping, mental and physical energy, happiness, and mental acuity. A deficiency of vitamin B2 can cause soreness and burning of the lips, mouth, and tongue; sensitivity to light; itching and burning eyes; and cracks in the corners of the mouth. Vitamin B2 can help curb the craving for sweets and is needed for the synthesis of B6.

Vitamin B2 is needed to convert the amino acid tryptophan to Niacin (B3). B2 is not absorbed very well, and any excess will turn the urine a bright fluorescent yellow. It is not toxic.

Vitamin B3 (niacin) plays an important role in mental health. Orthomolecular physicians have used niacin to treat schizophrenia, anxiety, and depression. It is a by-product of the metabolism of tryptophan. Some people have a genetic inability to breakdown or absorb tryptophan, and this can lead to aggressive behavior, restlessness, hyperactivity, and insomnia.

Large daily doses of niacin can decrease the bad LDL cholesterol and triglycerides while increasing the good HDL cholesterol. Niacin increases circulation, and this helps prevent blood clots and arteriosclerosis, which can lead to heart disease and stroke. A deficiency of niacin can cause weakness, dry skin, lethargy, headache, irritability, loss of memory, depression, delirium, insomnia, and disorientation. Large doses of vitamin B3 can cause a flushing of the skin, but this can be prevented by starting off with 25 mg. daily and gradually increasing the dosage over a period of days, because the flushing is due to the release of cellular histamine. Niacin acts as a wonderful sedative to calm nerves and help with sleep.

Daily doses of 1,000 mg. appear to be safe, and large doses are needed to treat high cholesterol. To treat high cholesterol, use timed-release Niacin. For psychiatric disorders, including anxiety, depression, and insomnia, use a special version of vitamin B3 known as niacinamide.

Vitamin B5 (pantothenic acid) is crucial for managing stress, boosts the immune system, is needed by all cells in the body, and is required for normal functioning of the GI tract. It converts carbohydrates, fats, and proteins into energy. It is also needed in order to produce adrenal hormones, which play an important role in stress management. In fact, **B5 is some- times referred to as the "antistress" vitamin.** Vitamin B5 can help reduce anxiety and may play a significant role in depression recovery. It helps convert choline into acetylcholine, which is responsible for memory.

A deficiency in vitamin B5 can lead to fatigue, depression, irritability, digestive problems, upper respiratory infections, dermatitis, muscle cramps, and loss of sensation in the extremities. Vitamin B5, along with vitamin C, helps to reduce uric acid levels (increased uric acid levels are associated with gouty arthritis). B5 helps boost endurance by manufacturing ATP, an essential chemical for cellular energy. Large doses may cause diarrhea.

Vitamin B6 (pyridoxine) may be the most important B vitamin. It is involved in more bodily functions than any other vitamin, and its benefits include:

• making neurotransmitters, including serotonin, epinephrine, and norepinephrine.
• inhibiting the formation of homocysteine, a toxic chemical associated with heart disease.
• helping to synthesize DNA and RNA.

- helping metabolize essential fatty acids.
- helping prevent the destruction caused by free radicals.
- helping produce hydrochloric acid (HCl), which is crucial for proper digestion.
- helping form hemoglobin.
- serving as a natural diuretic.
- alleviating carpal tunnel syndrome (tingling or pain in the wrists and hands).
- stimulating IgA antibodies, which help prevent tooth decay.

A vitamin B6 deficiency can cause anemia, even if iron levels are normal. Deficiency can also lead to PMS, depression, insomnia, fatigue, tingling and numbness in the extremities, increased susceptibility to infections, nausea, kidney stones, anemia, irritability, tension, headache, fluid retention, and acne. Vitamin B6 may be suppressed by certain medications, including oral contraceptives and estrogen.

Some asthmatics have a malfunction in the way they assimilate vitamin B6 and process tryptophan, so supplementing with 250–500 mg. of vitamin B6 a day may help with symptoms of asthma. Vitamin B6 is also needed for proper magnesium levels in red blood cells. Orthomolecular physicians use megadoses of vitamin B6 to treat schizophrenia. It's been found through clinical trials that individuals who do not dream have low levels of B6.

Some individuals can't adequately break down regular vitamin B6 and will need to take a special form known as pyridoxal-5-phosphate (P5P).

Vitamin B12 (cobalamin) is the only B vitamin stored by the body. A vitamin B12 deficiency occurs only in malnutrition, malabsorption, or other impediments to proper digestion.

Vitamin B12 is important in the growth of children. It is responsible for the replication of genetic material and so is essential for the development and maintenance of all the cells. Vitamin B12 helps form the myelin sheath that insulates nerve processes and allows rapid communication from one cell to another.

A deficiency of B12 can cause a reduction in mental acuity, evidenced by poor memory. Alzheimer's and senile dementia, two diseases associated with memory loss, confusion, and nerve damage, might both be attributed to a deficiency of B12 It is only found in animal products (especially liver), so vegetarians should supplement it. Antigout medications, anticoagulant drugs, and potassium supplements may interfere with B12 absorption, and taking antacids will block its absorption. Calcium is necessary for normal absorption of B12 High doses of folic acid can mask the symptoms of B12-deficiency anemia.

Because vitamin B12 deficiency is routinely seen in the elderly, I believe everyone over the age of 60 should be supplementing with vitamin B12. Vitamin B12 is not toxic.

Beta-carotene, found in dark green, dark orange, and yellow fruits and vegetables, can be converted into vitamin A. And beta-carotene is relatively nontoxic, whereas too much vitamin A can be quite dangerous.

It is a strong antioxidant with anticancer properties—one molecule of beta-carotene can destroy 1,000 free radicals. It protects the skin from harmful ultraviolet (UV) light. Women with low levels of beta-carotene in their cervical tissues are at risk for developing cervical cancer. A 19-year study involving 3,000 men shows that beta-carotene may significantly reduce the incidence of lung cancer in both smokers and nonsmokers. (Studies have also demonstrated a 45% reduction in lung cancer in those individuals who take vitamin supplements.) The only side effect of consuming too much beta-carotene is a yellowing of the skin, and this condition disappears once intake is reduced. Vitamin E and selenium enhance the role of beta-carotene.

Biotin is critical to the body's fat metabolism, and it aids in the utilization of protein, folic acid, B12, and pantothenic acid. Sufficient quantities are needed for healthy hair and nails. Biotin supplementation may help prevent hair loss in some men. Biotin is also important in promoting healthy bone marrow, nervous tissue, and sweat glands.

Saccharin inhibits the absorption of biotin. Raw egg whites, antibiotics, and sulfa drugs all prevent its proper utilization. Due to poor absorption, infants are susceptible to a biotin deficiency, and symptoms include a dry, scaly scalp and/or face.

A biotin deficiency is considered rare, and deficiency is usually seen in hospitalized patients on intravenous feeding tubes or patients taking large dosages of antibiotics. Symptoms of a deficiency include depression, dry skin, conjunctivitis, hair loss and color, elevated cholesterol, anemia, loss of appetite, muscle pain, numbness in the hands and feet, nausea, lethargy, and enlargement of the liver. Biotin is not toxic.

Vitamin C (ascorbic acid) produces and maintains collagen, a protein that forms the foundation for connective tissue, the most abundant tissue in the body. Benefits include:

- **increasing immune system function,**
- **helping the adrenal glands form important stress hormones,**
- fighting bacterial infections,
- helping wounds heal,
- preventing hemorrhaging,
- reducing allergy symptoms,
- helping prevent heart disease,
- helping prevent free-radical damage,
- acting as a natural antihistamine,
- helping to convert tryptophan to serotonin,
- reducing blood pressure in mild hypertension,
- preventing the progression of cataracts,
- helping regulate blood sugar levels,
- possibly improving fertility,
- lowering LDL (bad) cholesterol while raising HDL (good) cholesterol,
- helping prevent toxicity of cadmium, a heavy metal that can increase the risk of heart disease,
- and counteracting other heavy metals, including mercury and copper.

A deficiency in vitamin C can cause bleeding gums, loose teeth, dry and scaly skin, tender joints, muscle cramps, poor wound healing, lethargy, loss of appetite, depression, and swollen arms and legs. Aspirin, alcohol, antidepressants, anticoagulants, oral contraceptives, analgesics, and steroids can all interfere with vitamin C absorption. Ester C is absorbed four times faster than regular ascorbic acid. Pregnant women should not exceed 5,000 mg. of C a day. Large doses can cause diarrhea, so I—along with many other nutritional experts—recommend gradually increasing vitamin C until you have a loose stool. Then, reduce your intake 500 mg. at a time until your stools are normal to find your optimal dose.

Choline is essential for the health of the liver, gall bladder, kidneys, and nerves. It helps with fat and cholesterol metabolism. It prevents fat from accumulating while helping fight fat buildup in the arteries and liver. Our bodies can make choline from vitamin B12, folic acid, and the amino acid methionine. Choline is essential for brain development and proper liver function. A deficiency may cause poor memory and mental fatigue, and megadoses have been used to treat Alzheimer's disease, Huntington's disease, learning disabilities, and tardive dyskinesia with varying degrees of success. Choline is not toxic.

Vitamin D is produced by the body after exposure to sunlight. It is one of the oldest hormones, having been produced by life forms for over 750 million years. Phytoplankton, zooplankton, and most plants and animals that are exposed to sunlight have the capacity to make vitamin D. In humans, vitamin D is critically important for the development, growth, and maintenance of a healthy body, from birth until death. See more about vitamin D's role in the prevention and treatment of disease in the box on p. 389.

The Institute of Medicine brought experts together recently to explore the question of whether the recommended daily allowance (RDA) of vitamin D has been set too low. The impetus for the occasion was the mounting evidence for this vitamin's role in preventing common cancers, autoimmune diseases, type-1 diabetes, heart disease, chronic pain, and osteoporosis and the growing evidence that vitamin-D deficiency is common in the United States.

According to Michael F. Holick, MD, PhD, of the Boston University School of Medicine, the typical symptoms of vitamin-D deficiency are aching bones and muscle discomfort. **So vitamin-D deficiency is often misdiagnosed as fibromyalgia or chronic fatigue syndrome.** Too little vitamin D has also been implicated as the cause of various other health disorders, including influenza, psoriasis, gout, otosclerosis, interstitial cystitis, decreased pulmonary function, thrombosis, chronic kidney disease, pancreatitis, rheumatic diseases, hepatitis-B infections, hemochromatosis, and gastrointestinal diseases.

Should I be tested for a vitamin-D deficiency? After seeing some of the new research on vitamin D a few years ago, I began testing all my patients for a deficiency. I was surprised to see that many of them were far too low in this vital micronutrient! I originally only tested my patients who lived in the colder, more northern climates. Then I started testing my patients from the southeastern states. They began producing lab work showing low D levels. Now I recommend that anyone with a chronic illness—especially FMS or CFS—has her vitamin-D levels checked.

How much vitamin D do I need? In the summer, those with at least 15 minutes of sun exposure on their skin most days should take around 1,000 mg. of vitamin D3 each day. They should take more in the winter. Those who have darker skin, are older, avoid sun exposure, or live in the northern United States should take higher amounts, around 2,000 mg. a day in the summer and up to 4,000 mg. a day in the winter.

Are high amounts safe? Vitamin D is remarkably safe; there have been no deaths caused by the vitamin. People consuming only government-recommended levels of 200–400 IU per day often have blood levels considerably below 50 ng./ml. This means that the government's recommendations are too low and should be raised for optimal health function.

What kind do I need? High-dose vitamin D can be purchased at a number of health-food stores or major drug chains. However, not all vitamin D is equal. I recommend using only pharmaceutical grade, naturally occurring Vitamin D3.

Vitamin E is a major antioxidant that protects cells and tissues from oxidative stress. It also protects—from free-radical damage—the pituitary and adrenal hormones, fatty acids, and myelin sheaths

---

Vitamin D to the Rescue!

Autoimmune Illnesses: Autoimmune diseases include rheumatoid arthritis, diabetes, Reiter's syndrome, lupus, asthma, and ulcerative colitis. Researchers are discovering an increasing number of links between the immune, nervous, and endocrine systems. Hormones of the endocrine system, such as vitamin D, help the immune and nervous systems defend the body; defects in this intricate system lead to autoimmune disorders.

Autism: Research has shown that low maternal vitamin D3 has important ramifications for a baby's developing brain. Vitamin D is a steroid hormone with many important functions in the brain, mediated through the nuclear vitamin-D receptor (VDR). Dysfunctional VDR demonstrate altered emotional behavior and specific motor deficits.

Cancer: Vitamin D inhibits inappropriate cell division and metastasis, reduces blood-vessel formation around tumors, and regulates proteins that affect tumor growth. It also enhances anti-cancer actions of immune-system chemicals and chemotherapy drugs. A four-year study of 1,179 healthy, postmenopausal women showed that taking calcium along with nearly three times the U.S. government's recommendation of vitamin D3 resulted in a dramatic 60% or greater reduction in all forms of cancer. It's estimated that if vitamin-D levels were increased worldwide, a minimum of 600,000 cases of breast and other cancers could be prevented each year. Nearly 150,000 cases of cancer could be prevented in the United States alone! *Studies show that by taking vitamin D (about 2,000 IU per day), females can cut breast cancer incidence by half!*

Chronic Pain: In a study involving 150 children and adults with unexplained muscle and bone pain, almost all were found to be vitamin D deficient; many were severely deficient with extremely low levels of the vitamin in their bodies. Muscle pain and weakness was a prominent symptom of vitamin-D deficiency in a study of Arab and Danish Moslem women living in Denmark. In a cross-sectional study of 150 consecutive patients referred to a clinic in Minnesota for the evaluation of persistent, nonspecific musculoskeletal pain, 93% had serum levels indicative of vitamin-D deficiency.

Mental Function and Moods: Recent research indicates that vitamin-D deficiency is associated with low mood and cognitive impairment in the elderly. It has also been implicated in various psychiatric disorders, including anxiety and depression.

Type-2 Diabetes: Vitamin D helps maintain adequate insulin levels, and preliminary evidence suggests that supplementation can increase insulin levels in people with type-2 diabetes. Prolonged supplementation may help reduce blood sugar levels.

Immune Function: There is considerable scientific evidence that vitamin D has a variety of positive effects on the immune system. Additionally, there is growing evidence that maintaining vitamin-D levels in the body during the winter helps to prevent the flu and other viral infections by strengthening the immune system.

Heart Disease: Activated vitamin D has been shown to increase survival in patients with cardiovascular disease.

Hyperparathyroidism: Low plasma vitamin D3 has been found to be a major risk factor for hyperparathyroidism, which can result in calcium loss from bone and renal damage with frequent kidney-stone formation.

High Blood Pressure: Clinical and experimental data support the view that vitamin-D metabolism is involved in blood-pressure regulation and other metabolic processes.

Melanoma: An inability to tan is the number one risk factor for melanoma. Those who tan easily or who have darker skin are far less likely to develop the disease. A new theory is that melanoma is actually caused by sunlight (vitamin-D) deficiency and that safe sun exposure actually helps prevent the deadly disease.

Multiple Sclerosis: Vitamin-D supplementation may help prevent the development of MS as well as provide for additional treatment.

Osteoarthritis: Low intake and low serum levels of vitamin D appear to be associated with an increased risk for progression of osteoarthritis.

Osteoporosis: Maintenance of serum calcium levels within a narrow range is vital for normal functioning of the nervous system, for bone growth, and for the maintenance of bone density. Vitamin D is essential for the efficient utilization of calcium by the body. Vitamin-D deficiency is extremely prevalent in the elderly. Most often the first symptoms are muscle pain, fatigue, muscular weakness, and gait disturbances. More severe deficiency causes osteomalacia (bone weakening and loss) with deep bone pain, reduced mineralization of bone matrix, and bone fractures. A recent study found that supplementation of elderly women with 800 IU per day of vitamin D and 1,200 mg. per day of calcium for three months increased muscle strength and decreased the risk of falling by almost 50% compared to supplementation with calcium alone.

surrounding nerves and genetic material. A deficiency in vitamin E can lead to heart disease, muscular dystrophy, nervous system disorders, anemia, liver damage, and birth defects. Smokers need to take extra vitamin E, since research at the University of California shows that vitamin E and vitamin C levels are reduced by exposure to cigarette smoke. Studies done in Israel show vitamin E to reduce the symptoms of osteoarthritis. Its other benefits include:

- **increasing and maintaining proper brain function,**
- **effectively reducing tension in the lower extremities, which is associated with intermittent claudication and heart disease,**
- **relieving restless leg syndrome or "the fidgets,"**
- preventing abnormal blood clotting,
- increasing the efficiency of muscles—including the heart—by reducing oxygen requirements,
- helping to slow the aging process,
- and helping protect the body from the toxic effects of lead and mercury.

One study conducted at Columbia University revealed the ability of vitamin E to slow the effects of Alzheimer's. Researchers at Tufts University found that on a diet supplemented with 200 IUs of vitamin E, control groups had a 65% increase in immune-fighting abilities. In another study at Harvard School of Public Health, people who supplemented their diets with 100 IUs of vitamin E reduced their risk of heart disease by 40 percent (100 IUs is seven times the RDA). Researchers at Duke University have demonstrated that vitamin E acts as a potent antioxidant to counter the toxic effects of air pollution. (The amount needed to combat air pollution, including ozone and nitrous oxide, is six times the RDA.)

Selenium enhances the effects of vitamin E, and a zinc deficiency increases the need for it. Vitamin E is relatively nontoxic, but taken in very high doses, it can cause interference with vitamin K and lead to prolonged bleeding. Vitamin E is safe, however, taken in dosages several times higher than the RDA.

Folic Acid is "brain food." It is involved in energy production, synthesis of DNA, formation of red blood cells, metabolism of all amino acids, and production of the neurotransmitters, including serotonin. Folic acid needs B12, B3, and C in order to be converted into its active form. Low folic-acid levels are associated with an increase in homocysteine, an amino acid linked to cardiovascular disease (vitamin B6, folic acid, and vitamin B12 all help reduce homocysteine levels). A deficiency in folic acid (one the most common vitamin deficiencies), will produce macrocytic anemia, digestive disorders, heart palpitations, weight loss, poor appetite, headache, irritability, depression, insomnia, and mood swings. A sore, red tongue may also indicate a folic-acid deficiency. When taken by pregnant women, folic acid can improve an infant's birth weight, neurological development, and chances of escaping a neural tube defect. Women trying to get pregnant and expectant mothers should take a multivitamin with at least 400 mcg of folic acid. Large doses of folic acid can mask a vitamin B12 deficiency.

Inositol is important in the metabolism of fats and cholesterol, and in the proper function of the kidneys and liver. It is vital for hair growth and prevents hardening of the arteries. Inositol is needed for the synthesis of lecithin, which helps remove fats from the liver. Along with gamma-aminobutyric acid (GABA), inositol may help reduce anxiety. Caffeine may decrease inositol stores. There is no known deficiency or toxicity for inositol.

Para-aminobenzoic acid (PABA) is needed to form red and white blood cells, which in turn, form essential B vitamins. PABA is used in suntan lotion to help block harmful UV rays and prevent sunburn. It has antiviral properties and has been reported to help in treating Rocky Mountain spotted fever. PABA may help restore gray hair to its natural color. PABA and sulfa drugs cancel each other out. Doses over 1,000 mg. can cause nausea and vomiting.

RESOURCES
All the vitamins discussed in this chapter are contained in my Essential Therapeutics CFS/Fibro formula. See p. 461 to order.

FOR FURTHER READING AND RESEARCH
• The Vitamin D Council, www.vitamindcouncil.com.

· 27 ·
ROCK SOLID MINERALS

Boron is needed in trace amounts for the proper absorption of calcium. A recent study by the US Department of Agriculture showed that **women who consumed 3 mg. of boron a day lost 40% less calcium and one-third less magnesium in their urine.** **Toxicity:** Excessive amounts of boron can cause nausea, diarrhea, skin rashes, and fatigue.

Calcium is the most abundant mineral in the body. It comprises two–three pounds of total body weight and is essential for the formation of bones and teeth. Calcium regulates heart rhythm, cellular metabolism, muscle coordination, blood clotting, and nerve transmission. Adequate intake of calcium can help lower high blood pressure and the incidence of heart disease. **Calcium also contributes to the release of neurotransmitters and can have a calming effect on the nervous system.** A deficiency of calcium can result in hypertension, insomnia, osteoporosis, tetany (muscle spasm), and periodontal disease.

The ratio of calcium-to-magnesium and calcium-to-phosphorous is important. Recommended ratios are 2 to 1 (or 1.5 to 1) for calcium to magnesium and 2 to 1 (or 3 to 1) for calcium to phosphorous. Calcium absorption needs vitamin D and is decreased by high-protein, -fat, and -phosphorous (junk food) diets. Chelated calcium (which is bound to a protein for easier absorption) combined with magnesium can help reduce aluminum and lead poisoning. **Toxicity:** Excessive calcium intake (several grams a day) can cause calcium deposits in the soft tissue, including the blood vessels (causing arteriosclerosis) and kidneys (causing stones). Oyster shell or bone-meal calcium supplements often contain high levels of toxic lead. Use calcium citrate or calcium ascorbate instead.

Chromium is essential in the synthesis of cholesterol, fats, and protein. It also helps stabilize blood sugar and insulin levels, helping ensure proper protein production and reducing the chance for fat storage. A deficiency in chromium can cause type-2 diabetes, hypoglycemia, and coronary artery disease. **Ninety percent of the U.S. population is deficient in chromium!** Diets high in simple sugars increase the loss of chromium, and a deficiency can cause a craving for sugar. A normal dose of chromium is 200 mcg. taken 30 minutes before or after meals, two-three times daily. Chromium is not toxic in high amounts.

Type-1 and type-2 diabetics on the Essential Therapeutics CFS/ Fibro Formula (or any formula containing zinc) should consider taking chromium separately from their formula (at least a few hours apart) to maximize its efficiency in helping to balance blood-sugar levels.

Copper maintains the myelin sheath, which wraps around nerves and **facilitates nerve communication**. It plays a vital role in **regulating neurotransmitters** and helps maintain the cardiovascular and skeletal systems as well. It is part of the antioxidant enzyme supraoxide dismutase and may help protect cells from free-radical damage. Copper helps with the absorption of iron, and a deficiency in copper can lead to anemia, gray hair, heart disease, poor concentration, numbness and tingling in the extremities, decreased immunity, and possibly scoliosis.

Cadmium, molybdenum, and sulfate can interfere with copper absorption. A niacin deficiency can cause an elevation of copper. Zinc and copper impair the absorption of one another, so they should be taken separately. **Toxicity:** Intake of 20 mg. or more in a day can cause nausea and vomiting. Wilson's disease (not Wilson's syndrome) is a genetic disorder characterized by excessive accumulation of copper in the tissues, as well as liver disease, mental retardation, tremors, and loss of coordination.

Iron is important in the formation of hemoglobin, the use of oxygen, energy production, muscle function, thyroid function, and components of the immune system, protein synthesis, normal growth, and mental acuity. Excessive amounts of vitamin E and zinc interfere with iron absorption. Vitamin C helps with the absorption of iron, and B6 is needed to develop the iron-containing protein hemoglobin.

Iron should not be routinely supplemented; a blood test should first confirm an iron deficiency. The exception would be females who rigorously exercise. Studies show that only 8% of the U.S. population is deficient in iron. **However, 20% of premenopausal women and as much as 80% of women who exercise are deficient in iron. People suffering from** *Candida* **overgrowth or chronic herpes infection usually have a deficiency in iron.** If you suspect you have an iron deficiency, ask your health professional for a blood test.

Excessive amounts of iron are associated with an increased risk of heart disease and can lead to decreased immunity and to liver, kidney, and lung disorders. For this reason, iron is not included in my Essential Therapeutics CFS/Fibro Formula.

Magnesium is one of the most important minerals in the body. It is responsible for proper enzyme activity and transmission of muscle and nerve impulses, and it aids in maintaining a proper pH balance. It helps metabolize carbohydrates, proteins, and fats into energy. Magnesium also helps synthesize the genetic material in cells and helps to remove toxic substances, such as aluminum and ammonia, from the body. Magnesium and calcium help keep the heart beating; magnesium relaxes the heart, and calcium activates it. A deficiency of magnesium, then, may increase the risk of heart disease.

Magnesium also plays a significant role in **regulating the neurotransmitters. A deficiency can cause muscle pain, joint pain, headache, fatigue, depression, leg cramps,** high blood pressure, heart disease and arrhythmia, constipation, irritable bowel syndrome, **insomnia,** hair loss, **confusion,** personality disorders, swol-len gums, and loss of appetite. High intake of calcium may reduce magnesium absorption. **Simple sugars and/or stress can deplete magnesium.**

Magnesium is a natural sedative and can be used to treat muscle spasm, anxiety, depression, insomnia, and constipation. It is also a potent antidepressant. It helps with intermittent claudication, a condition caused by a restriction of blood flow to the legs. It's effective in relieving some of the symptoms associated with PMS, and women suffering from PMS are usually deficient in it.

New studies are validating what many nutrition-oriented physicians have known for years: a magnesium deficiency can trigger migraine headaches. Magnesium also helps relax constricted bronchial tubes associated with asthma. In fact, a combination of vitamin B6 and magnesium, along with avoidance of wheat and dairy products, has cured many of my young asthmatic patients.

Unfortunately, dietary magnesium intake in this country is steadily declining. It has been consistently depleted in our soils and further depleted in plants by the use of potassium- and phosphorus-containing fertilizers, which reduce a plant's ability to uptake magnesium. Food processing also removes magnesium, while high-carbohydrate and high-fat diets increase the body's need for it. Diuretic medications further deplete total body magnesium.

It is estimated that up to 80% of those with FMS/CFS are deficient in magnesium. Normal dosage is 500–800 mg. daily. **Toxicity:** Too much magnesium can cause loose bowel movements. If this occurs, reduce your dose.

Manganese aids in the development of mother's milk and is important for normal bone and tissue growth. It is involved in the production of cellular energy, metabolizes fats and proteins, and is essential in maintaining a healthy nervous system. Manganese is needed to synthesize thiamin, and **it works in coordination with the other B vitamins to reduce the effects of stress.** Many of my FMS/CFS patients are deficient in manganese.

A deficiency of manganese can cause fatigue, impaired fertility, retarded growth, birth defects, seizures, and bone malformations. Recommended dosage is 5–15 mg. daily. **Toxicity:** Manganese is not toxic in large doses, but since calcium, copper, iron, manganese, and zinc all compete for absorption in the small intestine, large doses of one nutrient may reduce the absorption of the others.

Molybdenum aids in the conversion of purines to uric acid and allows the body to use nitrogen. It is important in sulfite detoxification and promotes normal cell function. It also works with vitamin B2 in the conversion of food to energy.

Molybdenum can help reduce symptoms associated with **sulfite sensitivities.** I had a patient who broke out in a rash every time she ate foods containing the preservative sulfite, and sure enough, her tests revealed a molybdenum deficiency. Once her molybdenum levels were normalized, she was once again able to tolerate sulfites.

Recommended dosage is 50–150 mcg. daily. Molybdenum deficiency can cause stunted growth, loss of appetite, and impotence in older males. Excessive copper may interfere with molybdenum absorption. **Toxicity:** High dosages can cause symptoms similar to gout: joint pain and swelling.

Potassium helps regulate the nervous system. A deficiency of potassium manifests itself as irregular heart rate, sterility, muscle weakness, apathy, paralysis, and confusion. Potassium and magnesium are synergetic in lowering blood pressure and therefore should be taken together. (They are combined in good balance in my Essential Therapeutics CFS/Fibro Formula.)

Selenium is an important antioxidant that protects the body from free-radical damage. It is a component of glutathione peroxidase, an enzyme essential for detoxification of cellular debris. Selenium, along with other antioxidants, combats free radicals that can cause heart disease. It may also help prevent certain forms of cancer and help those suffering from autoimmune disorders such as rheumatoid arthritis. **Selenium is an important component of the immune system** and helps make thyroid hormones and essential fatty acids.

A deficiency can cause birth defects, certain cancers, and fibrocystic, heart, and liver disease. Recommended dosage is up to 200 mcg. daily. **Toxicity:** Doses above 600 mg. can cause side effects that include tooth decay and periodontal disease.

Zinc is important in over 90 enzymatic pathways. It facilitates alcohol detoxification within the liver and plays a role in producing and digesting proteins. Zinc is also important in maintaining normal blood levels of vitamin A, **boosting the immune system,** healing wounds, converting calories to energy, reducing low birth rates and infant mortality, controlling blood cholesterol levels, and producing the prostaglandin hormones that regulate **heart rate, blood pressure, inflammation,** and other processes. A deficiency of zinc can lead to bad taste in the mouth, anorexia nervosa, anemia, slow growth, birth defects, impaired nerve function, sterility, glucose intolerance, mental disorders, dermatitis, hair loss, and atherosclerosis.

Excess copper can cause a zinc deficiency, and vice versa. Pregnant women often accumulate excess copper and become zinc-deficient, which can lead to postpartum depression. Extra zinc, 50 mg. per day, should be consumed by pregnant females to help avoid postpartum depression. (I don't recommend prescription prenatal vitamins, because they are too low in the needed micronutrients, especially zinc and the B vitamins. Instead, I encourage my pregnant patients to take a high potency vitamin with a maximum of 10,000 IUs of vitamin A. Doses of vitamin A above 10,000 IUs should be avoided.)

It is estimated that 68% of the population is deficient in zinc. And a zinc deficiency can cause depression, since it's necessary for the production of dopamine. White specks on the fingernails are indicative of a zinc deficiency. Recommended dosage is up to 50 mg. daily.

Zinc lozenges have been shown to reduce the symptoms and duration of colds by 50 percent. If taking zinc for a cold, take it at least a few hours apart from your CFS/Fibro Formula, or any other formula containing chromium.

IV VITAMINS AND MINERALS

Individuals with chronic illnesses like FMS and CFS usually have problems with digestion: bloating, gas, indigestion, irritable bowel syndrome, malabsorption, leaky gut syndrome, and/or yeast overgrowth. Because of this, they sometimes don't digest and absorb the essential nutrients in their foods or supplements. Prescription medications often further deplete these nutrients. And without these essential nutrients, chronically ill patients stay chronically ill!

Using IVs to transport the vitamins and minerals bypasses the over-taxed digestive system and puts the nutrients where they should end up anyway: in the bloodstream.

Clinical experience has proven IV therapy to be quite effective in treating FMS and CFS patients. But if you can't tolerate or afford it, however, don't worry. You can attain improvements in absorption by following the correctional therapies in chapter 12. And at the same time, you'll be healing your gut, not just bypassing it.

RESOURCES
• All the minerals discussed in this chapter, unless otherwise indicated, are contained in my Essential Therapeutics CFS/Fibro formula. See p. 461 to order.

· 28 ·
AMINO ACIDS:
LIFE'S BUILDING BLOCKS

Amino acids are the building blocks of life. They help regulate our thinking, energy, moods, pain, mental functions, digestion, immunity, and more. Deficiencies can cause major problems.

There are 20 amino acids. Nine are known as essential amino acids. They can't be made by the body and must be obtained from our diet. Nonessential amino acids can be manufactured from within our own cells.

Individual amino acids are joined together in sequential chains to form proteins. Protein, the body's building material, is essential to every cell and makes up our muscles, hair, bones, collagen, and connective tissue.

Essential and nonessential amino acids are involved in every bodily function. They are the raw materials for the reproduction and growth of every cell. Amino acids are in every bone, organ (including the brain), muscle, and most every hormone. Amino acids are also needed to make enzymes.

Enzymes are protein molecules that coordinate thousands of chemical reactions that take place in the body. Enzymes are essential for breaking down and digesting carbohydrates, proteins, and fats.

Amino acids can occur in two forms: D-form and L-form, which are mirror images of one another. The L-form

Essential Amino Acids	Nonessential Amino Acids
• isoleucine	• glycine
• leucine	• glutamic acid
• lysine	• arginine
• methionine	• aspartic acid
• phenylalanine	• alanine
• threonine	• proline
• tryptophan	• serine
• valine	• tyrosine
• histadine	• cysteine
	• glutamine
	• asparagine

is available in the foods we eat and is the more easily absorbed. In a natural state, all amino acids are L-form. D-forms can be formed by bacteria, by tissue catabolism, or synthetically. (Most D-forms can be detrimental to normal enzyme functions; however, DL-phenylalanine is the exception. It inhibits the breakdown of endorphin- and enkaphalin-limiting enzymes.) The white, crystalline free-form amino acids derived from brown rice protein are the purest supplements available. Always supplement with free-form (L-form) amino acids.

Results of Amino-Acid Deficiencies

- fatigue
- poor immunity
- anxiety
- mental confusion
- dermatitis
- chemical sensitivities
- insomnia
- cardiovascular disease
- osteoporosis
- high blood pressure
- arthritis
- inflammatory disorders
- depression
- poor detoxification

Amino acids can be taken as a blend to shore up any underlying nutritional deficiencies. Taken individually, they act like drugs to produce specific reactions. It's best to take single amino acids on an empty stomach: 30 minutes before or one hour after eating. Individuals with malabsorption syndrome, irritable bowel, leaky gut, and chronic illnesses are wise to take an amino acid blend in addition to any single amino acids. The Essential Therapeutics CFS/Fibromyalgia formula contains all of the essential amino acids. Here are some of the amino acids and how they are used in nutritional medicine:

Carnitine increases energy. Produced by combining methionine and lysine, it helps transport fats into the cells for the mitochondria to use as energy. And since the mitochondria burn fatty acids during physical activity, carnitine is a valuable tool for reducing weight and the risk of fat buildup in heart muscle. Its efficient use of fats helps the body lower cholesterol, triglycerides, and possibly the risk of heart attack. The consumption of alcohol can cause a buildup of fat in the liver, but carnitine inhibits this buildup. **It also helps boost cellular energy and is helpful in reducing fatigue associated with CFS.**

Cysteine helps detoxify the body. It is formed from the amino acid methionine and plays an important role in detoxifying the body. Cysteine is the precursor to the most abundant and important amino acid in the body, glutathione. Glutathione is a combination of glutamine, cysteine, and glycine.

Cysteine destroys free radicals, removes heavy metals from the body, and guards cells—including heart and liver cells—from toxic chemicals like alcohol, xenobiotics, and other damaging substances. Glutathione and cysteine are effective in reducing or eliminating skin conditions such as psoriasis, acne, liver spots, and eczema. **Those with respiratory problems, asthma, bronchitis, and allergies may benefit from taking a specialized form of cysteine known as N-acetylcysteine.**

I prescribe cysteine and methionine, usually in a combination formula, to my patients with aluminum toxicity and poor liver function. By itself, cysteine should be taken on an empty stomach at 500–1000 mg. daily.

Gamma-aminobutyric acid (GABA) treats anxiety. It can be formed from the amino acid glutamine and has a calming effect on the brain similar to Valium and other tranquilizers, but without the side effects. Used in combination with the B vitamins niacinamide (a form of vitamin B3) and inositol, **GABA can alleviate anxiety and panic attacks.** Many of my patients are surprised by the effectiveness of GABA in treating their anxiety and panic attacks.

To treat anxiety, start with 500 mg. two–three times daily (or as needed) on an empty stomach. Some individuals may need up to 1,000 mg. two–three times daily.

Glutamine helps heal intestinal permeability. It is converted to glutamic acid in the brain. Glutamic acid increases neuronal activity, detoxifies ammonia (an abundant waste product in the body) from cells, and like glucose, is used to feed the brain. Glutamine plays an important role in intestinal maintenance and repair and is the major energy source of the intestines. It is one of the most important nutrients for the cells that line the colon.

Individuals with intestinal problems, including Crohn's disease, colitis, irritable bowel syndrome, intestinal permeability, yeast overgrowth, and food allergies, especially need glutamine supplementation. Studies in Britain and Canada show that when individuals with inflammatory bowel disease (IBD) were given glutamine, their symptoms, including abdominal pain and diarrhea, improved dramatically. In another study, children who took glutamine supplements showed increased mental abilities and tested higher on IQ tests. It also helps reduce sugar cravings and acts as an appetite suppressant.

Glutamine is one of the three amino acids that form glutathione. Glutathione is a powerful antioxidant and plays an important role in the detoxification system of the body. It helps clear unwanted toxins through the kidneys and liver. It is also the precursor to two very important neurotransmitters: glutamic acid (glutamate) and GABA (gamma-aminobutyric acid). Glutamate is excitatory; GABA is relaxing.

Usual glutamine dose is 500–1,000 mg. twice daily on an empty stomach. Higher doses are necessary to repair leaky gut syndrome.

Glycine helps detoxify the body. It is another inhibitory amino acid. **It can be used to reduce the symptoms of bipolar depression, epilepsy, and nervous tics.** It is also important in neutralizing toxic chemicals (especially alcohol). It helps synthesize glutathione and has been used in the treatment of depression and in the inhibition of epilepsy. It is usually taken in a combination formula.

Histidine improves digestion. A histidine imbalance can cause anxiety, schizophrenia, nausea (particularly in pregnant women), lethargy, fatigue, and anger. Histidine improves digestion by increasing the production of stomach acid.

Histidine is the precursor of histamine, which is known to play a role in allergic reactions. But histamine also acts as an inhibitory neurotransmitter by increasing alpha-wave activity within the brain. Alpha waves are associated with relaxation and when activated, help increase a person's resistance to stress and tension. Histidine is usually taken in a combination formula.

Lysine treats viral outbreaks. As the essential component of all proteins, it plays a major role in soft-tissue formation and repair. A lysine deficiency can cause a person to bruise easily and have a difficult time healing wounds. It is used for treating **cold sores** and is one of the most important and cost-efficient supplements I prescribe in treating **herpes.**

Lysine is also one of the most effective therapies for shingles. Cortisone reduces the itching but does nothing to rid the body of the skin lesions. In addition, steroids (such as cortisone) weaken the immune system and can cause further outbreaks. To treat shingles, use the natural antibiotic, antiviral herb echinacea along with 1,000 mg. of lysine and 25,000 IU of vitamin A, daily for two weeks or until the lesions disappear.

Methionine helps detoxify the body. An essential amino acid, methionine allows the body to digest fats, combat toxins, produce choline, and deal with allergic reactions. It's the precursor of cysteine, glutathione, and taurine and contributes to the production and regulation of insulin. Methionine is an excellent chelator, meaning it attaches itself to heavy metals (such as aluminum and lead) and escorts them out of the body.

I prescribe methionine to my patients with faulty detoxification systems. **People with chronic fatigue, fibromyalgia, liver problems, and heavy metal or xenobiotic overload need extra methionine.** The recommended dose is 500–1,000 mg. daily on an empty stomach. It may also be taken in a combination formula.

Methionine is the main component of s-adenosyl-methionine (SAMe), which is **involved in synthesizing neurotransmitters, so its deficiency can contribute to depression.** (For more information on SAMe and depression, see chapter 16.)

Studies involving FMS patients and SAMe have shown dramatic improvements in pain reduction. One study showed that patients taking SAMe for a period of six weeks had an improvement of 40% in pain reduction and 35% in depression. Recommended dose for SAMe is 400–800 mg. daily.

DL-phenylalanine assists pain control. This is a combination of the D- and L-form of phenylalanine, which acts as a natural pain reliever. It blocks the enzymes responsible for the breakdown of endorphins and enkaphalins, which are substances within the body that help relieve pain. Endorphins are similar in chemical structure and far more powerful than the drug known as morphine. They are produced in small cells located throughout the nervous system.

DL-phenylalanine acts as an appetite suppressant and mild stimulant. It has also shown to be effective in helping patients afflicted with Parkinson's disease.

DL-phenylalanine is an effective supplement in treating musculoskeletal pains, including those associated with FMS. Many of my fibromyalgia and chronic pain patients have benefited from taking DL-phenylalanine. **A clinical study shows subjects taking DL-phenylalanine saw a remarkable improvement in their condition:** improvements were seen in 73% of lower-back pain sufferers, 67% of those with migraines, 81% with osteoarthritis, and 81% with rheumatoid arthritis.

For pain control or as an antidepressant, take 1,000–4,000 mg. twice daily on an empty stomach. Phenylalanine can elevate blood pressure, and very high doses cause rapid heartbeat. Start with a low dose and increase to higher doses only as needed and only if no side effects are noticed.

L-phenylalanine fights depression. It is an important amino acid that is involved in the production of the neurotransmitter catecholamines. Catecholamines stimulate mental arousal, positive mood, and the fight-or-flight response to stress. **It creates several neurotransmitters:** adrenaline, epinephrine, norepinephrine, and dopamine. These help to elevate mood and reduce depression, pain, fatigue, and lethargy. Phenylalanine also curbs the appetite by stimulating a hormone known as cholecystokinin (CCK), which tells the brain when you've eaten enough.

Phenylalanine is converted to the nonessential amino acid tyrosine. Individuals with a rare but life-threatening illness known as phenylketonuria (PKU) can't make this conversion. The thyroid hormone thyroxin is made from tyrosine (see below). So supplementing with phenylalanine and tyrosine helps increase the thyroid gland and rate of metabolism. This in turn helps mobilize and burn fat.

As an antidepressant, use 1,000–4,000 mg. twice daily on an empty stomach. Phenylalanine can elevate blood pressure, and very high doses cause rapid heart beat. Start with a low dose and increase to higher doses only as needed and only if no side effects are noticed.

Tyrosine boosts thyroid function, so it can be a lifesaver for those suffering from depression that has been resistant to all other medications. **It elevates mood, drive, and ambition by stimulating the neurotransmitters** norepinephrine, epinephrine, and dopamine. Tyrosine also helps those suffering from fatigue and asthma.

Tyrosine, which can be produced from phenylalanine, aids in the production of the adrenal, thyroid, and pituitary hormones. Many of my patients with low thyroid function have benefited from taking a special supplement that contains L-tyrosine. Low energy, brittle nails, and cold hands and feet can mean a person is suffering from adrenal hormone insufficiency. These people may benefit from taking tyrosine along with an adrenal extract supplement.

Tyrosine can also raise blood pressure, so use with caution. To treat low thyroid, supplement with 1,000 mg. twice daily on an empty stomach. For depression and fatigue, use phenylalanine (see above).

Tryptophan...well, you already know what it does so well! If you've forgotten, then reread chapter 10.

RESOURCES
- All the amino acids discussed in this chapter are either contained in my Essential Therapeutics CFS/Fibro Formula or your body can make them from the ingredients in the Formula. See page 461 to order.
- SAMe is also available from my office, or it can be found in many health food stores. Make sure that any SAMe you use is enteric-coated for maximum potency.

· 29 ·
THE REAL SKINNY ON FATS AND FATTY ACIDS

Fat provides energy, produces certain hormones, insulates us from cold, and makes up cellular membranes. It is the primary source of fuel for the muscles, including the heart.

Fats have gotten a bad rap in our society. Low-fat diets have been the rage for years, promising weight loss and improved health. But this line of thinking has contributed to yo-yo dieting, heart disease, and type-2 diabetes. In fact, researchers at the National Institute of Health have recently shown that while our consumption of fat and cholesterol have drastically declined over the last several years, we've actually gained an average of ten pounds per person. Statistics show that during the years between 1960 and 1980, one-quarter of the population was overweight. But that number has grown to 60% of the population. Researchers and health officials are still scratching their heads over these statistics. It is now estimated that by the year 2010, over 80% of the U.S. population will be overweight. The "fat-free" mantra has proven to be the most misguided medical blunder since bloodletting.

The fear of fat and its derivative, cholesterol, has spawned a multibillion-dollar industry of low-fat foods, but it's not turning the tide. We trust medical intervention, but drugs that lower fats and cholesterol have been shown to increase the risk of certain cancers. Dieters dutifully avoid fat, but hidden sugars in our processed foods are being turned into fat right under our noses (and our belts!).

The truth is that fat is in all natural foods. It is an essential nutrient that plays a vital role in our overall health. We can't live without fat in our diet. Fat provides over twice the amount of energy of carbohydrates and 70% of the energy needed just to keep the body warm.

Fats make up 70% of the brain. The fat insulates the brain cells and allows the neurotransmitters to communicate with one another.

Cholesterol and fats make up each and every cell. Cholesterol helps keep cell membranes permeable, and this permeability allows good nutrients in and toxic waste products out. Over 8% of the brain's solid matter is made up of cholesterol, and cholesterol is essential for proper brain function and normalized neurotransmitters such as serotonin. A deficiency in cholesterol can result in mood disorders including depression, anxiety, irritability, and fibro-fog. Cholesterol is also involved in the production of such essential hormones as DHEA, testosterone, estradiol, progesterone, and cortisol. Because it is essential to our very survival, cholesterol is manufactured by the body on a daily basis. Eliminating cholesterol from our diet only triggers the body to make more!

WHAT ABOUT CHOLESTEROL AND HEART DISEASE?

Believe it or not, your body needs cholesterol. It's not some foreign element to be avoided. It's a valuable nutrient. Consider these facts about cholesterol, taken from my book *Heart Disease: What Your Doctor Won't Tell You.*

• Cholesterol is so important that the body manufactures 800–1500 mg. each day. This is about twice as much as you take in through diet!

• Cholesterol and other fats are the very building blocks that make up each and every cell.

• Cholesterol is an important fat that helps keep cell membranes permeable, allowing good nutrients to get in and toxic waste products to get out.

• Cholesterol makes the bile salts required for the digestion of fat.

• Cholesterol is the precursor to vitamin D.

• Cholesterol is essential in proper hormone production. Testosterone, dehydroepiandrosterone (DHEA), progesterone, estradiol, and cortisol are all made from cholesterol.

• Fats make up 70% of the brain, and over 8% of the brain's solid matter is made up of cholesterol. The fat and cholesterol insulates brain cells and allows for proper functioning of neurotransmitters.

- Cholesterol levels have been repeatedly linked to decreased brain function, including **depression.** Those with low cholesterol are three times more likely to suffer from depression as normal adults. The *British Medical Journal* has published research showing that the lower the cholesterol, the more severe the depression.

- Low cholesterol levels are also linked to an increased risk of **suicide.** One study, reported in the *British Medical Journal,* showed that of the 300 people studied who had committed suicide, all had low cholesterol levels. Another study reveals that men whose cholesterol levels are lowered through the use of prescription lipid-lowering medications double their chances of suicide.

- Low cholesterol (below 180) has been linked to an increased risk for **heart attack.** Yes, you read this correctly. Low cholesterol increases the risk of a heart attack.

> I hope I've made my point; *please* don't rush to take cholesterol-lowering drugs, which can cause some of the very symptoms associated with fibromyalgia and CFS—including muscle aches and pain, mental confusion, fatigue, poor memory, and depression.
>
> And *please* eat fat, including saturated fats.

WHAT ABOUT DIETARY FAT AND HEART DISEASE?

By 1998, there were a total of 30 different studies—involving more than 150,000 people—investigating the relationship of dietary fat to the risk of heart disease. These studies revealed that there was no difference in the risk of heart disease in those who ate animal fats and those who did not.

What's more, research shows that there is no evidence that saturated fats are bad for health and plenty of evidence that saturated fats prevent both cardiovascular disease and stroke. In fact, the fatty acids found in clogged arteries are mostly unsaturated (74%), of which 41% are polyunsaturated.

THE SKINNY ON FATS

Fats are a type of lipid (meaning they can't be dissolved in water) that are made up of fatty acids: saturated, unsaturated, and polyunsaturated.

- **Saturated fatty acids (SFAs)** are found in butter, shortening, coconut oil, eggs, meat, and cheese. They consist of long, straight chains of molecules packed tightly together, and they are solid at room temperature. A diet too high in SFAs may contribute to atherosclerosis, heart disease, and stroke. However, even saturated fats are part of a balanced diet.

- **Monounsaturated fatty acids (MUFAs)** are found in almond oil, avocados, canola oil, oats, peanut oil, and olive oil. Monounsaturated oils are usually liquid at room temperature but may become cloudy or hardened in the refrigerator. MUFAs have one kink or bend in their structure, so they are more flexible than SFAs.

- **Polyunsaturated fatty acids (PUFAs)** are found in corn oil, primrose oil, flaxseed oil, borage oil, certain fish, and sesame, sunflower, safflower, and wheat germ oil. PUFAs are liquid at room temperature. They have many bends in their chains and are quite flexible. Although a person needs all types of fat, PUFAs are generally considered the healthiest.

PUFAs are further divided into two families of essential fatty acids (EFAs): omega-6 and omega-3.

The omega-6 family can be found in pure vegetable oils, including sunflower, safflower, and corn oil. It includes:

- linoleic acid (LA)
- gamma-linolenic acid (GLA)
- dihomo-gamma-linolenic acid (DGLA)
- arachidonic acid (AA)

The omega-3 family can be found in some nuts, meats, and especially in deep cold-water fish. It's also in flax seed, soy- bean, walnut, and chestnut oils, as well as some dark-green leafy vegetables. It includes:

- alpha-linolenic acid (LNA)
- stearidonic acid (SDA)
- eicosatetraenoic acid (ETA)
- eicosapentaenoic acid (EPA)
- docosahexaenoic acid (DHA)

Essential fatty acids are, as their name implies, essential for our existence, but our body can't make them. We have to take them in by food. We can't live without them, because they make up the outer membranes of each cell. The membranes of healthy cells can resist entry by viruses and other pathogenic agents and, at the same time, facilitate the entry of nutrients.

But when EFAs are deficient, cell membranes are weakened in their abilities, and the wrong substances are allowed into the cell. A deficiency in EFAs can cause some of the very symptoms associated with FMS and CFS: fatigue, depression, malabsorption, muscle pain, insomnia, poor mental function, and lowered immunity. It's estimated that at least 25% of the population suffers from some amount of EFA deficiency. Sixty percent of the population is deficient in omega-3. But we're not all terrible eaters, right? Why are we so deficient in EFAs? Well, certain groups of people have inherited a need for more EFAs and especially GLA (gamma-linolenic acid): those of Irish, Scottish, Welch, Scandinavian, Danish, British Columbian, and Eskimo decent.

WHY ARE WE EFA DEFICIENT?

Even for those without special EFA needs, obtaining enough EFA can be challenging. Here's why:

Dramatic changes in our agricultural, food processing, and food preparation methods in the past several decades have helped deplete the soil and our foods of valuable nutrients. For instance, changes in flour milling technology have resulted in the elimination of essential fatty acids from most machine-processed grains. Even our meat is less nutritious. One hundred years ago, our ancestors ate real butter, unprocessed grains, flax seed oil (a rich source of EFAs), and free-range cattle and chickens. Today's farmer, in most cases, keeps cattle and chickens caged and feeds them processed grains devoid of EFAs. Consequently, the meat is significantly less nutritious to humans. Free-range cattle, chicken, and dairy products can have over five times the omega-3 and omega-6 fats in their tissues as industrially raised animals.

Man-made trans fats have replaced healthy EFAs in many of our processed foods, so these foods are not only devoid of life-giving, health-building EFAs, but they also prevent what EFAs are present from being absorbed and effectively utilized.

How are these trans fats toxic? There are receptor sites on cell membranes where neurotransmitters—such as serotonin—attach themselves. Trans fats block and harden these sites, preventing nutrients from entering and exiting the cell. The neurotransmitters are then unable to attach themselves to the cell membrane, and the results can include depression, insomnia, anxiety, fatigue, ADD, or any disorder that involves the brain hormones.

Alcohol and caffeine can also block the conversion of EFAs to anti-inflammatory prostaglandin hormones (see below for more about prostaglandins).

Increased ingestion of toxins in our food, water, and air depletes our EFAs.

Lack of breastfeeding can create EFA deficiencies, as omega-3 fats and DHA (docosahexanoic acid) are not present in many infant formulas or in commercial cow's milk.

Excessive consumption of omega-6 fats (too many grains) may interfere with the absorption of omega-3 fats.

RESULTS OF EFA DEFICIENCIES

EFA deficiency can contribute to a number of health problems. Without enough EFAs, the body can't produce prostaglandins— short-lived, hormone-like chemicals that regulate cellular activity from moment to moment. They stimulate and relax uterine muscles, reduce swollen nasal passageways, help regulate the "happy hormones" like serotonin, and are intimately involved in the immune system. They play a role in healthy blood pressure, air passageways, blood vessels, and fat metabolism. They help stimulate steroid production and reduce appetite, and since they can cause or reduce inflammation, they are involved in regulating allergic reactions.

Insufficient EFAs can keep your body from properly reducing inflammation. Many FMS patients have been on NSAIDs for years by the time I see them in my clinic. **But while these medications block the prostaglandins that cause inflammation, they also block those that stop inflammation.** A safer way to reduce chronic inflammation is to increase consumption of EFA, especially omega-3. This is because **the fats you eat largely determine your body's ability to fight inflammation.**

Conversely, too much of the EFA (omega-6) called arachidonic acid (AA) can put you in a *pro*imflammatory state. AA is found in corn and corn-oil products. And these products are used as the prominent foodstuff in westernized livestock. Consequently, U.S. land-animal food products (meat, eggs, and cheese, for instance) have a high AA content. Several research articles have demonstrated that the more animal fats a human eats, the more AA they have in their blood and cell membranes *and* the more likely they are to have inflammation.

Omega-6 fatty acids, while essential for optimal health, do generate AA. AA comes from excessive consumption of vegetable oils and grains (which is the typical diet of livestock). Therefore when battling inflammation, its best to avoid overconsumption of wheat-based products including breads, pasta, crackers, etc. and corn-based products. As for meat, grass-fed livestock is your best option. Many of my fibromyalgia patients find that they feel considerably better when they avoid wheat and dairy products.

A diet high in fish oils promotes the opposite: *less* inflammation and a *lower* level of inflammatory chemicals. Fish oils (omega-3 fatty acids) increase our natural anti-inflammatory prostaglandin hormones.

The balance of fats in our bodies is significant, too. Consider the importance of the ratio between AA and eicosapentaenoic acid

(EPA). An AA/EPA ratio of 1.5 to 1 is ideal. But the average AA/EPA ratio of Americans is 11:1. In those patients with inflammatory conditions and neurological disorders, the ratio is 20:1 or more. The Japanese population, on the other hand, comes very close to the ideal ratio, and they have the highest life expectancy and the lowest rate of cardiovascular disease on the planet!

Since most Americans are carrying around at least 10 pounds of excess fat, it is no wonder that arthritis and other inflammatory diseases are out of control in our country.

I recommend you reduce your inflammation-producing AA intake by reducing your intake of wheat, corn, vegetable oils, and grain-fed livestock. Increase your consumption of deep cold-water fish (such as salmon, tuna, and Mahi Mahi). Have a minimum of two servings of such fish a week. You should also supplement with pure fish-oil capsules, up to nine grams a week.

Depression is strongly linked to EFA deficiencies. A deficiency of omega-3 fat is one the main cause of depression and other mental disorders. This is because omega-3 fats work to keep us mentally and emotionally strong in three ways: as precursors for preprostaglandins and neurotransmitters; as the substrate for B vitamins and coenzymes to produce compounds to regulate many vital functions, including neurotransmitters; and in providing energy and nourishment to our nerve and brain cells.

Omega-3 deficiency is related to *Candida* (yeast) overgrowth. In a healthy digestive tract, *Candida* and other yeasts and fungi are kept in check by healthy flora—that is, bacteria. But when a person becomes deficient in omega-3 fatty acids and other vital nutrients, the normally benign yeast changes into an aggressive form and—out of starvation—attacks the walls of the digestive tract in search for nutrients. The integrity of the intestinal walls are then compromised. (This condition is known as intestinal permeability, or more frankly, "leaky gut" syndrome.) Nutrients from within the digestive tract—along with *Candida* secretions—are then able to penetrate through the lining and enter the bloodstream. These poisons then circulate throughout the body, causing everything from allergies to depression to a heightened susceptibility to *staph* infections.

Lack of EFAs means a greater susceptibility to viruses. EFAs have direct antiviral effects and are lethal at surprisingly low concentrations to many viruses. Specifically, the body's production and utilization of the hormone interferon, a chemical our immune system produces to kill viruses, is dependent on EFAs and compromised in their absence. (The antiviral activity of human mother's milk seems to be largely attributable to its EFA content.)

EFAs are also the major components of all cellular membranes in the body, and the integrity of these membranes is the key to preventing infection. Our skin, digestive tract, mouth, sinuses, lungs, and throat are covered with trillions of bacteria, viruses, parasites, and yeasts. So a membrane's capacity to recognize what is beneficial and to keep out what is harmful is vital for the immune system. But without enough EFAs, these membranes are compromised.

This helps explain why some people get sick and others don't when exposed to the same virus. In the case of the Epstein-Barr virus, for example, a good 90% of the U.S. population carries this virus, yet only a fraction become ill from it. One theory is that those who actually develop symptoms have below-normal levels of EFAs and their derivatives. A study investigating sufferers of the EBV particularly confirms this: Both eight and 12 months into the study, subjects who had recovered from the virus showed normal or near normal EFA blood levels. In contrast, those who were still clinically ill from the EBV showed persistently low levels.

Insufficient EFAs in the bloodstream can lead to fatigue. In a Scottish trial, patients with chronic fatigue syndrome were given EFA supplements with great success. After six months, 84% of the patients in the group receiving EFA supplements—and only 22% of those in the placebo group—rated themselves as better or much better. In another study, 74% of CFS patients taking EFA supplements—compared with 23% of those on placebo—assessed themselves improved.

A malfunction of essential fatty acid metabolism has been solidly established to be a major, if not the principle, cause of eczema. Many people report substantial improvement in eczema when they eliminate refined and processed oils and supplement with flax seed and sometimes primrose oil.

Other conditions associated with EFA deficiency include acne, psoriasis, PMS, Sjögren's syndrome (dry eyes and mouth), some forms of cancer, arthritis, heart disease, and asthma.

EFA LEVELS DURING PREGNANCY

EPAs (omega-3) are important to both mommy and baby during pregnancy. We know that low EPA levels can cause depression, and pregnancy draws severely on a person's store of EPAs. (This could explain many of the cases of postpartum depression.) A University of Minnesota study shows that omega-3 fats decreased in a woman's blood during pregnancy, and they stayed decreased for six weeks after birth. Subsequent pregnancies made the deficiency even worse.

The study also demonstrates the importance of omega-3 fats for fetal development. EPA is so important that the mother's brain shrinks three percent in order to provide enough fuel for fetal development. Quoting the study's authors, "Long chain fatty acid deficiency at any stage of fetal and/or infant development can result in irreversible failure to accomplish specific brain growth."

If you are pregnant, consider taking EPA (fish oil) supplements. Diaper rash, eczema, and cradle cap are also all associated with a deficiency in EFAs in children, so make sure your children receive plenty of good fats in their diets. And seriously consider breastfeeding, which is an excellent source of EFAs for your infant.

TIME FOR AN OIL CHANGE

For our purposes, food oils aren't defined by how they start out in nature, but rather how they end up. Let's call the two types "processed" and "natural."

Processed oils have undergone deodorization, bleaching, and/or hydrogenation. These processes remove lecithin, beta-carotene, EFAs, and vitamin E. Hydrogenation is the process of adding hydrogen atoms to oils for the purpose of creating solid fats like margarine. In order to make a hydrogenated oil, natural oils are heated under pressure for six to eight hours at 248–410°F and reacted with hydrogen gas by the use of a metal such as nickel or copper. (Both of these heavy metals have been linked, incidentally, to depression and fatigue.)

Most of the cooking oils found on store shelves today—including corn, sunflower, and others—have been processed to increase their shelf life. The oil then smells bad (go figure!) and must be "deodorized" at a high temperature. The results are oils devoid of nutrition and loaded with poisonous trans fats.

Trans fats prevent the omega-6 EFAs from attaching to their receptors on cell membranes. The membranes then becomes impermeable and, because nutrients can't get in and toxins can't get out, the cells begin to die. Neurotransmitters (serotonin and others) are also blocked from attaching themselves to the cell, and this can lead to depression, insomnia, anxiety, fatigue, and ADD. In addition, trans fats also increase the amount of LDL—bad cholesterol—in the blood and decrease the amount of HDL—good cholesterol.

Natural oils are derived from pressing seeds and nuts. Extra-virgin olive oil and other nonrefined seed and nut oils have not undergone processing and retain their nutritious ingredients. Choose cold processed, nonhydrogenated, polyunsaturated oils, which haven't been heated to the high temperatures that create trans fats.

Still, all oils can turn into trans fats, and some at relatively low heat. As a result, we can actually create trans fats in our own kitchens. So cook with extra-virgin olive oil or organic canola oil, as they withstand higher temperatures without producing trans fats. Avoid lard, coconut oil, and palm oils. Use real butter or cold-pressed margarine—organic when possible. Avoid nonorganic cottonseed oil, as cotton is one of the most heavily pesticide-treated agricultural crops.

If you suffer from rheumatoid arthritis or other inflammatory-related illnesses, avoid peanut oil, as it's high AA levels and can cause more inflammation. Also reduce other sources of AA: red meat, dairy, vegetable oils, and seed oils; use olive oil instead.

For healthy fats, snack on nuts and seeds, such as almonds, walnuts, cashews, pecans, and pumpkin seeds—but not peanuts. Also enjoy guacamole, olives, lean (preferably free-range) meats, cold-water fish, and tofu. All these contain poly- and monounsaturated fats.

Consult your nutritionally oriented physician about supplementing omega-3 and -6 fatty acids, flax seed oil, and primrose oil. Most individuals who need to supplement need a higher ratio of omega-3 to omega-6, at least initially. This is because most people get omega-6s through grains on a daily basis. I recommend starting with an EFA blend containing two–four times as much omega-3 as omega-6. The Essential Therapeutics formula contains 1,000 mg. of cold-pressed pure fish oil per packet.

I also recommend that my patients have a fatty acid profile. This lab test measures the body's different fatty acids and their ratios. For more information about this test, see Appendix B.

RESOURCES
- All the essential fatty acids are contained in my Essential Therapeutics CFS/Fibro formula. To order, see page 461.

FOR FURTHER READING AND RESEARCH
- P.O. Behan and W.M.H. Behan, "Effective high doses of essential fatty acids in the post-viral fatigue syndrome," *Acta Neurol Scand* 82 (1990): 209–16.
- C.L. Broadhurst et al., "Rift valley lake fish and shell fish provided brain specific nutrition for early homo," *British Jour of Nutr* 79 (1998): 3–21.
- Bruno Bertozzi et al, correspondance, *British Medical Journal* 1(312) (1996): 289–99.
- Galland, "Leaky gut syndromes: breaking the vicious cycle," The Third International Symposium on Functional Medicine, Vancouver, British Columbia, 1996.
- D.F. Horrobin, "Post-viral fatigue syndrome, viral infections, and atopic eczema and essential fatty acids," *Medical Hypotheses* 32 (1990): 211–17.
- R.T. Holman, "The slow discovery of the importance of omega 3 essential fatty acid in human health," *Jour Nutr* 128 (1998): 4275–335.
- U. Ravnskov, "The questionable role of saturated fat and polyunsaturated fatty acids in cardiovascular disease," *Journal of Clinical Epidemiology* 51 (1998): 443–60.
- L.L. Williams et al., "Serum fatty acid proportions are altered during the year following acute Epstein-Barr virus infection," *Lipids* 23(10) (1988).

· 30 ·
CHIROPRACTIC
AND OTHER
PHYSICAL MEDICINE

Chiropractic health care is a 110-year-old profession, licensed and practiced in all 50 states as well as most countries around the world. Chiropractic health care originated in America in 1895 and is now the third largest (and the fastest-growing) health profession in the country, serving over 25 million Americans each year.

When Daniel David Palmer, a successful, self-taught healer in Davenport, Iowa, founded chiropractic as a health profession, it was a pretty dark time for health care and medicine in particular. We hadn't yet discovered antibiotics, and bloodletting and folk medicine ruled the day. Palmer emphasized a more natural approach, teaching that nerve interference or "nerve tone" was the cause of all disease. He focused on finding misalignments (subluxations) in the spinal column and realigning (adjusting) them to restore proper nerve flow.

More recently, chiropractic has doggedly overcome an aggressive campaign by the American Medical Association to contain and eliminate chiropractic care. Through sheer determination, a sometimes militant belief that chiropractic should stay separate from conventional medicine, and the popularity chiropractic was enjoying among its ever-growing crowd of supporters, it prevailed.

In the 1980s, the U.S. Supreme Court upheld a previous verdict stating that the AMA had, for political and economic reasons, illegally and maliciously sought to destroy the chiropractic profession. Later the AMA rescinded its ban on referring to chiropractors. Today, chiropractic and the medical profession work together at many medical facilities around the country. Dozens of hospitals have chiropractors on staff, and most insurance companies, including Medicare, cover chiropractic services.

CHIROPRACTIC TODAY

A minority of chiropractors still believe in a one-cause, one-cure philosophy: they seek to heal all diseases through chiropractic adjustments. However, most of today's chiropractors focus on musculoskeletal conditions, primarily low-back pain, sciatica, neck pain, and headaches.

Of today's chiropractic treatments, 95% are for musculoskeletal problems. And there are more randomized clinical trials of chiropractic adjustments for spine-related disorders than for any other single approach. Affirmative backing by such highly respected organizations as the U.S. Agency for Health Care Policy and Research

Education of Chiropractors

Doctors of chiropractic are not only trained in problems of the spine but are formally educated in clinical examination and diagnosis of the entire human body. The chiropractic degree bestows the title of doctor of chiropractic (DC), and it usually takes four–five years and 4,805 clinic and classroom hours to earn. Over 70% of those entering chiropractic college already have one or more college degrees. And DC students receive about the same amount of total educational hours as do medical students. See a comparison below:

Subject	Chiropractic hours	Medical hours
Anatomy	520	508
Physiology	420	326
Pathology	271	335
Chemistry	300	325
Bacteriology	114	130
Diagnosis	370	374
Neurology	320	112
X-Ray	217	148
Psychiatry	65	144
Ob/Gyn	65	198
Orthopedics	225	156
Specialty	1,598	1,492
Total:	**4,485**	**4,248**

(AHCPR), the RAND corporation, the Canadian Government, and others have allowed chiropractic to continue to grow and flourish around the world.

Along with chiropractic adjustments, chiropractors may incorporate diet, exercise, nutritional supplements, and physical therapies to treat most musculoskeletal conditions. Still a firm believer that the power that made the body heals the body, today's chiropractor is often a leading thinker in 21st century medicine, integrating conventional approaches with alternative therapies that have been clinically proven effective. For low-back pain and leg pain, both acute and chronic, scientific studies recommend chiropractic as the first line of management.

Still, some critics would have the public believe that chiropractors are witch doctors. But chiropractic has proven itself through numerous studies and inquiries to be the safest health profession, when compared to dentistry and traditional medicine. There is a 0.000001% risk of severe complications from spinal manipulation. And 94% of the complications that do occur are from osteopaths, medical doctors, and physical therapists attempting spinal manipulation procedures.

Compare this to the staggering amount of patients who die each year from medical complications. There are approximately 225,000 deaths per year due to iatrogenic causes—meaning induced in a patient by a physician's activity, manner, or therapy. This means that deaths due to conventional medical treatment is the fourth leading cause of death in the United States![1]

Used properly, manipulation can help a range of health problems including low back pain, sciatica, neck pain, headaches, carpal tunnel syndrome, and symptoms of FMS and CFS.

CHOOSING YOUR CHIROPRACTOR

It isn't always easy to find just the right chiropractor. Sometimes the doctor or the therapy just doesn't connect with the patient. When this happens, just find another DC with whom you feel comfortable.

Some chiropractors specialize in family medicine, some in nutrition, and some in sports chiropractic. Although I've not found many chiropractors who specialize in FMS/CFS like I do, this shortage is beginning to change. **But a DC who doesn't specialize in FMS/CFS can still help you heal from it.**

Chiropractic treatments should never hurt. Occasionally, your chiropractic physician might need to use certain techniques that can leave you sore for a few days. However, this shouldn't be a common occurrence.

I like what applied kinesiology (AK) has to offer for FMS/CFS patients. This technique, when carried out in conjunction with other gentle adjusting techniques, has benefitted the majority of my patients. So ask your DC about applied kinesiology. I've found that with most of my FMS/CFS patients, gentle techniques result in the best responses.

Just remember that you are the consumer, and the doctor provides a service. If something is not going right, tell your doctor. An open dialogue is extremely helpful and will be appreciated.

MASSAGE THERAPY

Massage therapy is one of the oldest health-care techniques in existence. Chinese medical texts show that massage has been used for over 4,000 years. Modern massage therapy was introduced in America in the mid-1800s.

Massage therapy uses soft-tissue body manipulations to help restore proper musculoskeletal function. It is made up of hundreds of different techniques. Massage therapy continues to grow and now plays an important role in today's health care. There are many different types of massage, and some are better known than others in the United States:

Swedish massage is based on long gliding strokes along stressed muscles. This form of massage is rarely uncomfortable and is probably for everyone, including those with FMS/CFS.

Deep tissue massage is used to release chronic patterns of muscular tension. It uses slow and sometimes very firm pressure to restore normal muscle function. It is usually not comfortable for individuals with FMS/CFS, though there are always exceptions.

Neuromuscular massage is deep massage applied to an individual muscle. It might be too uncomfortable for individuals with FMS or CFS.

Acupressure is based on Chinese meridians and is administered by applying finger- or thumb-pressure to specific locations around the body.

Shiatsu is a form of acupressure. It might be too uncomfortable for individuals with FMS or CFS.

Craniosacral therapy is a method for finding and correcting disturbances in the flow of spinal fluid. This form of therapy is extremely gentle, and in the hands of an experienced therapist, patients are known to experience tremendous relief.

Myofascial release technique seems to offer a good deal of relief for our FMS/CFS patients. It's a gentle therapy used to remove unwanted restrictions within the fascial system. See more about this technique below.

MYOFASCIAL RELEASE TECHNIQUE

John Barnes, PT, has trained many thousands of therapists around the world to treat a system of our body ignored in medical training: the fascial system. This technique, MFR, is used especially to treat headaches, TMJ syndrome, myofascial pain syndrome, CFS, FMS, neck pain, chronic pelvic pain, and low-back pain

Fascia is a densely woven connective tissue that actually exists from head to toe without interruption, kind of like a pair of nylon tights or a spider's web. The fascia system covers every cell—every nerve, artery, and vein, and all of the brain, the spinal cord, muscles, organs, and bones. In fact, we wouldn't be able to remain upright without this structure, which is able to tighten to a tensile strength of 2,000 psi and then relax to totally reshape itself. Visualize it this way: if our body were a tent then fascia is like the ropes that hold up the tent poles. If the ropes become too tight they will pull the tent to one side making it less stable, should the wind blow.

In a normal healthy state, the fascia is relaxed and has the ability to stretch and move without restriction. But physical trauma, scars, poor posture, spinal misalignments, stress, and inflammation all cause the fascia to tighten. It then becomes restricted and creates unwanted tension on the rest of the body. Repetitive traumas and stress have a cumulative effect; they can cause the fascia system to exert excessive pressure to the point of inflammation and pain.[2]

Fascial restrictions can then cause sudden or chronic pain syndromes including headaches, carpal tunnel syndrome, frozen shoulder, sciatica, tennis elbow, and neck, back, knee, foot, and hip pain.

MFR, as taught by Barnes, is designed to find and release any fascial restrictions that may be contributing to a person's pain. Many patients describe the therapy as a gentle but effective massage. The therapist analyzes the patient's posture, palpates and locates fascial restrictions, and then through gentle techniques, releases these restrictions.

Touching the fascia through the skin sets off a piezoelectric effect. This is where physical touch affects cellular energy. A therapist, utilizing the gentle, sustained pressure of myofascial release through compression, stretching, or twisting of the myofascial system, generates a flow of bioenergy throughout the mind/body complex. This flow starts at the cellular level and is transferred to large areas of tissue through a tubular system, recently discovered to also carry neurotransmitters. Remember that neurotransmitters are brain chemicals, linked strongly to emotions. This means that an injury in your body can actually carry "memories" of the injurious event. I know it sounds strange, but it's true. Just ask someone who has had MFR for the first time and burst into tears from strong emotion the minute that a certain facial restriction was released. We may not completely understand the amazing mind-body connection, but MFR is one way to see it at work.

Every individual is different, and length of treatment depends on the length of time the problem has been present and the patient's willingness to practice home stretching exercises. In general, pain and fascial restrictions that are new or less than several months old may resolve in one–three treatments. Conditions that have developed over a number of years would benefit from that many treatments per week. If your fascial restrictions are extensive, you'll work with your therapist to develop a self-treatment stretching program to do at home to minimize the chances of your facial retightening.

TREATING FMS WITH MFR

When someone has fibromyalgia, many systems of her body are involved, and the fascial system is often a primary site of abnormal function. One result can be temperomandibular syndrome (TMJ), which also increases restriction in the neck, shoulder, arms, and even the pelvic area. Bowel and bladder problems can result: urgency, diarrhea, and constipation. As the therapist opens up these areas with gentle techniques, such patients might see dramatic improvement. Some of these techniques can be taught to you as well, so that you can treat yourself for flare-ups.

When to Avoid MFR

I don't recommend MFR if you have any of these conditions:

- malignancy
- acute rheumatoid arthritis
- cellulitis
- sutures
- febrile state
- hematoma
- localized infection
- healing fracture
- osteoporosis
- acute circulatory condition
- osteomyelitis
- anticoagulant therapy
- aneurysm
- advanced diabetes
- obstructive edema
- hypersensitivity of skin
- open wounds

If you ever feel pain during an MFR treatment, tell your therapist, because pain will result in the fascia tightening even more to protect the body. Soft, gentle pressure allows the fascia to return to a normal state. Sometimes you may feel pain for one–two days after treatment. As the fascia is opened, the metabolic waste that was trapped can be released, so drink lots of water to flush your system.

Many massage therapists are given some training in myofascial release, but the technique described above is a system developed over a number of years that requires gentle sustained holds of at least two–three minutes. So seek out a therapist trained in Barnes's method.

CRANIOSACRAL THERAPY

Craniosacral therapy is included in Barnes's MFR training, and John Upledger, DO, has also trained thousands of therapists in this technique. The craniosacral system includes the tissue and fluid that surround the brain and spinal cord, as well as the structures related to production of this fluid. Many systems of the body influence and are influenced by the craniosacral system: the brain, the spinal cord and all other nerves, the muscles, blood vessels, and endocrine and respiratory systems. Just as our heart usually beats 68–72 beats per minute, our fluid through-out this system flows at a 6–12 cycle per-minute rate. TMJ syndrome—with its constant clinching—can especially alter this system, as can fibromyalgia.

> ### When to Avoid Craniosacral Therapy
>
> I don't recommend craniosacral therapy if you have any of these conditions:
>
> • acute intracranial hemorrhage
> • brain aneurysm
> • medulla oblongata
> • recent skull fracture
> • acute systemic infection

Massage of this area requires gentle techniques with hands resting on various parts of the head and sacrum. Many people describe their experience of craniosacral therapy as a feeling of "floating." For more information, you can visit www.myofascialrelease.com.

NOTES

1. Source: *JAMA* 284(4) (2000): 483–5. Number of deaths is subdivided this way: 12,000 due to unnecessary surgery; 7,000 due to medication errors in hospitals; 20,000 due to other errors in hospitals; 80,000 due to infections in hospitals; and 106,000 due to nonerror negative effects of drugs.
2. Currently there are not diagnostic tests that demonstrate this phenomenon. However, MRI may someday be able to demonstrate the restrictions that cause you so much pain.

· 31 ·
REPLENISHING LOW SEX-HORMONE LEVELS

A dysfunctional HPA-axis can cause estrogen, testosterone, and progesterone levels to become imbalanced, causing the same symptoms associated with fibromyalgia and CFS.

The overwhelming majority of fibromyalgia and CFS patients who walk through my office door are women. This is an intriguing trend. I'd like to chalk it up to my winning personality and rugged good looks, but then I suppose they'd have to start filing this book in the fiction section! Let's examine some more realistic explanations!

Many researchers, in fact, are grappling with this very question: why are so many more women than men getting diagnosed with FMS/CFS? Well, men and women are hardwired a little differently. When depressed, men tend to be low in dopamine and norepinephrine, while depressed women are usually low in serotonin. (Now this isn't based on hard data mind you, just 10 years of treating mood disorders.)

Hormones are another obvious place to look for clues. Women are certainly more vulnerable to the ebb and flow of the sex hormones estrogen, progesterone, and testosterone. A large portion of my fibromyalgia patients have had a hysterectomy or have been on birth control pills for a number of years, which makes me suspect a link between sex hormones and fibromyalgia.

HOW A WOMAN WORKS

OK, let me apologize ahead of time for any insults to your intelligence that might surface in this chapter. You women out there probably know your own bodies better than any doctor, but allow me to lay a foundation for our discussion of gender-specific hormones by defining a few terms.

The uterus is a muscular organ that holds a baby for nine months. Located in the pelvic cavity, it is made up of three distinct layers: the outer peritoneum, the middle myometrium, and the inner endometrium. The endometrium thickens each month in preparation for the implantation of a fertilized egg.

The fallopian tubes are located at the top of the uterus, one on the left and one on the right. They are the site of fertilization and act as a passageway for a mature egg until it is deposited to the uterus for implantation.

The two ovaries, positioned just outside the uterus, are the sites of egg production. They contain sack-like follicles, which hold immature eggs. Each month (or so), one egg (or rarely, more than one) is released for maturation. The ovaries also produce estrogen and progesterone.

HORMONES

Remember that hormones are compounds that act like keys to unlock cellular doors to facilitate chemical reactions. The shape of the key (hormone) determines which doors (cells) open.

You're familiar, no doubt, with the sex hormone **estrogen.** What you may *not* know is that there are actually three main forms of estrogen: estrone (E1), estradiol (E2), and estriol (E3). This is an important distinction, as we'll see later in this chapter. **Estradiol** encourages the thickening of the endometrium every month.

Of the three estrogens, estradiol (E2) is the most predominant. Produced by the ovaries prior to menopause, it's also the most biologically active of the three. After menopause, the main estrogen in the body is estrone (E1). Before menopause, it is made by body fat, adrenal glands, the liver, and the ovaries. Estrone is also produced from converted estradiol. Estriol (E3) is the weakest estrogen and is produced by the placenta during pregnancy. Estriol is not normally measurable in nonpregnant women.

Estrogen has many tasks:

• It increases the production of and life of serotonin,

- helps regulate body temperature,
- helps regulate sleep-wake cycles (circadian rhythms),
- increases pain tolerance,
- inhibits monamine oxidase (MAO) enzymes, which are responsible for breaking down serotonin, norepinephrine, and dopamine (MAO inhibitors were some of the first antidepressant drugs; St. John's Wort is considered an MAOI),
- increases mental clarity and memory,
- helps reduce body fat,
- and slows bone loss.

Progesterone is produced by the **corpus luteum,** which was formed from the follicle by which the mature egg was released. Progesterone is responsible for making the endometrium lining more receptive to implantation of a fertilized egg. It also prevents further growth from the follicles.

Progesterone also has its tasks:

- It acts as a sedative,
- may act like the benzodiazepines (prescription tranquilizers) Xanax and Ativan, without the side effects,
- decreases the conversion of testosterone to its active form,
- decreases the release of norepinephrine and dopamine,
- reduces the production of growth hormone,
- may stimulate carbohydrate cravings,
- helps promote deep sleep,
- increases insulin levels,
- may increase body fat,
- and helps build bone.

Gonadotrophin releasing hormone (GnRH) is produced by the hypothalamus. GnRH controls the production and levels of estrogen in your body. When estrogen levels begin to decline (at the end of your cycle), this hormone kicks in until high levels of progesterone turn it off.

Follicle stimulating hormone (FSH) and **luteinizing hormone**

(LH) are produced by the pituitary gland in response to the hypothalamus's production of GnRH. FSH stimulates the follicles—causing the egg to be produced—and raises estradiol levels. LH works with the follicles to produce testosterone.

Testosterone is made in the ovaries and testicles. It promotes sex drive and is converted in the ovary from DHEA. It also helps build bone and promotes healthy muscle tone. Low levels are associated with depression, fatigue, thin hair or hair loss, and dry, thin skin.

Do you remember when I explained that sex hormones are controlled by the HPA-axis? That means that a disruption in the HPA-axis may adversely affect the sex hormones. The question is: *Could a disruption of the HPA-axis and the sex hormones they control cause some of the symptoms of fibromyalgia?* **Absolutely!** Read on.

THE MENSTRUAL CYCLE

Beginning: A women's menstrual cycle can last 25–35 days, with an average length of 28 days. The first day of the cycle (and the end of the previous cycle) begins with the first day of bleeding, which is really the shedding of the uterine lining that occurs because there is no fertilized egg to nourish. As the lining is shed, the body is preparing for the next cycle. Progesterone and estrogen are at their lowest levels.

Follicular Phase (until ovulation): From day one until ovulation, estradiol and—to a lesser extent—estrone rise with the growth of several follicles, which are being stimulated by FSH. Estrogen levels reach a certain point, and all but one of the follicles shrink and then die off. The remaining follicle then becomes the egg to be released at ovulation.

Progesterone levels remain very low. Rising estradiol levels stimulate the pituitary to release LH, and ovulation occurs when estradiol reaches its peak—typically at day 14 of the cycle. LH then signals the follicle to be released as an egg, and estradiol levels drop. It has been theorized that migraine headaches are triggered by this sharp drop in estradiol. The drop may also contribute to mood disorders, poor sleep, and increased pain.

Luteal/Secretory Phase (after ovulation): During this phase, the egg is developing into the corpus luteum. The corpus luteum produces progesterone, which prepares a woman for sustaining pregnancy. Progesterone levels typically reach their peak in the third week around day 21 or 22 of the menstrual cycle.

If the egg becomes fertilized, progesterone levels stay high. If not, the corpus luteum begins to die off, and progesterone levels rapidly drop. This drop in progesterone triggers uterine bleeding and possibly anxiety and sleep disorders. Estrogen is also low at this time, which can lead to headaches, mood disorders, increased pain, and disturbed sleep.

See below for a simple summary of your average estradiol and progesterone levels for any given cycle.

Hormone	Cycle Day	An Average Level
Estradiol	1–4	85 pg./ml.
	4–14	200 pg./ml.
	14	425 pg./ml. (peak)
	15–28	225 pg./ml.
Progesterone	1–14	.6 ng./ml.
	15–28	15 ng./ml.
	20–22	17.5 ng./ml. (peak)

HORMONE-REPLACEMENT THERAPY

More and more, we are beginning to understand the effects that low levels of certain hormones can have on a woman's body. It may very well be that there is a causal relationship between low hormone levels and the symptoms of FMS and CFS. More research on this is needed.

Still, doctors have known for a while that low hormone levels can lead to a host of problems for women. Thus the advent of hormone replacement therapy (HRT). It seemed like a great idea, but the disturbing truth about HRT was brought to light in 2002, when the Women's Health Initiative (WHI), a study of PremPro (a mix of Premarin and Provera), was halted three years early due to a clear increase in serious risks. The study, which analyzed 16,000 women aged 50–79, found that after using PremPro for only five years, participants showed a 29% increased risk of breast cancer, a 26% increased risk of heart disease, and a 41% increased risk of stroke.

If we project these numbers to include all women currently taking PremPro, the number of sufferers is quite scary. And this doesn't count the millions on other forms of synthetic HRT. The study caused a bit of a scare, and millions of women abandoned their synthetic HRT. But after the dust settled, many in the medical profession began to recommend synthetic HRT once again. Funny how we have such a short-term memory sometimes.

Many women are happy to take these synthetic hormones, in spite of the risks. On the one hand, this seems incredible, even absurd. But on the other hand, it just shows how extreme is the discomfort for a woman when her hormones are out of balance.

If you're considering HRT, please consider the following information about synthetic hormones:

PREMARIN AND OTHER SYNTHETIC ESTROGENS

This synthetically manufactured compound contains small amounts of estradiol and estrone. It is over 90% horse hormones, derived from the urine of pregnant mares. Never mind the inhumane conditions these horses are exposed to; horse hormones are for horses, not humans! Equine (horse) estrogens have several components that attach more strongly to the estradiol receptor than does human estradiol, so some of the equine hormones stay in the body far longer than human estrogens—up to three months longer. The liver has to work rather hard to break down estrogens and even harder to break down these equine estrogens. This may be one reason there have been so many problems with mainstream synthetic HRT.

PROVERA AND OTHER SYNTHETIC PROGESTINS

Synthetic progestins are associated with a variety of side effects including birth defects, blood clots, stroke, breast tenderness, depression, nausea, insomnia, breakthrough bleeding, fatigue, hair loss, and more. But before you begin to feel like treatment of your low hormone levels is hopeless, read on about a better, more reasonable treatment.

BIOIDENTICAL HORMONE REPLACEMENT THERAPY

Bioidentical Estrogen: Bioidentical (pronounced BY-oh-identical) hormones are generally made from the oils of plants such as soy or Mexican yam. They are specifically made (usually by a compounding pharmacy) to mirror the body's own sex hormones. BHRT therapy may offer the benefits of hormone replacement without the many potential side effects of synthetic HRT. Biestrogen contains estriol with estradiol, and Triestrogen contains all three estrogens. They do require a prescription.

Bioidentical Progesterone: Progesterone USP is a form of progesterone made from chemicals found in wild yams and soybeans. Along with this specially compounded prescription, there are dozens of over-the-counter progesterone creams, including Pro-Gest and Restored Balance.

Unfortunately, there has not been enough research conducted on the safety of BHRT. However, the dangers of synthetic HRT are real and indisputable. And many doctors and pharmacists who recommend BHRT are convinced that plant oil–compounded hormones, in combinations typical of the body's own natural ratios, offer a safe and effective way to combat the symptoms of hormonal imbalances. Visit www.johnleemd.com for more information about BHRT.

So what do I need to replace?

If you're wondering where to start in your replacement of low hormones, consider this: Estrogen and progesterone each have their pro's and con's. And some hormone experts have taken up one hormone's cause over the other. This is certainly true in the case of two highly respected hormone experts: Dr. John Lee and Dr. Elizabeth Vliet.

Dr. Lee is a vocal advocate for using natural progesterone replacement therapy. The idea that progesterone is more important than estrogen is counter to the message that a generation of women have heard. Dr. Lee believes that most of the unwanted symptoms of perimenopause and menopause—including weight gain, mood swings, fatigue, poor sleep, and water retention—are due to low progesterone. Dr. Vliet, however, recommends estrogen replacement. She believes estrogen boosts mood, improves sleep, and increases mental and physical energy. Both doctors have published popular books on their findings.

No matter…we can all agree that a balance of these hormones is essential for optimal health. I've had patients who've found their sleep improved by replacing natural progesterone alone. Others report that estrogen replacement reduced their depression and improved their pain. Generally though, I've found that where HRT (or BHRT) is concerned, *balancing* the hormones is the key.

Standard blood tests can offer a base-line reading of your hormone levels. However, taking one sample one day out of a 28-day cycle has its limits. Even in menopause, one-sample tests may be misleading. I prefer my patients to use 28-day urine and saliva samples instead. Unfortunately, some labs don't accept all insurance, and the tests can cost as much as $400. Yet if a patient is still struggling after her jump-start plan and the other protocols in this book, this test can turn out to be a fantastic resource. Ask your doctor for a referral to Genova Labs, or see p. 461 to order from my office.

PLANT-BASED AND HERBAL REMEDIES

• **Phytoestrogens** are plant-based compounds that mimic the effects of natural estrogen. There are four families of phytoestrogens: isoflavones, stibenes, lignans, and coumestans. **Soy** is an isoflavone compound. A number of studies have shown that phytoestestrogens are somewhat effective at maintaining healthy bone-mineral levels in postmenopausal women. Other studies show that phytoestrogens reduce LDL (bad) cholesterol and raise HDL (good) cholesterol, and improve mental clarity, attention, memory, and concentration. Many of my patients have found that phytoestrogens, especially soy-based products, reduce their hot flashes, night sweats, and other symptoms of perimenopause and menopause. Dose is typically 60–90 mg. a day.

- **Black Cohosh** is a native North American perennial plant. The American College of Obstetricians and Gynecologists reports that at least a dozen studies involving this herb have shown beneficial effects for postmenopausal women suffering from sleep disorders, hot flashes, and mood disorders.

- **Chasteberry** has been used successfully to treat PMS and menopausal symptoms including breast tenderness and mood disorders.

- **DIM Plus** by Nature's Way contains diindolylmethane, a phytonutrient found in broccoli and Brussels sprouts. It supports the activity of enzymes that improve estrogen metabolism. This product has been helpful for some of my menopausal patients.

RESOURCES
- At-home hormone-level testing is available by referral from your doctor to Genova Labs or by contacting my office. See page 461.

FOR FURTHER READING AND RESEARCH
- S.E. File et al., "Eating soy improves human memory," *Psychpharm* 157(4) (2001): 430–6.
- "Food, Nutrition, and the Prevention of Cancer: A global perspective," American Institute for Cancer Research, 1997.
- L. Francisco, "Bio-identical hormone therapy: fact or fairy tale?" *Nurse Pract* 28(7pt1) (2003): 39–44.
- M. Halaska et al., "Treatment of cyclical mastalgia with solution containing Vilex agnus-castus extract: results of a placebo-controlled double-blind study," *Breast* 8(4) (1999): 175–81.
- A.F.M. Kardinaal et al., "Phytoestrogen excretion and rate of bone loss in postmenopausal women," *Eur J Clin Nutr* 52(11) (1998): 850–5.
- E.G. Loch et al., "Treatment of premenstrual syndrome with phytopharmaceutical formulation containing Vitex agnus-castus," *J Womens Health Gend Based Med* 9(3) (2000): 315–20.
- "Use of botanicals for management of menopausal symptoms," Clinical Management Guidelines for Obstetricians-Gynecologists, ACOG Committee on Practice Bulletins, *Obstet Gynecol* 97(6, suppl.) (2001) :1–11.
- K.E. Wangen et al., "Soy isoflavones improve plasma lipids in normocholesterolemic and mildly hypercholesterolemic postmenopausal women," *Am J Clin Nutr* 73(2) (2001): 225–31.

PART FIVE

PUTTING IT ALL TOGETHER

· 32 ·
TWENTY STEPS TO WELLNESS

So, what are you to say when people ask you, "What caused your illness?" You can tell them, "There are myriad causes, really, but basically it's due to dysfunction in my HPA-axis and a depleted stress-coping savings account."

"What?" they might ask, puzzled. "Well, basically, my body is falling apart and my hormones are out of sync." If they have any more questions, then lend them this book. What if they ask, "Can't you take a pill for it?" Just politely explain that conventional medicine alone has proven very effective in treating your particular illness. While prescription medications are often helpful, they aren't natural to the body, they have potential side effects, and they may actually be causing some of your present symptoms. You are treating and beating your fibromyalgia or CFS by getting healthy from the inside out, by using the natural chemicals that make up your body to repair your body. Then you can add, "I'll be a whole lot better in a couple of months. Check back with me then!"

> "Progress, however, of the best kind, is comparatively slow. Great results cannot be achieved at once; and we must be satisfied to advance in life as we walk, step by step."
>
> —Samuel Smiles

Remember that FMS/CFS (two sides of the same coin) are biochemical problems manifesting as physical ailments. Vitamins, minerals, amino acids, and essential fatty acids provide the building blocks you need to get well and stay well. Sure it can be a hassle to take all these supplements. But individuals with complex chronic illnesses must take supplements to get well. Stay on your supplements, especially a good comprehensive multivitamin and mineral formula for at least a few months—maybe even years. Don't stop when you start to feel better.

Discovering and correcting the causes of fibromyalgia and chronic fatigue syndrome take time and commitment. Remember, you are peeling away dysfunction and its symp-toms—one layer at a time. It's easy to lose faith. You *will* feel better, but it *will* take time.

I know that I've given you a substantial amount of information in this book, and your head might be swimming from all the instructions, recommendations, supplementations, and innovations! Below is a simplified list that breaks down the general order of all I've discussed in this book. Consider it the Cliff's Notes version of you get-well plan.

Please, please, please don't sacrifice your health by taking cheap, inexpensive vitamin-and-mineral supplements. They don't work! I know this from years of experience consulting with thousands of patients who have tried numerous fad remedies and cheap one-a-day supplements. Use the best, most complete formulas that you can find. You don't have to buy my Essential Therapeutics brand, but use their ingredients are your guide in choosing supplements. My protocols are based on quality supplements, and you won't get results from puny RDA-based formulas.

> Victory becomes, to some degree, a state of mind. Knowing ourselves superior to the anxieties, troubles, and worries which obsess us, we are superior to them.
>
> —Basil King

1. **Begin the Jump Start Plan (see chapter 13) right away.**
   This includes boosting serotonin levels with 5-HTP, correcting adrenal fatigue with adrenal cortex glandular supplements, ensuring proper digestion by taking a digestive enzyme with each meal, supplementing with an optimal daily allowance high-dose multivitamin-and-mineral formula with fish oil, extra magnesium (700 mg.), malic acid, and free-form amino acids. To find a doctor or a health food store near you that carries my Essential Therapeutics products, including the CFS/Fibro Formula, call my office or visit my web site. See p. 461.

2. **Make it your highest priority to get eight or more hours of deep, restorative sleep each night.** Follow the instructions in chapter 10, and don't quit until you are an Olympic sleeper! Start with 5-HTP and use melatonin if needed. If you're taking a prescription drug for sleep, make sure it is one that promotes deep, restorative sleep.

3. **Commit to reducing stress in your life.** Don't be afraid to make some drastic changes. Consider getting help from a counselor who can help you look critically at your lifestyle and how it might be contributing to your symptoms. Improve your daily stress-managing skills. See more in chapters 8 and 9.

4. **Seriously critique any prescription medicines that you are currently taking.** Consider natural alternatives, or even safer prescriptions, recommended in this book. Talk to your prescribing doctor about the possibilities of weaning off some or all of your medications, including antidepressants and sleep aids (see chapter 6). If you are on antibiotics, supplement with probiotics starting immediately. If you are on hormone replacement therapy, talk to your doctor as soon as possible about bioidentical or herbal options (see chapter 31).

5. **Test yourself for low thyroid, and treat it if necessary.** See chapter 14.

6. **Treat your pain—including any arthritis—with effective, natural supplements.** See chapter 15.

7. **Start the two-week elimination diet and the one-month nightshade-avoidance diet.** After the completion of the elimination diet, begin to test and slowly reintroduce (through a rotation diet) any allergic foods. These will get you on the road to repairing any digestive abnormalities, including intestinal permeability, malabsorption syndrome, and food allergies. See chapters 12 and 18.

8. **Take a good, long look at what you're requiring of your liver.** See chapter 19. Work to reduce the toxins in your immediate environment.

9. Treat any active urinary tract infection or interstitial cystitis according to the protocols in chapter 21. Remember to always supplement antibiotics with probiotics!

After you have *consistently* followed the above steps for about a month, then consider these further steps to help you heal even more. Use the self-tests in this book, as well as your understanding of your own body, to guide you.

10. Take the Brain Function Questionnaire, and treat any depression or anxiety that still plaques you. Use natural, amino acid–based treatments if possible. See chapter 16.

> Never, never, never give up!
>
> —Winston Churchill

11. Treat any opportunistic bugs, including viruses, parasites, and bacteria/yeast overgrowth. See chapters 20 and 22.

12. Build up your immune system for present and future wellness. See chapter 17.

13. If self-tests reveal that you continue to suffer from low adrenal function, add DHEA to your adrenal extracts. See chapter 11.

14. Implement a healthy diet for a lifetime. Avoid simple carbohydrates (see chapter 23). Increase your intake of good fats (see chapter 29). Stop smoking. Eliminate or greatly reduce alcohol, caffeine, and preservative-rich foods.

15. If you continue to suffer from recurrent urinary tract infections, follow the recommendations in chapter 21 for avoiding them.

16. Begin to exercise daily. Start slow; follow chapter 24.

17. Avoid future yeast infections (if you are prone to them) by implementing the recommendations in chapter 22, including the *Candida* diet.

18. Find a chiropractor and massage therapist who are knowledgeable about FMS/CFS. See chapter 30.

19. **Find—and listen to—your inner self.** Practice a daily quiet time. Journal your thoughts. What is this illness trying to show you? Is God giving you an opportunity to reevaluate your life? Become skilled in sifting through mind chatter, keeping the positive thoughts and responses and letting go of the negative disease-causing thoughts. See chapter 25.

20. **Keep in touch.** I want to hear your story of wellness.

I wish you joy, peace, and optimal health.

www.TreatingAndBeating.com

1-888-884-9577

· APPENDIX A ·
SYMPTOMS PROFILES

Yeast Symptoms Profile

Check any of the symptoms below that you experience on a regular basis. If you check more than five of the symptoms, you might be suffering from a yeast overgrowth. See chapter 22.

____ fatigue or lethargy
____ depression or manic depression
____ pain and/or swelling in joints
____ abdominal pain
____ constipation and/or diarrhea
____ bloating or excessive belching or intestinal gas
____ indigestion or heartburn
____ prostatitis
____ impotence
____ loss of sexual desire or feeling
____ endometriosis/infertility
____ cramps and/or menstrual irregularities
____ premenstrual tension (PMS)
____ attacks of anxiety (nerves) or crying
____ sore throat
____ recurrent infections or fluid in ears
____ cold hands or feet; low body temperature
____ hypothyroidism
____ chronic hives (urticaria)
____ cough or recurrent bronchitis
____ nasal congestion or post-nasal drip
____ nasal itching
____ laryngitis (loss of voice)

____ eczema, itching eyes
____ sensitivity to milk, wheat, corn, or other foods
____ mucus in stools
____ psoriasis
____ shaking or irritability when hungry
____ cystitis or interstitial cystitis
____ incoordination
____ pressure above ears; feeling of head swelling
____ tendency to bruise easily
____ troublesome vaginal burning, itching, or discharge
____ rectal itching
____ dry mouth or throat
____ mouth rashes, including "white tongue"
____ bad breath
____ foot, hair, or body odor not relieved by washing
____ pain or tightness in chest
____ wheezing or shortness of breath
____ urinary frequency or urgency
____ burning upon urination
____ spots in vision or erratic vision
____ burning or tearing eyes
____ ear pain or deafness

Wilson's Syndrome Symptoms Profile

Check any of the symptoms below that you experience on a regular basis. If you check more than five of the symptoms, you might be suffering from Wilson's Syndrome. See chapter 14.

___ fatigue
___ abnormal throat sensations
___ headaches
___ sweating abnormalities
___ migraines
___ heat and/or cold intolerance
___ PMS
___ low self-esteem
___ irritability
___ irregular periods
___ fluid retention
___ severe menstrual cramps
___ anxiety
___ low blood pressure
___ panic attacks
___ frequent colds and sore throats
___ hair loss
___ frequent urinary infections
___ depression
___ lightheadedness
___ decreased memory
___ ringing in the ears
___ decreased concentration
___ slow wound healing
___ decreased sex drive
___ easy bruising
___ unhealthy nails
___ acid indigestion
___ low motivation
___ flushing

___ constipation
___ frequent yeast infections
___ irritable bowel syndrome
___ cold hands or feet
___ inappropriate weight gain
___ poor coordination
___ dry skin
___ inhibited sexual development
___ dry hair
___ infertility
___ insomnia
___ hypoglycemia
___ falling asleep during the day
___ increased skin infections/acne
___ arthritis and joint pain
___ abnormal swallowing sensations
___ allergies
___ changes in skin pigmentation
___ asthma
___ muscle aches
___ excessively tired after eating
___ itching
___ carpal tunnel syndrome
___ high cholesterol
___ dry eyes/blurred vision
___ ulcers
___ hives
___ increased nicotine, caffeine use
___ bad breath

Adrenal Fatigue Risk Profile

Social readjustment scale: Add up all points applying to the following events that have occurred in your life over the past 12 months. Read about adrenal dysfunction in chapter 11.

Event	Points	Event	Points
1. Death of spouse	100	24. Trouble with in-laws	29
2. Divorce	73	25. High personal achievement	28
3. Marital separation	65	26. Spouse begins or stops work	26
4. Jail	63	27. Beginning or end of school	26
5. Death of a close family member	63	28. Change in living conditions	25
6. Personal injury or illness	53	29. Revision of personal habits	24
7. Marriage	50	30. Trouble with boss	23
8. Fired from work	47	31. Change in work conditions	20
9. Marital reconciliation	45	32. Change in residence	20
10. Retirement	45	33. Change in schools	20
11. Illness of family member	44	34. Change in recreation	19
12. Pregnancy	40	35. Change in church activities	19
13. Sexual difficulties	39	36. Change in social activities	18
14. Addition of new family member	39	37. Small mortgage	17
15. Business adjustment	39	38. Change in sleeping habits	16
16. Financial change	38	39. Change in number of family reunions	15
17. Death of a close friend	37	40. Change in eating habits	15
18. Change to a different line of work	36	41. Vacation	13
19. Increased arguments with spouse	35	42. Christmas	12
20. Large mortgage	31	43. Minor violation of law	11
21. Foreclosure of loan or mortgage	30		
22. Change of work responsibilities	29		
23. Your child leaving home	29		

(Continued on next page)

Adrenal Fatigue Risk Profile
(continued)

200 points or more in one year's time is indicative of a weakened immune system and increases the risk for serious illness.

A score of 100 or above is enough to bring on adrenal fatigue, especially if you would answer "yes" to any of the following:

___ I've been under stress for long periods of time.

___ I work or my spouse works over 50 hours a week.

___ I work full-time.

___ I have one or more children living at home.

___ I've been unhappy for more than two months.

___ I'm unhappy at work.

___ I'm overweight.

___ I have a chronic illness.

___ I have a nervous stomach.

___ I have been on a low-fat or low-calorie diet in the past year.

___ I don't exercise.

___ I exercise more than 14 hours per week.

___ I drink more than two cups of coffee per day.

___ I drink sodas on a daily basis.

___ I smoke.

___ I drink two or more alcoholic beverages per day.

___ I can't sleep at night.

___ I get fewer than seven hours of sleep each night.

___ I eat sugary foods on a regular basis.

___ I've had surgery in the past year.

___ I've had more than one surgery in the past two years.

___ I'm a professional or family caregiver.

___ My spouse doesn't understand my illness.

___ I take prescription or over-the-counter medicines to lift me up.

Brain Function Questionnaire
(also found in chapter 16)

The "O" Group

If three or more of these descriptions below apply to your present feelings, you are probably part of the "O" group. Read about **opioid neurotransmitters** on on page 254.

- Your life seems incomplete.
- You feel shy with all but your closest friends.
- You have feelings of insecurity.
- You often feel unequal to others.
- When things go right, you may feel undeserving.
- You feel something is missing in your life.
- You occasionally feel a low self-worth or -esteem.
- You feel inadequate as a person.
- You frequently feel fearful when there is nothing to fear.

The "G" Group

If three or more of these descriptions below apply to your present feelings, you are probably part of the "G" group. Read about **gamma-aminobutyric acid (GABA)** on page 256.

- You often feel anxious for no reason.
- You sometimes feel "free-floating" anxiety.
- You frequently feel "edgy," and it's difficult to relax.
- You often feel a "knot" in your stomach.
- Falling asleep is sometimes difficult.
- It's hard to turn your mind off when you want to relax.
- You occasionally experience feelings of panic for no reason.
- You often use alcohol or other sedatives to calm down.

The "D" Group

If three or more of these descriptions apply to your present feelings, you are probably part of the "D" group. Read about **dopamine** on page 258.

- You lack pleasure in life.
- You feel there are no real rewards in life.
- You have unexplained lack of concern for others, even loved ones.
- You experience decreased parental feelings.
- Life seems less "colorful" or "flavorful."
- Things that used to be "fun" aren't any longer enjoyable.
- You have become a less spiritual or socially concerned person.

(continued on next page)

Brain Function Questionnaire
(continued)

The "N" Group

If three or more of these descriptions apply to your present feelings, you are probably part of the "N" group. Read about **norepinephrine** on page 260.

- You suffer from a lack of energy.
- You often find it difficult to "get going."
- You suffer from decreased drive.
- You often start projects and then don't finish them.
- You frequently feel a need to sleep or "hibernate."
- You feel depressed a good deal of the time.
- You occasionally feel paranoid.
- Your survival seems threatened.
- You are bored a great deal of the time.

The "S" Group

If three or more of these descriptions apply to your present feelings, you are probably part of the "S" group. Read about **serotonin** on page 263.

- It's hard to go to sleep.
- You can't stay asleep.
- You often feel irritable.
- Your emotions often lack rationality.
- You occasionally experience unexplained tears.
- Noise bothers you more than it used to; it seems louder than normal.
- You flare up at others more easily than you used to; you experience unprovoked anger.
- You feel depressed much of the time.
- You find you are more susceptible to pain.
- You prefer to be left alone.

Parasite Symptoms Profile

Check all the questions to which you would answer "yes."

____ Have you ever traveled outside the US?

____ Do you have foul-smelling stools?

____ Do you experience any stomach bloating, gas, or pain?

____ Do you experience any rectal itching?

____ Do you experience unexpected weight loss with increased appetite?

____ Do you experience food allergies that continue to get worse despite treatment?

____ Do you feel hungry all the time?

____ Have you been diagnosed with irritable bowel syndrome?

____ Have you been diagnosed with inflammatory bowel disease?

____ Are you plagued by an itchy nose, ears, or anus?

____ Do you have sore mouth and gums?

____ Do you experience chronic low-back pain that's unresponsive to treatment?

____ Do you have digestive disturbances?

____ Do you grind your teeth at night?

____ Do you own a dog, cat, or other pet? Or are you frequently around animals?

If you checked three or more of the above symptoms, you might be suffering from a parasitic infection. See chapter 20.

· APPENDIX B ·
TESTS AND THEIR RESULTS

Described below are many of the numerous medical tests used by doctors for evaluating the health of fibromyalgia and chronic fatigue syndrome patients. This list is intended for general reference, and the descriptions are far from exhaustive. It should not be used to diagnose or treat any condition. An increased or decreased level in any area should not be assumed as an indication of illness. Your doctor will take many other factors into account before diagnosing you.

Adrenal Cortex Stress Profile: This test uses saliva samples taken throughout the day and night to measure levels of the adrenal hormones cortisol and dehydroepiandrosterone (DHEA). These adrenal hormones play a vital role in balancing a person's response to stress. They allow us to adapt to and manage stress appropriately.

Abnormal cortisol levels have been observed in patients suffering from CFS, FMS, depression, panic disorders, male impotence, infertility, PMS, menopause, and sleep disorders. **Low levels of DHEA** are associated with fatigue, insomnia, depression, decreased libido, and lowered immunity.

I like this test because it shows how these two hormones perform throughout the day—a single sample doesn't provide much information. Cortisol levels ebb and flow throughout the day in accordance with our circadian rhythms (sleep/wake cycle). I've found cortisol and DHEA to be extremely valuable in correcting many of the problems associated with CFS and FMS. See chapter 10.

An adrenal cortex stress profile is available by referral from your doctor to Genova Diagnostics or by contacting my office (see p. 461).

Antinuclear Antibodies (ANA): This is a blood test that measures autoimmune reactions. A positive finding may indicate rheumatoid arthritis, scleroderma, or lupus (if accompanied by glucoronic acid) in the liver. Increased in hepatitis (liver disease). Decreased in hemolytic (blood) disease.

Bilirubin: Bilirubin is the main bile pigment. Free bilirubin is released into the blood as a result of RBC breakdown and is the conjugated form.

Blood Urea Nitrogen: This blood test measures urea. Urea is the end product of protein metabolism and is formed in the liver. It is excreted by the kidneys. Increased in kidney damage or urinary tract obstruction. Decreased in liver failure or pregnancy.

C Reactive Protein: C reactive protein is a substance present in tissue destruction and inflammation. Positive may indicate rheumatic fever or myocardial infarction (heart disease). Also is a warning sign of increased risk for heart disease, cancer, and inflammation.

Complete Blood Count (CBC): The CBC test usually includes a red blood cell (RBC) count, a white blood cell (WBC) count, hemoglobin, hematocrit, indices mean corpuscular volume (MCV), platelet count, and WBC differential.

- **RBC count:** The amount of RBCs per cubic millimeter is used to assess the degree or presence of anemia. Increased in polycythemia. Decreased in anemia.
- **WBC count:** The WBCs are the main defense against invading microorganisms. WBCs destroy most bacteria. Normal range: 5,000–10,000 cubic units. Increased in various infections, certain blood disorders, and emotional distress. Decreased in overwhelming infections.
- **Hemoglobin:** Hemoglobin is the oxygen-carrying portion of RBCs. Normal range: female: 12–15 mg.%; male: 13–16 mg.% Increased in polycythemia and dehydration. Decreased in all anemias and late pregnancy.
- **Hematocrit:** This is a measure of the volume of settled RBCs per 100 ml. of blood. Normal range: female: 40–48%; male: 42–50%. Increased in polycythemia. Decreased in anemia.

- **Indices MCV:** MCV is calculated by dividing the hematocrit result by the RBC count. Increased in macrocytic anemia. Decreased in microcytic anemia.
- **Platelet count:** Blood platelets strengthen the resistance of the vessel walls against trauma and are the initial factor in coagulation (clotting). Increased in trauma, blood loss, and polycythemia. Decreased in anemia, thrombocytopenia, and severe burns.
- **WBC differential:** Neutrophils are active and increased in acute bacterial infections. **Lymphocytes** are particularly active in fighting off viruses and are increased in acute viral infections, lymphocytic leukemia, and multiple myaloma. They are decreased in Hodgkin's disease. **Eosinophils** are increased in allergies and parasitic infections. **Monocytes** are active in chronic infections and Hodgkin's disease. **Basophils** release heparin to prevent clotting in inflammation. They are increased in polycythemia and decreased in acute infections.

Comprehensive Parasitology Profile: This profile checks for parasite as well as bacterial and yeast overgrowth. The test also uncovers harmful bacteria or yeast inhabiting the intestinal tract and measures the amount of good bacteria there. The test requires a stool sample.

Most people, including physicians, don't realize how common parasites infect Americans. We think of parasites as being a "third world" phenomenon, and that's true in a sense. Up to 99% of those living in undeveloped countries have one or more parasites. But world travelers have spread many of these parasites, and it is not uncommon for those in developed countries to be stricken with parasitic infections. In a study of outpatients at the Gastroenterology Clinic in Elmhurst, NY, a 74% incidence of parasites was found. Genova Diagnostics in Asheville, North Carolina, is arguably the stool-testing lab in the world. They report that 30% of all examined specimens are positive for parasites.

Parasites can cause a wide range of health problems, including irritable bowel, ulcers, gastritis, malabsorption, fatigue, autoimmune reactions, colitis, low back pain, irregular bowel movements, and abdominal cramps. See chapter 20.

Creatinine: Creatinine is a waste product usually eliminated by the kidneys. It is increased in possible kidney disease or urinary obstruction; it is decreased in possible muscular dystrophy.

DHEA: Normal test range: 12–379 mcg./dl. This is a very broad range, and I like to see DHEA levels above 200. DHEA is a very important hormone, and most FMS and CFS patients are very low (less than 100 mcg./dl.) and need replacement therapy. Treatment of females is usually 25 mg. a day; of males, 50 mg. a day. I prefer a special sublingual form of DHEA. I've tried several different types of DHEA, but sublingual (absorbed under the tongue) DHEA (and this brand in particular) seem to yield the quickest results.

EBV (Epstein–Barr Virus AB and Cytomegalovirus) Panel: This blood test measures the antibodies immunoglobulin M (IGM) and immunoglobulin G (IGG). A measure of IGM describes the acute (active) phase of a virus, and a measure of IGG describes its dormant (inactive) phase. An EBV panel also measures Epstein-Barr nuclear antigen (EBNA) antibodies. If the IGM is normal (low) but the IGG and EBNA are elevated, then the Epstein-Barr virus or cytomegalovirus is causing CFS.

We often see a reactivated virus in CFS patients. The person was exposed to the virus in the past and was able to get over the acute infection. But later in life, when the immune system was compromised, the virus became active again.

If IgM is normal (low) but the IgG is high and the EBNA is high: indicates that the virus is again active. (This criteria is also useful in testing for the cytomegalovirus.)

Erythrocyte Sedimentation Rate (ESR): This test is used to detect inflammatory conditions. It is relatively nonspecific and is used as a screening tool. If levels are abnormal, further testing might be needed. Increased in heavy metal poisoning, all collagen diseases (autoimmune arthritis), some cancers, gout, infections, and other inflammatory diseases. May be decreased in sickle-cell anemia and congestive heart failure.

Fibrinogen: Fibrinogen is formed in the liver. In the presence of thrombin, it is converted to fibrin as part of the clotting mechanism. Increased in kidney disease. Decreased in liver disease. Fibrinogen has been implicated as a possible contributing cause of FMS and CFS.

Food and Inhalant Allergy Testing: Food and inhalant allergies have been implicated in a wide range of health problems. There are several ways to test for allergies, including blood tests, scratch tests, Electro acupuncture according to Voll (EAV), muscle testing or Applied Kinesiology (AK), provocation/neutralization, and elimination diets. I usually recommend blood tests that combine Radio Allergo Sorbent (RAST) testing with Enzyme-Linked Immunoabsorbant Assay (ELISA) testing. RAST testing is very useful in uncovering inhalant allergies like pollen, ragweed, and molds. ELISA testing is more accurate in measuring reactions to foods. See chapter 18.

An ELISA food allergy test is available by referral from your doctor to Genova Diagnostics or by contacting my office (see p. 461).

Glucose: Glucose (blood sugar) can be measured by either a blood or urine test. This test is usually conducted after a period of fasting, since blood levels are naturally effected by eating. **Normal test range:** 80–120 mg./dl. Increased in diabetes and Cushing's disease. Decreased in hypoglycemia and Addison's disease.

Hair Elemental Analysis: This test should only be used to access the levels of heavy metals. It's not an accurate test for mineral levels and shouldn't be used to measure mineral stores. Still, an inexpensive screening test like a hair analysis is an ideal way to uncover any potential contributors to poor health.

Heavy metals include cadmium (in smokers), aluminum, lead, mercury, tin, silver, and arsenic. Heavy metal toxicity can present a host of unwanted symptoms, and we commonly find heavy metals in FMS and CFS patients. See chapter 19.

Human Growth Hormone (HGH) and Insulin-like Growth-factor 1 (IGF1): HGH helps increase muscle mass, decrease adipose (fat), repair damaged tissues (especially muscle), build stronger bones, increase energy, and improve sleep. Insulin-like growth factor-1 levels are an indication of how much HGH is circulating in the body.

I have found FMS and CFS patients improve much faster when HGH levels are over 200—over 250 is ideal. Restoring HGH to normal or above-normal levels can often provide dramatic relief for insomnia and the symptoms associated with it: fatigue, depression, and achy muscle pain.

Intestinal Permeability Profile: This is a functional medical test that measures the permeability of the cells that line the intestinal tract. These cells are known as mucosal cells. They act as a barrier to help prevent toxic substances from leaking into the rest of the body. Increased permeability of the intestinal tract is associated with a number of health problems, including food allergies, malabsorption, irritable bowel syndrome, and rheumatoid arthritis. See chapter 12. An intestinal permeability profile is available by referral from your doctor to Genova Diagnostics or by contacting my office (see p. 461).

Lipase: Lipase is a fat-digesting enzyme produced by the pancreas that is increased in inflammation of the pancreas (acute pancreatitis), obstructed pancreatic duct, and pancreatic cancer.

Liver Detoxification Profile: This test evaluates the ability of the liver to properly detoxify foreign substances. Standard blood liver panels are used to uncover elevated liver enzymes and gross liver diseases. Functional medical tests like this one are designed to access the body's or organ's performance when challenged with a potentially harmful substance. The test uses saliva and urine samples to measure the liver's ability to detoxify potential harmful substances. Our liver's detoxification system can be measured by challenging it with caffeine, aspirin, and acetaminophen. See chapter 19.

A liver detoxification profile is available by referral from your doctor to Genova Diagnostics or by contacting my office (see p. 461).

Prothrombin Time: Prothrombin is produced in the liver and is converted to thrombin in the clotting process. Therefore, clotting ability decreases with an increase in the prothrombin time. Increased in vitamin-K deficiency and in liver and biliary disease.

RA Latex Agglutination: A positive test indicates rheumatoid arthritis.

Serum Glutamic Oxalacetic Tranaminase (SGOT):
SGOT is an enzyme present in large amounts in muscle and liver tissue. It is also in heart muscle. It's primarily used as a marker for heart disease, but elevation may also be due to liver disease or muscular dystrophy.

Serum Glutamic Pyruvic Transaminase (SGPT):
Primarily an indicator of liver disease (hepatitis) and myocardial infarction.

Thyroid Stimulating Hormone (TSH): The pituitary gland is responsible for secreting TSH, which then prompts the thyroid gland to release thyroid hormones. **If T3 and T4 are low and TSH is elevated:** indicates hypothyroidism. **If T3 and T4 are low and TSH is also low:** indicates pituitary gland dysfunction (secondary hypothyroidism).

Thyroxine (T4): T4 is a thyroid hormone that is converted into T3. It is increased in hyperthyroid and decreased in hypothyroid.

Triiodthyronine (T3): T3 is a thyroid hormone increased in hyperthyroidism and decreased in hypothyroidism.

Uric Acid: This is increased in arthritic gout and kidney insufficiency and decreased in acute hepatitis.

Other tests available by referral from your doctor to Genova Diagnostics—or by calling my office—include:

• female hormone panel
• melatonin panel
• EFA profile
• yeast overgrowth stool test
• comprehensive parasitology test

· APPENDIX C ·
RESOURCES AND CONTACT INFORMATION

TO ORDER SUPPLEMENTS AND MEDIA
• order online at www.TreatingAndBeating.com,
• call toll-free 1-888-884-9577,
• or in Birmingham, call (205) 879-2383.

HEALTH NEWS YOU CAN USE
Contact Dr Murphree for a free trial of *Health News You Can Use,*
a monthly publication containing the latest breakthrough therapies
and ideas on FMS, CFS, and other health issues.

CONSULTATIONS AND ENGAGEMENTS
Dr. Murphree is available for conference and convention events and,
as of printing, is still accepting new patients.

DIAGNOSTIC TESTING
Genova Diagnostics: Your licensed healthcare provider may order
a female hormone panel, melatonin panel, intestinal permeability
profile, liver detox profile, yeast overgrowth stool test, comprehensive parasitology test, hair analysis, essential fatty acid profile, amino
acid profile, adrenal cortex profile, food allergy test, and other tests
from:

Genova Diagnostics
63 Zillicoa Street
Asheville, NC 28801.
1-800-522-4762.
Fax (828) 252-9303.
www.gdx.net

· INDEX ·